D1317314

BOTTOM LINE'S

FIT AND FLEXIBLE
AFTER 50

The experts' guide to building your strength...maintaining your balance... and staying active for life

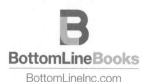

BottomLineBooks

BottomLineInc.com

Fit and Flexible After 50: The experts' guide to building your strength…
maintaining your balance…and staying active for life

Copyright © 2020 by Bottom Line Inc.

10 9 8 7 6 5 4 3 2 1

ISBN 0-88723-843-2

Bottom Line Books® is a registered trademark of Bottom Line Inc.,
3 Landmark Square, Suite 201, Stamford, CT 06901

BottomLineInc.com

Bottom Line Books® is an imprint of Bottom Line Inc., publisher of print periodicals, e-letters and books. We are dedicated to bringing you the best information from the most knowledgeable sources in the world. Our goal is to help you gain greater wealth, better health, more wisdom, extra time and increased happiness.

Printed in the United States of America

Contents

Contents

PART II: HEALING FITNESS STRATEGIES

10. BETTER BALANCE AND BONE HEALTH

Contents

14. FOR WOMEN ONLY

15. EXERCISES FOR BETTER VISION

PART III: THE FIT AND FLEXIBLE WEIGHT-LOSS GUIDE

16. BETTER WAYS TO WEIGHT LOSS

Contents

Preface: How to Use This Book

Fit and Flexible After 50 is a result of Bottom Line Inc.'s ongoing research and connection with a wide variety of leading fitness experts—and is a distillation of their latest findings and advice. We trust that you will glean helpful and actionable information about the fitness topics that concern you most…and find vital topics of interest to family and friends as well.

How to use this book: Fit and Flexible After 50 is an extensive collection of fitness routines and important information on exercise and general fitness. The book features heart-pumping and strength-building workouts, as well as balance, agility, functional fitness, stretching…and pose-movement disciplines, such as yoga and tai chi. Every individual has different fitness needs and goals, whether you want to improve your golf game, up your workout based on moves used by Olympic athletes, vary your strength-training with kettlebells or relieve minor back or knee pain. If your concerns are that specific, we suggest you turn to the Index and look up the various topics of interest and dig in.

It you'd like to start a simple exercise program and need some inspiration: We suggest you begin with chapter 1, "Create Your No-Fail Start-Up Program." We also suggest you review chapters 5 and 12, "Everyday Ways to Stay Fit" and "Routines That Heal Pain," to discover simple ways to stay fit and heal any nagging minor pain or stiffness that's keeping you from an active and full life.

If you'd like some structured discipline… included with this hardcover collection of fitness information is *The Fit and Flexible 28-Day Success Planner* that will guide you through a progressive, full-body workout program that you can do at your own pace.

If you'd like to lose weight: See chapter 16, "Better Ways to Weight Loss." You'll also find weight-loss suggestions featured throughout the book, such as pages 123 and 129 in chapter 7, "Best, Easy Ways to Strength Train." See also "Recipes for Staying Fit and Flexible," in *The Fit and Flexible 28-Day Success Planner* that accompanies this book.

If you'd like to prevent falls: See chapter 10, "Better Balance and Bone Health" to build agility.

If you have chronic pain or stiffness: See chapter 12, "Routines That Heal Pain."

If you have limited mobility: See chapter 8, "Anyone Can Exercise."

If you have a chronic condition such as diabetes or Parkinson's disease: See chapter 13, "Exercises for Special Conditions."

If you want exercises that help with daily living such as lifting groceries or moving furniture: See chapter 5, "Everyday Ways to Stay Fit." Also review neck, shoulder and hand exercises in chapter 12,

"Routines That Heal Pain" and "Exercises for Real Life" on page 116.

If you want a detailed strength workout specifically tailored to women: See chapter 14, "For Women Only."

Please note that we've included information from a wide selection of experts. Some favor group classes, others do not. Some favor dumbbells for weight lifting…other experts turn to resistance bands and yoga to build muscle and bone health. Go with what you enjoy and what feels safe to you. Overall, all our experts agree that if you feel any pain at any moment in your exercise routine, relax your pace or stop what you're doing.

As a reader of a Bottom Line book, be assured that you are receiving well-researched information from a trusted source. But please use prudence in health matters. Always speak to your physician before taking supplements or any medications… changing your diet…or beginning an exercise program.

Be well,

The Editors, Bottom Line Inc.

Stamford, Connecticut

PART I:

Get Started
and Stay Motivated

1

Create Your No-Fail Start-Up Plan

Why Walking Is the #1 Way to Exercise

Mark Fenton, MS, adjunct associate professor at the Friedman School of Nutrition Science and Policy of Tufts University, Boston, and author of *Pedometer Walking: Stepping Your Way to Health, Weight Loss, and Fitness.* He is a national public health, planning and transportation expert who advocates for and consults with local agencies to provide more bicycle- and pedestrian-friendly communities.

I s it really necessary to exert yourself in such an intense way to greatly improve your health and fitness? Many people believe that the answer is yes—and for this reason, these people don't exercise.

And that's a tragedy.

Because in fact, the best exercise for most people is one that's already quite familiar and quite enjoyable—and much less physically taxing than those sweat-till-you-drop workouts that some people put themselves through.

GET BACK TO BASICS

What's this amazing exercise? Walking! *Here's why…*

•**You're less likely to feel pain or get hurt.** The reason is that you're operating within a very natural range of motion for your body. You're not asking your muscles or joints to do anything that they're not used to doing, and so the likelihood of soreness or injury is very low. Plus, unlike running and other high-impact sports, walking is low-impact, so the load that you're putting on your body's joints when you walk is much less.

•**It's convenient.** Walking is probably the most flexible activity. You can do it anytime and anywhere. You don't need a partner or teammates. It's also easy to fit walking into a busy schedule because you don't have to do the entire workout at once. Unlike taking, say, a 30-minute fitness class, where you truly need to spend 30 consecutive minutes exercising, you don't have to do 30 consecutive minutes of walking. You can break it up into three 10-minute walks and still get the benefit.

•**It's free.** Perhaps best of all, you don't need to pay for a personal trainer, fancy equipment, a gym membership or anything else. You just need a comfortable pair of shoes.

•**It's suitable for any fitness level.** If the last time you broke a sweat was in high school gym class, then walking is the perfect workout for you. For inspiration, just look at Michael Moore, the documentary filmmaker who is famous for (among other things) his, well, potato-like look. Even someone as overweight and out of shape as he is has been able to commit to walking—and has grown to love the activity. In fact, he shared on Twitter (#walkwithmike) that he's been walking 30 minutes a day, every day, and that walking has had a healthy domino effect on his life, helping him sleep better, feel better and take better care of himself.

• **Walking is also great for people who are already moderately active.** That's because you can speed up your walks, walk uphill or walk for longer periods of time whenever you want to intensify the workout.

What about people who are already quite active and fit—is walking good for them, too? Admittedly, if you're already, say, an avid runner or tennis player, then a typical walk may not be enough of a workout to make you even fitter. But that describes a small fraction of people, and even those people could benefit from about one day a week of gentle walking to give their muscles a break—especially in the early stages of training for a race or tournament, when doing too much too soon is a common cause of injury. However, walking at high intensity is actually an effective workout for more fit individuals. For example, racewalkers cruising at six to 10 miles per hour—yes, a jogging pace for most people—burn as many calories as someone taking a jog. And elite racewalkers have aerobic fitness levels comparable to elite runners. So walking truly can take your fitness to any level.

• **You're more likely to stick with it.** For all of the reasons above!

A Foolproof Walking Program

Jamison Starbuck, ND, a naturopathic physician in family practice, Missoula, Montana, and writer and producer of "Dr. Starbuck's Health Tips for Kids," a weekly program on Montana Public Radio, MTPR.org. DrJamisonStarbuck.com

Not long ago, I saw a patient who had started walking regularly to lose weight. "Walking is now the best part of my day!" he proudly announced. He did lose weight—and a significant body of scientific research shows that walking also reduces the risk for cardiovascular disease (includ-

ing heart attack and stroke) as well as diabetes, breast cancer and colon cancer. Walking also helps fight osteoporosis, anxiety, depression and memory problems. It even improves immune health, reducing the frequency and duration of colds and flu.

For thousands of years, walking—at a speed of about three miles per hour, on average—was our primary mode of transportation. Now, nearly 40% of Americans don't walk beyond the bare minimum needed to get through the day. If this describes you, you are not letting your body do what it was designed to do. *My advice…*

• **Make walking a priority.** Set aside specific times to walk five days per week. If you keep a daily calendar, write down when you plan to walk. Also, invest in a good pair of walking shoes. Depending on where you live, you also may need rain gear as well as warm, but not restrictive, clothing and a head covering for cold weather. In hot weather, try to avoid the hottest part of the day—and wear a hat to avoid excessive sun exposure. In harsh weather, you can walk in a shopping mall.

• **Start slowly.** Many people are far too ambitious when they first start walking. In the beginning, walk only five minutes up to five days a week. Then increase your time by five minutes per session each week. If possible, work up to 30 minutes per day, five days per week within six weeks.

• **Walk outside whenever possible.** Walking is most enjoyable when it exposes you to fresh air, sunlight and views of nature—even urban trees and flower boxes. The varied terrain of outdoor walking, including uneven sidewalks or the slope of a trail, improve proprioception—the brain's awareness of body position and balance—and will make you more agile and less vulnerable to falls. To prevent injury, pay attention to the terrain, your surroundings and to how your body feels as you walk. If your balance is poor, invest in a walking stick, available at most outdoor-sports stores starting at $20.

• **Get the right amount of fluid and take supplements.** Drink one-half ounce of water per pound of body weight throughout the day—and at least 12 ounces of water just before walking. In addition, ask your doctor about taking daily mineral supplements containing 300 mg of magnesium and 99 mg of potassium. Following these steps will help you avoid muscle cramps, which are usually caused by dehydration, a deficiency of magnesium and/or potassium or lack of strength.

Caution: If you are taking blood pressure medication or have kidney disease, be sure to discuss potassium supplementation with your doctor before trying it.

Even if you don't need to lose weight, as my patient did, I'm betting that walking will make you feel healthier and stronger.

faster gait is associated with higher survival rates in older adults. But don't rush out to buy jogging sneakers just yet. Researchers found that everyone has her own best natural walking speed. Since walking uses various vital organ systems, including the circulatory and respiratory systems, slowing down with age may indicate that one of these systems is damaged.

So: Instead of focusing specifically on increasing your walking speed to live longer, commit to improving your overall health through a nutritious diet and regular moderate exercise. By doing so, your natural walking speed most likely will increase as well.

Faster or Farther?
Walk This Way

Stephanie A. Studenski, MD, MPH, is a professor in the division of geriatric medicine at the University of Pittsburgh School of Medicine and director of clinical research for the University of Pittsburgh Institute on Aging.

If you are just beginning an exercise routine—whether your goal is to lose weight, improve cardiovascular health or build muscle—you should definitely concentrate on distance first. One important reason is that you will be less likely to get injured.

Also, by focusing on distance, you'll probably burn more calories overall. That's because you will be able to sustain a moderate walking pace (about three miles per hour) longer than you could sustain a faster pace. You may be surprised to learn that the average person burns about 120 calories per mile no matter how quickly she or he covers that mile. So, if you can walk three miles at a moderate pace, it will take you about an hour and you'll burn about 360 calories. But if you walk at a very brisk pace of four miles per hour yet are unable to keep it up for more than two miles, you will spend only 30 minutes walking and will burn just 240 calories.

You may have heard of a study in *The Journal of the American Medical Association* that found that

Have a Love Affair
with Exercise...

Mark Stibich, PhD, behavior change expert and faculty member at the University of California, San Diego School of Medicine.

Some people just seem to adore exercise. You see them at the gym or jogging around the neighborhood—sweating, smiling, looking fit. But if you would rather dive into a cauldron of boiling oil than work out on a regular basis, you probably wonder how other people can possibly enjoy exercise ...and wish that you could, too.

Fact: You can learn to love exercise. Several simple behavioral changes can, within seven weeks, result in a major shift in the way you feel about physical activity.

WEEK ONE...

•**First, do nothing.** The number-one obstacle to exercise is lack of time. To overcome this, commit to a one-week predecision phase. You don't actually exercise yet—the purpose is to prove that your schedule can accommodate three 30-minute chunks of workout time per week. How? Wake up a half-hour earlier than usual on, say, Tuesday, Thursday and Saturday...or take 30 minutes after work on Monday, Wednesday and

From Small Steps to Running a Half-Marathon: A Specific Plan for Fitness

Motivational speaker and former publisher of *Success* magazine, Darren Hardy likes to tell this story to illustrate the power of starting small and steady:

One of the women that worked for me—her name was Beverly—just returned to work after having her second child. She was having a hard time losing her "baby weight" and was chatting with a friend who just signed up to run a half-marathon. I overheard Beverly saying how much she wished that she could run a half-marathon.

"Beverly, you could run a half-marathon," I said. "Oh, there's no way," she replied. "I get winded just going up a small flight of stairs."

So I said: "Beverly, if I could show you how to run a half-marathon with little or no pain during the process, would you take me up on it?"

"That's impossible," she replied. "The very idea of a half-marathon gives me pain." "Okay," I told her, "I will create a plan that will have you running a half marathon in nine months—and you will never experience any pain." "You're on," she said. *And here's the plan I created for her…*

I asked Beverly to get in a car and map out a one-mile loop around her house. Then I asked her to walk this loop just three times over a period of two weeks. And she did that easily.

Then I told her to walk it three times per week for an additional two weeks. And she had no trouble doing that.

Then I told her to start a slow jog until you become breathless. "As soon as you become breathless, just walk the rest of the way," I said.

Using this technique, Beverly was able to jog a quarter of a mile. In a short time, she was able to jog a half-mile. It took her three weeks to get up to three-quarters of a mile; and almost two months before she could run a full mile.

Now, a half-marathon is more than 13 miles. And if it took Beverly two months to run a mile, you're probably thinking that she is never going to make 13 miles. But you'd be wrong.

I asked Beverly to just increase her distance by 1/8 of a mile each time she went out for a jog. That's only 300 steps. Well, at the end of six months, she was running nine miles. And at the end of nine months, she was running 13½ miles. Result? She ran her half-marathon.

Since then, Beverly has run four full marathons—and she lost 50 pounds in the process. Running is her new passion and she can't wait to lace up her Nikes. It has changed everything in her life. She looks fantastic…has energy to spare for her kids…she's sexy and attractive to her husband…and she is loaded with self-confidence!

From The 30-Day Diabetes Cure *by Jim Healthy and Russ Canfield, MD. Bottom Line Books. Copyright Brainstorms Inc. Reprinted with permission.*

Friday. During these times, do not make phone calls, check email, pay bills or pick up clutter. Instead, just relax and imagine yourself doing different kinds of physical activities. *While you daydream…*

•**Open your mind.** Maybe you learned to hate exercise in your junior high school gym class when you were chosen last for a volleyball game or puffed around the track in an ill-fitting gym suit. That's understandable—but you don't have to let past unpleasantness poison your possibilities now. Instead, try to remember what you did enjoy as a youngster, such as riding a bike, jumping rope or playing softball. Or imagine doing something entirely new to you—for instance, a tai chi class or a boxing workout. Notice how the thought of each option makes you feel. When an imagined activity gets you excited, write it down on a list.

WEEKS TWO AND THREE...

•**Start moving.** For the next two weeks, continue carving out your thrice-weekly half-hour periods, but instead of just visualizing exercise, do a little. Don't push yourself too hard—if you vow to "go to the gym for two hours" or "run a 10K race," you'll feel achy and uncomfortable and will want to quit. Instead, take it easy. Go for a stroll...try some stretches...splash around in a pool.

Important: During this phase, do not look for results. Do not weigh yourself, take measurements of body parts or worry about whether an exercise is intense enough. Your purpose now is simply to let go of doubts.

WEEKS FOUR THROUGH SIX...

•**Experiment.** Now take a few weeks to try out all the intriguing activities on the list you made previously. Hike in the woods, go ice-skating, rent an aerobics video, try the Pilates class at a friend's club.

Helpful: Many gyms and recreation centers let guests pay by the visit or buy a one-week pass rather than committing right away to (and paying for) a year-long membership. *As you experiment...*

•**Identify favorite activities.** Keep track of what's fun and what's not, looking for patterns. Do you prefer working out at home, or are you inspired by the discipline of going to a health club? Do you like exercising alone or with others? Indoors or outdoors? Consider ways to enhance your enjoyment—for instance, by listening to a portable music player as you walk, watching a movie while using the Stairmaster or buying a new exercise outfit. Within a few weeks, you'll know what you like and what you don't like.

WEEK SEVEN AND BEYOND...

•**Commit.** Now that you've found some enjoyable activities, it's time to decide on a minimum number of workouts you'll do per week—perhaps two or three—and commit to never going below that minimum. Whenever possible, do more than the minimum. Even when you're traveling, you can fit in a half-hour walk or do some yoga poses in your hotel room.

•**Appreciate your progress.** As your exercise habit becomes more ingrained, notice the many positive changes it brings. You feel more energized and less stressed. You sleep more soundly. Your clothes fit better, your weight is easier to control and your posture is straighter. Your muscles are stronger, and everyday tasks are easier. You feel proud of yourself and more in control of your health. Let these benefits serve as reminders of the many reasons why you now love to exercise.

ALTERNATIVE WAYS TO WORK OUT

To keep your workouts fun and fresh, try some activities that you've never done before. *Options to consider...*

•**Core training.** The muscles in the center of your torso, which keep you balanced and support your spine, can be strengthened using equipment developed for this purpose.

Examples: The bosu is an inflated half-sphere that challenges core muscles as you stand on it... the kettlebell is a weighted iron ball with a handle to grip while doing various twists, lunges and other moves. Such equipment usually is available at gyms.

Best: Ask a trainer to help you develop a program using the apparatus.

•**Spinning.** Exercise on a stationary bike, led by an instructor, usually is done to music that fits the pace of the cycling.

•**Video games.** You can do these at home using a game console and your television. In Dance Dance Revolution, you stand on a special mat and move your feet in time to music, following visual cues to perform a series of specific steps. In Wii Fit, you stand on a balance board and get feedback on your technique as you do yoga, strength training, aerobics and balance games.

•**Zumba.** This fusion of Latin rhythms and easy-to-follow dance moves creates a fun fitness workout. For classes near you, visit Zumba.com.

Tricks to Make Yourself Exercise: Simple Ways to Stick with Healthy Activity

Robert Hopper, PhD, a Santa Barbara–based exercise physiologist and author of *Stick with Exercise for a Lifetime: How to Enjoy Every Minute of It!*

I f you're like most people, those exercise resolutions you made at New Year's are just a distant memory. In fact, seven out of 10 Americans can't make exercise a habit, despite their best intentions. That's because the most common reasons for starting an exercise program—to lose weight in time for a reunion, for example—are weak long-term motivators.

But you can learn to motivate yourself to make exercise a regular part of your life. Elite athletes as well as everyday people who have made a successful commitment to lifelong fitness use these insider tips. *Here are their secrets…*

• **Make your first experience positive.** The more fun and satisfaction you have while exercising, the more you'll want to pursue it and work even harder to develop your skills. Even if your first experience was negative, it's never too late to start fresh. Choose a sport you enjoy, and work to improve your skill level.

The key is finding a strong beginner-level coach who enjoys working with novices. For instance, the YMCA offers beginner swim lessons, and instructors are armed with strategies for teaching in a fun, nonintimidating way.

If your friends have a favorite dance class, play racquetball or practice karate, ask them for a referral to an approachable teacher. City recreation departments also often host beginner-level classes for a variety of indoor and outdoor activities. You might also try a private lesson. The confidence you gain will motivate you to try it out in a group setting next.

• **Focus on fun, not fitness.** Forcing yourself to hit the gym four times a week sounds like a chore, and you'll likely stop going before you have the chance to begin building your fitness level. But

lawn bowling, dancing, Frisbee throwing, hiking, even table tennis—those all sound fun, and you'll still be getting physical activity that helps promote weight control…reduced risk for heart disease, diabetes and cancer…stronger bones…and improved mood. As you start to have more fun, you'll want to become more involved and your fitness level will improve over time.

No strategy is more crucial than this: Get hooked on the fun, and you'll get hooked on the activity for life.

• **Find your competitive streak.** We all have one, and you can tap into it, no matter what activity you choose. Jogging outside? Make it a game by spotting landmarks in the near distance, like trees or homes, and push yourself to pass them in a certain number of seconds. Swimming laps? Try to match the pace of the slightly faster swimmer in the next lane. Or keep track of the time it takes to swim 10 laps, and try to beat your time. Even riding the recumbent bicycle at the gym can be turned into a competition by moving your workout to the spin studio, where you can privately compete against other class members for pace or intensity.

• **Practice the art of the con.** If you've ever overheard a pair of weight lifters in the gym, you'll recognize this tip: The spotter encourages the lifter, "One more, just one more!" and then after the lifter completes one more lift, the spotter again urges, "Now one more!" Make this tip work for you by learning how to self-con. Let's say you're too tired to work out. Tell yourself, *I'll just drive to the gym and park. If I'm still tired, I can leave.* This is often enough to kick-start your workout. And while swimming laps, tell yourself you'll just do five, then two more, then just three more.

• **Cultivate a mind-set of continuous improvement.** Tennis great Jimmy Connors once shared what keeps athletes motivated—"Getting better." Lifelong exercisers have a yearning to improve that acts as both a motivator and a goal.

Help yourself get better by educating yourself about your sport. To do this, read books by or about professional athletes…read articles about them in magazines, newspapers and online…and even book a private lesson to have your running gait/golf swing/basketball shot analyzed.

Also, offer yourself rewards for hitting certain benchmarks. Treat yourself to a massage after your first three months of walking your dog nightly for 30 minutes…or book a trip to a luxury ski lodge to celebrate your first year of skiing. You earned it!

If You're Starting to Exercise, Expect to Be Miserable… and Why You Should Keep At It

Tyler C. Cooper, MD, MPH, a preventive medicine specialist at the Dallas–based Cooper Aerobics Center (Cooper Aerobics.com) and founder of Cooper Ventures, which helps people incorporate healthy living into every aspect of their lives. He is coauthor, with his father, Kenneth H. Cooper, MD, MPH, founder and chairman of Cooper Aerobics Center, of *Start Strong, Finish Strong*.

We all know that exercise is perhaps the single most beneficial action we can take to protect our health, and millions of people vow each January 1 to start—and stick with—a program of regular physical activity.

So why are two of every three American adults still "sedentary"—meaning they get little or no exercise?

LIVE THREE YEARS LONGER!

Most people who want to start exercising do so because it's "good" for them. But to stay motivated, you should know exactly why you want to start exercising.

For example, compared with people who exercise regularly, sedentary people are three times more likely to develop metabolic syndrome—a constellation of risk factors including high blood pressure (hypertension), elevated "bad" cholesterol, high blood sugar and obesity. Regular physical ac-

tivity also has been found to reduce risk for cognitive decline.

And if that doesn't keep you motivated, consider this: People who regularly exercise briskly live an average of three years longer than those who are sedentary. "Briskly" means exercising at an intensity that makes you perspire and breathe a little heavily while still being able to carry on a conversation. This is known as the "talk test."

HOW MUCH EXERCISE?

It's a common misconception that you must exercise daily to achieve significant health benefits.

In a study of 10,000 men and 3,000 women conducted at the Cooper Aerobics Center's clinic, we found that walking just two miles in less than 30 minutes three days a week is all that's needed to achieve a "moderate" level of fitness, which lowers risk for all causes of death and disease.

For a less demanding workout that confers the same benefits, you could walk two miles in 35 minutes four days a week…or walk two miles in 40 minutes five days a week. If you prefer other forms of exercise, such as biking or swimming, use these frequency guidelines, plus the talk test (described above) to achieve a moderate fitness level. By increasing the frequency and/or intensity, you'll achieve even greater health benefits.

HIT THE SIX-WEEK MARK

If you have not exercised regularly in the last six months and/or are overweight (for women, having a waist size of 35 inches or more…for men, 40 inches or more), the basic exercise requirement described above may be too much. You may want to start by walking only to the end of the block for a few days, then gradually increase the distance. Aim for an increase of up to 10% weekly—for example, from 10 minutes per week to 11 minutes the next week and so on.

Helpful: Expect the first few weeks to be miserable—you'll feel some muscle soreness for a while. Accept it—but make the commitment to keep going.

Important: If your muscle pain doesn't go away within several weeks, see your doctor to rule out an underlying condition, such as arthritis.

We've found at the Cooper Aerobics Center that few people quit after they've performed a program of physical activity for six weeks. Once people reach the four- to six-month mark, adherence to an exercise program approaches 100% for the long term.

DETERMINE YOUR BASELINE

If you've been sedentary, be sure to get a comprehensive medical checkup before starting an exercise program. This is particularly important for men age 40 and older and women age 50 and older—cardiovascular disease risk rises at these ages.

People of any age with underlying health problems or a family history of diabetes, hypertension, high cholesterol or heart disease also should get a checkup before starting to exercise.

Ask your doctor—or a fitness trainer—to give you baseline measurements for strength, flexibility and aerobic capacity, which will enable you to track future changes.

Checking these measurements (along with such markers as blood pressure, cholesterol and blood sugar) again in about three months will give you tangible evidence of your progress and can motivate you to keep exercising.

Get Fit Together: The Benefits of Exercising as a Couple

John S. Raglin, PhD, sports psychology researcher, professor in the department of kinesiology and director of graduate studies at the School of Public Health at Indiana University–Bloomington. He is author of a published paper titled "Factors in Exercise Adherence: Influence of Spouse Participation" and dozens of other studies on sports psychology.

You know all about the motivational advantages to working out with an exercise buddy, but are they the same when the buddy is your spouse or life partner? The answer is yes and perhaps more so. Working out with your spouse or partner can strengthen your relationship along with your muscles. Here's how to start off on the right foot.

COMMIT TO AN EXERCISE PLAN

Sticking with an exercise program isn't easy. The average dropout rate is 50%, most often after just a few months. But exercising with your significant other can change that. I studied married people who joined a fitness program by themselves and as a couple. After 12 months, the couples had a better-than-90% adherence rate—that's remarkably high when you consider average adherence is about 50% after 12 months for people joining without their spouse. Most interesting was that they didn't need to be doing the exact same exercise program, provided they went to the gym together, so the issue of "he's stronger than I am" or "I don't like the same machines" doesn't matter. You don't have to work out side by side—you just have to make the commitment to exercise at the same time and place.

For busy working couples, it even can create date-night closeness. It's a terrific alternative to sitting silently in a movie.

KEYS FOR EXERCISE SUCCESS

•**Account for your differences.** Most couples have different fitness levels, and you need to create a plan that accounts for those. If you're working out with machines in a gym, it's easy to simply go together for a set period of time or go to a class together. But if you want to go running or biking together and one of you can handle a greater pace and distance than the other, you'll have to make accommodations.

Try this: Agree to separate distance goals. Start off together at the same speed, but pick a point where the person with less stamina will stop and allow the other to continue or where the one who is in front will pause and wait for his/her partner.

Hint: Make your route a repetitive loop that goes past your car or your home to make it convenient for one person to stop if needed. Don't put yourselves in the position of having to navigate differences on the fly when one of you suddenly runs out of gas at the midway point of the route.

•**Introduce your partner to the workouts you like.** If you are already in a class and want your partner to join (kickboxing, for example), make sure he will feel comfortable joining. If your partner thinks of the activity as being for the opposite sex, don't force it. On the other hand, if your spouse is open to trying it, help him avoid feeling awkward with the activity itself. Do this with a preview—demonstrate how to do key moves and use any equipment. It's like hosting friends in an unfamiliar city—you make the right introductions and give them the lay of the land so that they'll be more comfortable and confident.

●**Create a backup plan.** People drop out of fitness programs for many reasons—from a brief illness to changes in work schedules. To avoid getting derailed, preemptively take steps to create workarounds should speed bumps occur.

Example: If one spouse has to miss a week of exercise for a business trip, agree that the other will do it alone rather than sit it out—it's easier for one partner to rejoin activities than for two people to both do a reboot. And if one continues on his own, the other will be more likely to jump back into the routine. Have a list of alternate activities in case neither of you can get to a scheduled class. Switch to an after-dinner walk, for example.

●**Set and reset goals.** Initially, your shared aim might be to exercise a certain number of times a week for a certain length of time. After a while, each partner might add individualized goals. Maybe one wants to build more muscle, while the other wants to boost cardiovascular fitness. That's all OK. In fact, it gives each partner an additional opportunity to be supportive—cheer each other on and celebrate as you reach personal goals. ("Show me your muscles!") Just remember that if you get to your goal first, take time to reinforce all the progress your spouse has made, too. Being at different fitness levels becomes a problem only if one partner feels inadequate or believes that he is falling too far behind. Note that classes in gentle disciplines such as yoga and tai chi will have you both going at the same steady pace, no matter what your respective fitness levels are. Spin and Pilates also allow for different levels in the same class.

●**Consider a personal trainer.** If you're having trouble coming up with a fitness plan, consider signing up with a professional trainer who can take each partner's skill set into account, as well as make adjustments so that you're both doing the same type of program but at your own pace.

Important: Shop around for a trainer who has experience working with couples—ask friends, the manager at your gym and coaches at your local schools for recommendations. See the box at left for ideas on exercises you can do together.

●**Train together for an event.** When you set a competitive goal, such as running a 5K, you train harder and more regularly, and you can revel in the accomplishment of the goal. This can be very exciting for both partners. If you won't be side by side during the actual event, you still will be able to support each other before and after the event.

Do This Move Together…

Mona Xu, PhD, assistant professor of experimental psychology at Idaho State University (ISU) and director of the ISU Social, Health and Neuroscience Lab, which studies the interplay between close interpersonal relationships and behavioral health. She is coauthor of a recent study in *Psychology of Sport and Exercise* on the ways that others influence our exercise habits.

Try this fun "full-body" move with your partner. It gives your shoulders, arms, back and legs a nice stretch, which improves flexibility before or after exercise…

What to do: Warm up with a few minutes of easy walking, then begin by sitting on the floor. Face your partner and place the bottoms of your feet against his/her feet. Each of you should grab one end of a towel or resistance band. Slowly lean backward, gently pulling the towel or band so that your partner must lean forward until he feels a stretch in his hamstrings. Hold for 10 to 30 seconds, then return to the starting position and have your partner lean back. Repeat the entire sequence three to five times.

Caution: If you've had hip or back surgery, check with your doctor before trying this stretch.

An Exercise Program for Every Attitude

Wayne Westcott, PhD, professor of exercise science and chair of the exercise science program at Quincy College in Quincy, Massachusetts. He is the author or coauthor of 20 books, including *Strength Training Past 50.*

Pilates…yoga…aerobics…stairmaster…treadmill…jogging…water aerobics…the list of exercise options goes on and on. For people who are starting an exercise program, it is easy to get discouraged if they pick a program that doesn't work well for them. Once discouraged, it may be bye-bye exercise.

NO ONE SIZE FITS ALL

When it comes to weight loss, we all have different diet and exercise personalities. And if there's one mantra that virtually every fitness professional has come to embrace, its the one that says, no one program works for everyone. One size simply doesn't fit all. What works for your neighbor may not work for you, and what your neighbor hates most may be number one on your own personal hit parade. So, how do we choose the right diet and exercise program for our own personal situation?

There are a number of ways to accomplish weight loss. How you approach weight loss depends on your exercise attitude, of which there are several types.

Attitude Type One: I hate to exercise. If this is your attitude, Dr. Wayne Westcott, professor of exercise science and researcher, makes these recommendations…

Diet: Reduced-calorie diet (typically 1,600 calories or less per day for women, 1,800 for men).

Strength training: Only two times per week, 15 minutes per session (see strength training circuit below for specifics).

Aerobic exercise: Only two times per week, 15 minutes per session (aerobics can be anything that gets the heart rate up to 50% to 75% of maximum heart rate for your age—running, jogging, walking, swimming, spinning class, etc.). Target heart rates can be found at the American Heart Association website at Heart.org (search "target heart rate").

That minimum amount of exercise just one hour per week will actually maintain muscle and cardio fitness, says Dr. Westcott.

Attitude Type Two: I like exercise but don't like strength training much…

Diet: Less calorie restriction than Type One (1,700 to 1,750 for women…1,900 to 1,950 for men).

Strength training: Same as Type One above (two times per week, 15 minutes each session).

Aerobic exercise: Four times per week, 15 minutes per session (or twice a week, 30 minutes per session).

The extra aerobic exercise allows you to eat slightly more than Type One.

Attitude Type Three: I like to exercise hard…

Diet: Continue what you normally eat.

Strength training: Two to three times a week, 30 minutes per session (circuits).

Aerobic exercise: Two to three times a week, 30 minutes per session.

Those strength-training circuits burn a lot of calories. Remember that the more vigorously you exercise, the more calories you burn.

STRENGTH TRAINING: WHAT TO DO

Dr. Westcott recommends a circuit of exercises. A circuit is performed by doing an exercise and moving on to the next with minimum rest in between. When you've performed each exercise in the series, you've done one circuit. You can repeat the circuit up to three times in a session. Studies have shown that unfit people performing just one hard circuit, twice a week with a one-minute or less rest between exercises will get measurable results from this routine. Those who are more fit and conditioned to begin with have to up the ante a bit in order to get serious improvement—either by performing more circuits or using heavier weights.

TWO ACTUAL CIRCUITS

Here are two recommended strength-training circuits (for more easy ways to get started with strength training see chapter 7, page 114). Weight for each exercise should be enough that you can complete eight to 12 repetitions. If 12 is too easy, and you feel you could continue, raise the weight. If you cannot complete eight, lower the weight until you can finish the set.

The first circuit is composed of exercises that use multiple muscles (called compound exercises). The second includes specific arm exercises. Either is effective, and you may alternate. They can be performed at home or at the gym. (*Note:* For an excellent illustrated explanation of how to perform these exercises with correct form, see *Weight Training for Dummies* by Liz Neporent and Suzanne Schlosberg.)

STRENGTH TRAINING: CIRCUIT ONE

1. **Leg press or squat**
2. **Dumbbell bench press (if at home) or chest press machine (if at the gym)**
3. **Bent-over row (home) or rowing machine (gym)**
4. **Dumbbell shoulder press (home) or shoulder press machine (gym)**
5. **Chin-up (home: have someone assist you) or assisted chin-up (gym)**
6. **Incline dumbbell bench press (home) or incline chest press machine (gym)**
7. **Crunches**

STRENGTH TRAINING: CIRCUIT TWO

1. **Leg press or squat**
2. **Chest press**
3. **Bent-over row (home) or seated row (gym)**
4. **Shoulder press**
5. **Lat pulldown (gym only)**
6. **Triceps press**
7. **Biceps curl**
8. **Crunches**

PICKING AEROBIC EXERCISES

As for the aerobic portion of your workout, the key is to make it enjoyable. Be sure to choose an activity that is fun for you and remember that it doesnt have to be the same one every time. In fact, your muscles will respond better if you mix it up, so that you exercise slightly different muscle groups each time you work out. You can ride a bicycle one day…use a cross-country ski machine another…

and swim on a third. Or take an aerobics or dance class. In good weather, kayaking will give you a good upper body workout, while cycling or a fast walk will exercise your lower body on alternating days.

If a certain exercise gives you pain, then don't continue. Pick a different one that doesn't strain your trouble spot(s).

How I Stay Motivated to Exercise

Ruth Heidrich, PhD, a certified fitness trainer and eight-time gold medalist in the US Senior Olympics. She is the author of several books, including *Lifelong Running* and *Senior Fitness.*

I'm in my mid 80s, and I've completed more than 60 marathons (26.2-mile races) in recent decades. Today, I continue to compete frequently at shorter distances such as half-marathons. Even though I was diagnosed with breast cancer at age 47, I now have no signs of cancer in my body.

What keeps me going? It's really quite simple—I want to remain robust and vigorous. This desire helps me overcome the excuses that many people use for not exercising. Even if you're not interested in running a marathon, my strategies work amazingly well—regardless of your current fitness level. *Five secrets that can keep your exercise program on track…*

1. Visualize yourself as fit and healthy. A combination of regular aerobic exercise (such as walking or jogging)…strength training (with hand weights or exercise machines)…and stretching (including touching your toes to loosen the hamstring muscles in the back of the thigh) will increase your energy and help keep your weight down, your bones and muscles strong, and your blood vessels healthy.

But if these benefits are not enough to motivate you, try visualizing how you will look as a fit, healthy person. Close your eyes and see yourself as lean and strong, with firm, toned legs, a flat stomach and a bounce in your step. Imagine how you will move and feel once you start exercising regularly.

For best results: Do this visualization for a couple of minutes whenever you feel the need for some extra motivation.

2. Make a "rewards" list. Write down all the ways that exercise will improve your life. Don't give general answers, such as "better health." Be specific. Include rewards that will be meaningful to you, such as not needing as many (or any) medications…saving money on health-care expenses…or gaining the stamina to travel anywhere you like.

For best results: Keep this list on your desk or refrigerator where you'll see it every day.

3. Be sure that your goals are complete. Just "wanting to" start exercising is not enough of a goal. Goals must include four key parts—they must be specific, measurable and attainable—and you must create a timeline for achieving them. For example, your goal may be to "walk for 30 minutes at least three times a week for two months." Consult your doctor to ensure that your goals are appropriate and realistic.

For best results: Sign up to participate in an event that is several months away, such as a walk-a-thon or an organized bike race. Flyers for such activities are posted on the bulletin boards of many gyms, health-food stores and bookstores.

4. Get a new calendar. You say you don't have time to exercise? That's one of the oldest excuses in the book. If you decide that there's something you must do, you make an appointment—and then do it!

For best results: Find a calendar (I like the large wall calendars that are sold in office-supply stores for about $10) that has enough space for each day so that you can write not only the time that you will exercise, but also what each workout will include.

For example: For Mondays, Wednesdays and Fridays, you might write "20-minute weight workout at 8 am." For Tuesdays, Thursdays and Saturdays, it might be "30 minutes of walking at 7 am."

Also helpful: On the same monthly calendar, make a check mark next to each exercise session you complete or add a brief summary if your workout was shorter or longer. This journal will keep you honest in terms of the amount of exercise you're actually doing.

5. Share your goals. To stay motivated, share your goals with a friend, then set up regular times to exercise together. Between the support of your training partners and your desire to not let them down, your exercise program will flourish.

For best results: Join an organized exercise class or group. This can be especially helpful if the group has a coach or teacher who can help you set and reach your goals.

2

Limber Up with Stretching, Yoga, Tai Chi and Qigong

How Limber Are You? Take Our Quiz!

Diana Zotos Florio, licensed physical therapist and certified yoga teacher, New York City.

Marla Altberg, certified personal trainer and Pilates mat instructor, New York City.

H ere's an unusual resolution that you probably have never made.

Become more flexible this year—literally!

For anyone who wants to have a fit, healthy body, building more endurance and strength are common goals, but you rarely hear someone say, "By the end of the year, I want to be able to touch my toes with the palms of my hands while standing—and do it smiling!"

But improving and/or maintaining flexibility is key to your health, because being loose and limber makes it easier to build strength and endurance…it makes everyday activities, such as tying your shoes or reaching behind the driver's seat in a car, less painful…and it makes you less prone to injury.

And it just feels great.

So, how flexible are you?

Take our quick quiz to find out…and then, if you discover that you're not exactly like Gumby,

don't worry—here are some easy tips from an expert that'll make you flexible in no time.

YOUR QUICK FLEXIBILITY TEST

To get an idea of how limber you are (or aren't), take this simple test created by Diana Zotos Florio, a physical therapist and yoga instructor in New York City.

●**Shoulder Stretch.** Standing, place your right forearm behind your waist and then raise your hand as far up as you comfortably can. Repeat this move with your left forearm. *Can you…*

a. Reach your shoulder blades with your fingertips?

b. Reach your middle back?

c. Reach your lower back?

●**Trunk Rotation.** Sit up straight in a chair with your arms crossed lightly across your chest, hands touching opposite shoulders. Stare straight ahead. When you gently twist your upper body and head from side to side, can you…

a. Turn your torso to about the 3:00 position on your right side and 9:00 on your left?

b. Turn not quite as far—only to 2:00 and 10:00?

c. Turn only to 1:00 and 11:00, or not much further than your starting position?

●**Leg Reach.** Stand up straight with feet hip-distance apart. When you bend forward and simultaneously slide both of your hands as far as you can down your legs (with your right hand on your right leg and your left hand on your left leg), can you…

a. Reach below the knee?

b. Reach the knee?

c. Reach mid-thigh?

•**Toe Touch.** Sit on the floor with your back straight and your legs extended straight in front of you. *When you bend over, can you…*

a. Touch your toes?

b. Reach your ankles but no further?

c. Get only as far as your shins?

If you answered mostly As, good job—you're lithe and limber. Just keep stretching a couple of times a week. If you fall into the B range, you're getting a bit stiff and could benefit from stretching more often, three to five times a week. If you answered primarily Cs, watch out! You may not be moving around as much as you should, and as a result, you're losing a lot of flexibility—but it's never too late to reclaim it! Doing the following stretches can help you open up your muscles and start to see improvement in your flexibility in as little as one to two weeks.

LIMBER UP!

Marla Altberg, a certified personal trainer and Pilates mat instructor in New York City, explains that even if you have spent weeks (or longer) on the couch, you can easily loosen up again by performing this 10- to 15-minute stretching routine…

ON YOUR BACK: To perform the following stretches, lie on your back with your knees bent, feet slightly apart and flat on the floor and arms by your sides with palms facing downward.

•**Triangle Stretch** (For hamstrings, quads, inner thighs and hips)…

1. Make a triangle by crossing your left foot over your right knee.

2. Grasp your right leg behind your thigh, and inhale as you bring it in toward your chest.

3. Take your left elbow and press it gently against your left knee.

4. Breathe naturally as you hold the stretch for 20 seconds.

5. Return to your starting position and repeat on the other side.

•**Leg Raise** (For hamstrings, quads and back)…

1. Leaving your left leg where it is, bring your right knee to your chest as you inhale, and then slowly raise your right foot straight up to the ceiling as you exhale.

2. Using both hands, grab hold of your right leg behind your thigh, and climb up your leg, hand over hand, as far as you can toward your foot.

3. Keeping your hands as close as possible to your right foot, pull your right leg toward you, keeping it as straight as possible while your knee moves toward your face, gently but carefully—never to the point of pain. At the same time, push the leg against your hands in the opposite direction. Hold this pose for a count of 10, if possible.

4. Walk your hands back down, and repeat on the other side.

•**"T" Stretch** (For back and side abdominals)…

1. Join your knees together and tilt them both over to the left side until they touch the floor (or come as close to the floor as possible).

2. Spread your arms out to your sides, so your body forms the letter "T," and turn your head and torso to the right.

3. Hold for 20 seconds, breathing naturally and deeply into the stretch. Repeat on the opposite side.

ON YOUR TUMMY: To perform the next set of stretches, roll over onto your stomach.

•**Ab Contraction** (For abs and back)…

1. Make a pillow with your hands, rest your forehead on it and position your feet hip-width apart.

2. Inhale deeply, and then exhale as you draw your abdominal muscles in and up. Hold for 5 to 10 seconds and release. Pause for just a few seconds and then repeat twice.

3. Next, make the same muscle contraction but, as you do so, slightly raise your head (keeping your forehead glued to your hands) and chest **off the floor.** Hold for five seconds and release. Pause for just a few seconds and then repeat twice.

•**Fly Like Superman** (For back, abs, butt and shoulders)…

1. **Still lying on your stomach, extend your arms above your head, shoulder-width apart, with the palms of your hands facing downward.**

2. **Inhale deeply.** Exhaling, contract your abs and raise your right arm and left leg slightly off the floor simultaneously.

3. **Hold for a count of 3 to 5 and then release.** Repeat on the other side, and then do one more set.

•**Cat Stretch** (For back and abs)…

1. **Get on your hands and knees.**

2. **Inhaling, pull your stomach in, tip your pelvis forward and arch your back like a cat.** Hold for 3 to 5 seconds.

3. **Exhaling, gradually relax back into your original position.** Pause for just a few seconds and then repeat twice.

Note: If you have a health issue such as a bad back, joint problems or heart disease, consult your primary care provider before beginning any new exercise program.

Stretches for Body Parts You Didn't Know Needed It!

Jessica Matthews, DBH (doctor of behavioral health), a certified yoga teacher, professor of kinesiology at Point Loma Nazarene University in San Diego and 2017 IDEA Fitness Instructor of the Year. She is author of *Stretching to Stay Young: Simple Workouts to Keep You Flexible, Energized, and Pain-Free.*

Even if stretching is part of your regular workout routine, there are probably body parts that need stretching and aren't getting it. But if you want to keep your whole body flexible, energized and pain-free, you need to keep those ignored areas limber, too.

Regular stretching enhances flexibility and range of motion in joints, which helps the body move with greater ease when doing other kinds of exercise as well as during daily activities, while also helping to prevent injuries such as muscle strains and falls. Stretching also can help to reduce pain and stiffness. And when paired with mindful breathing, stretching can help mitigate stress and reduce mental tension.

However, most people tend to leave some muscles out of stretching routines because they're not aware of them, such as the quadratus lumborum and the tibialis anterior…and other muscles they may exercise to strengthen but not know they also need to be stretched, such as the biceps and obliques.

The American College of Sports Medicine recommends that flexibility exercises be performed at least two to three days per week, with daily stretching being most effective. The following passive static stretches should be held to the point of mild tension or slight discomfort to enhance joint range of motion, but never to the point of pain. Each stretch should be held for 15 to 30 seconds per repetition. *Some commonly ignored muscles and the stretches that keep them limber…*

•**Biceps stretch.** The biceps brachii is located at the front of the upper arm and is the primary muscle involved in flexing the elbow and moving the

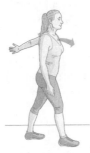

forearm. Biceps exercises tend to focus on concentrically engaging (shortening) the muscles in order to build them up. Even when followed by lengthening motion, the lengthening is created by tension and doesn't really stretch the muscles. Stretching the biceps helps maintain their ideal length and range of motion and minimizes risk for injury.

Bonus: Biceps stretches may support improved posture, countering a rounded shoulder position by also stretching the shoulders and pectoral muscles.

How to do it: Stand facing a wall, as close as you can get to it. Extend your left arm along the wall straight out to shoulder height and place your palm flat against the wall, thumb pointing up. Keep your right arm relaxed at your side. Keeping your left palm on the wall, rotate your body clockwise (to the right) by pivoting on your feet to assume a position with shoulders and hips perpendicular to the wall and your right foot slightly ahead of your left foot. Complete the stretch by rotating your hips and shoulders away from the wall while your feet stay firmly in position. Hold the stretch for three to five breaths (approximately 30 seconds). Switch sides and repeat. Complete two repetitions per side.

•**Quadratus lumborum and obliques stretch ("standing crescent moon").** The quadratus lumborum (QL) is a deep abdominal muscle that con-

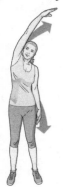

nects your lower spine to your pelvis. The QL gets taxed by extended periods of sitting, poor posture and also strain from repetitive day-to-day movements, leading to tightness and pain in the lower back. The obliques—internal and external—are muscles found on the sides of the rectus abdominis (the "six-pack" muscles) and run from hips to rib cage. They help stabilize the spine and aid in flexion (the ability of the spine to bend), lateral flexion (bend to the side) and rotation (twist). Tight obliques can pull the spine out of alignment and lead to poor posture. Research also shows that when lateral flexion is restricted, it increases risk for low-back pain. Lateral flexion of the spine is often neglected in daily exercise routines.

How to do it: Stand with feet hip-width apart, arms at your sides. Keeping your left arm relaxed at your side, inhale and sweep your right arm out to the side and up, fingers pointing toward the ceiling and your palm facing to the left. Next, exhale while reaching your right arm over your head toward your left side, keeping your fingertips pointed out, as you lean your torso to the left to stretch the right side of your body. Hold the stretch for three to five breaths (approximately 30 seconds). Switch sides and repeat. Complete two repetitions per side.

•**Tibialis anterior stretch.** Your tibialis anterior is located on your outer shin and is involved in moving the foot and ankle, specifically pointing your foot up. You're probably familiar with tight tibialis anterior muscles—commonly called "shin splints." Lengthening the muscle helps avoid this potential pain. Exercises that stretch the backs of the legs, such as runners do to warm up, put the foot and

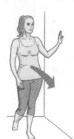

ankle in a position that tightens the tibialis anterior. To stretch this muscle, you need to do the opposite—point your toes forward, a move that is not part of many exercises.

How to do it: Stand barefoot next to a wall or chair on your left side with your feet together. Bracing your left hand on the wall or holding a chair for support, bend your right knee and extend your right leg back, pointing the toes of your right foot so that you can place the tops of your tucked-under toes on the floor behind you. Keeping the tops of your toes on the floor, shift your weight slightly forward to create a stretch in the front lower part of your leg (shin). Hold this stretch for three to five breaths (approximately 30 seconds). Switch sides and repeat with your left leg. Complete two repetitions per side.

Illustrations of stretching figures: Copyright © Christian Papazoglakis/Illozoo

6 Common Stretching Mistakes That Can Hurt You

Karl Knopf, EdD, director of fitness therapy and senior fitness for the International Sports Sciences Association and retired director of adaptive fitness at Foothill College in Los Altos Hills, California. He is author of many fitness books including *Stretching for 50+* and a board member of Sit and Be Fit, a nonprofit organization dedicated to healthy aging.

We now know that stretching is key to staying limber and flexible. But did you know that it also could be dangerous?

Many people stretch improperly, overstressing muscles and even tendons in ways that lead to strains and sprains. An injury can come on gradually as a result of cumulative "insults" from performing a stretch a certain way over and over again. You don't know you're hurting yourself…until you're really hurt.

Other people don't stretch wrong—they just don't stretch at all or only once in a while. Many people focus more on cardiovascular exercise and weight training, yet often neglect stretching—until they get hurt. To benefit from a flexibility program, you need to practice it regularly, ideally every day.

As we age, stretching becomes even more important. Our bodies undergo changes that result in lack of elasticity. Women tend to be more flexible than men, but starting in their 50s, both genders start to lose flexibility and range of motion, especially in the shoulders and low back, which can lead to shoulder and back issues. The good news is that this age-related decline can be slowed through a regular stretching program.

By learning to stretch properly, you'll maximize your mobility…greatly reduce the risk for pain and injury…perform better at any sport you engage in…and look younger. (*One caution*: If you've had a recent fracture, sprain, injury or surgery, or if you suspect that you have osteoporosis, speak to your doctor/physical therapist first.)

Here are common stretching mistakes that can hurt you—and how to steer clear of them…

HOLDING YOUR BREATH

One common stretching mistake is holding your breath as you hold a stretch. Muscles need oxygen throughout a stretch—plus, holding your breath can elevate your blood pressure. Breathe slowly and consistently throughout each phase of a stretch—especially when you're holding one.

Simple stretches, such as shoulder rolls (see "Safe, Effective Stretches You Can Do Anywhere" on the next page), don't require that you hold them. But most do. These stretches should be held for at least 20 seconds—and recent studies suggest that for older adults, 60 seconds is even better. Breathe throughout.

STRETCHING COLD

Not that long ago, we were instructed to stretch before playing sports when our muscles were "cold." Now we know that's a bad idea. Think of your muscles and tendons as taffy. Then imagine trying to stretch and bend cold taffy. It can snap. On a micro level, that's like stretching a cold, tight muscle. Ouch!

Much better: Warm up for five minutes or more first, before you do any stretch that you hold. Try light running…a few minutes in a steam room or sauna…or, if you're home, a warm bath.

GETTING INTENSE

Too many people follow the old paradigm that the more intense the exercise, the better. They overdo it with weights, aerobics—and stretching. In my opinion, no pain, no gain is…insane. If you feel sore a few hours after exercising, you overdid it.

Much better: When stretching, move slowly and gently, and stay within your comfort zone. You should feel mild tension in your muscles and joints. Don't push past it. Listen to your body, especially your neck, back, shoulders and knees. If you have tightness or joint pain, take some time off. If it continues, see your doctor or a physical therapist before it turns into a real issue.

GOING OLD SCHOOL—FAST AND BOUNCY

If you played a sport in high school, it's time to unlearn some things you learned, including bouncing toe touches. These moves weren't safe then, and they are even riskier now that you're older. Those neck circles you started every gym class with? Terrible! They strain supporting ligaments and can lead to pinched nerves.

That hurdler stretch where you sit with one leg out in front of you and the other bent behind you? It stresses the meniscus and the medial collateral ligament of your knee—an injury in the making. Fast toe touches? No! Bending and rotating at the same time is a recipe for trouble.

Red flag: Avoid stretches such as the hurdler that make your knees twist or move in an unnatural position. Be careful about back bends that call for you to raise both hands over your head and lean back. That can pinch the facet joints of the spine. Go slow in any yoga moves that use this bend.

Much better: Always keep knees "soft" (slightly bent) when stretching. When turning, move your body slowly, as a unit, and pivot your feet.

STRETCHING ONLY WHEN YOU EXERCISE

Chances are that if you stretch, you do so only before working out or playing a sport. Big mistake! To maintain flexibility, your muscles need to be worked just about every day.

Much better: Think of stretching as part of your daily routine, like brushing your teeth. You don't need a designated area or even to wear gym clothes. Spend a few minutes doing a body-flexibility session daily, especially in high-risk areas such as the hamstrings, shoulders and lower back.

NOT BEING WELL-BALANCED

The body is designed with opposing muscle groups, and each group needs to be worked equally. Weight training can unbalance muscles, so you need stretching to get you back into balance.

Example: If you do a movement such as a bench press that rolls your shoulders forward, you should do a stretch that pulls them back. My golden rule is, *Do unto the front as you do unto the back, and do unto the left as you do unto the right.*

Conversely, being too flexible can be a problem, especially if you don't have muscles that are strong enough to support your joints. I once taught a dancer who kept dislocating her shoulder joints because her muscles weren't strong enough to keep her shoulders in place. It's all about balance.

One final tip—enjoy your stretching session. It's a great time to integrate the mind and the body.

SAFE, EFFECTIVE STRETCHES YOU CAN DO ANYWHERE

Here are two different kinds of stretches—no-hold stretches that you can do anywhere anytime and standard stretches for which you warm up for five minutes and then hold for at least 20 seconds, ideally 60.

Together, these stretches work on your upper and lower body. Repeat each one at least three times.

Upper-body no-hold stretches…

•**Elbow touches (for the chest).** Place your hands on your shoulders (left on left, right on right), elbows pointing forward as much as possible. Slowly move your elbows out to the side as far as is comfortable, pinching the shoulder blades together, and hold for just a few seconds. Bring your elbows back to the starting position and repeat.

•**Shoulder rolls (for the upper back).** With your arms hanging down naturally, shrug your shoulders up and squeeze them back, as if attempting to touch them together…then relax them.

•**Apple pickers (for the shoulders).** Place your hands on your shoulders (left hand on left, right on right). Then slowly raise your right hand as high up as is comfortable—reach for that apple! Return to the start position, and repeat with the left hand. Keep good posture throughout.

These are standard "hold 'em" stretches…

•**Chest stretch (for the chest and shoulders).** Stand facing a corner. Place one hand on each side wall, with your elbows in a push-up position. Lean gently into the corner until you feel a stretch across your upper chest. Hold for at least 20 seconds.

•**Seated knee to chest (for the lower back and gluteal muscles/butt).** Sit on a stable chair with your feet flat on the floor. Clasp your hands beneath your left leg. Pull your left knee toward your chest with your hands and hold for at least 20 seconds, feeling the stretch in the gluteal and low-back area. Return to start position, and repeat with other leg.

•**Rear calf stretch (for your calves).** Stand facing a wall, with both hands on the wall at shoulder height. Your knees should be slightly bent. Keeping the heel down, slide your right leg back until you feel the stretch in the calf area. Hold for at least 20 seconds. Switch sides and repeat.

A Personal Trainer for Olympians Shares His Favorite Stretches

Joel Harper, a New York City–based personal trainer whose clients include several Olympic medalists. The creator of the PBS DVD *Firming After 50*, he designed all of the personal workout chapters for Drs. Mehmet C. Oz and Michael F. Roizen's YOU series of books and accompanying workout DVDs. JoelHarperFitness.com

You may not be surprised if you feel a little stiff or achy after doing something you ordinarily don't do—such as sleeping on one side all night long…playing an especially tough match of tennis or round of golf…or hunching over a computer for long hours.

What does surprise most people is the long-term effect of habitually doing any of these things. The result is out-of-balance muscles—an often hidden cause of chronic pain and tightness in the back, knees, hips, shoulders and/or ankles.

Muscle imbalances don't happen overnight, but if certain activities are repeated day in and day out, the pain often goes undiagnosed and may drive sufferers to take potentially dangerous medications or even get surgery.

Joel Harper, a leading New York City–based personal trainer, knows how harmful muscle imbalances can be and has created specific muscle-balancing stretches for the Olympic medalists and other clients he works with. *Here are the habits that most often cause muscle imbalances—and the simple daily exercises that help…**

•**Sleeping on the same side every night.** This habit compresses one shoulder and hip.

The fix: Remind yourself when you go to bed that you want to start alternating sleeping sides throughout the night. After a while, your habit may change. Also, do the passive spinal twist below each morning upon waking to elongate the muscles on both sides of your body.

What to do: While lying on your back in bed, interlock your fingers behind your head. Keep your elbows out, and lift your knees into a 90-degree angle. Then, keeping your torso flat and level, gently drop both of your knees to one side as far as you comfortably can, while looking straight up, and take five deep breaths. Repeat on the other side. If you notice more tightness on one side, repeat the stretch on that side for a few more breaths.

Also: Place a pillow between your knees when sleeping to help keep your hips and spine aligned.

•**Too much sitting.** Sitting for hours on end at a desk, while traveling or even on the couch tightens the hip flexors (the muscles that contract when lifting your knees to your chest) and weakens the opposing muscles of the buttocks, or "glutes." As a result, your pelvis tilts downward, stressing your lower back muscles.

The fix: Walk around for at least five minutes every few hours. Also, try the seated airplane stretch.

What to do: Sit in a chair with your feet flat on the floor. Then, place your right ankle on your quad, about an inch above your left knee. Next, rest your right elbow on top of your right knee and place your right hand on your right ankle. Gently lean forward, until you feel a comfortable stretch, while looking ahead, not down, and keeping your back straight. Hold for 30 seconds, then switch sides.

•**Repeated one-sided activities.** Stand shirtless in front of a full-length mirror. If one shoulder appears slightly lower than the other, it may be because you always keep your computer mouse on the same side…favor your right or left leg when crossing your legs…or always wear a purse, backpack or other bag on the same side. These activities cause a muscle imbalance in which your back becomes overworked on one side but underused on the other. Sports in which one side is dominant, such as tennis, golf or bowling, also can cause this type of muscle imbalance.

The fix: Alternate the shoulder on which you carry your bag, the way you cross your legs and, yes, even the side of the computer where you place your mouse (this will help you become ambidextrous). Then, try a stretch for your chest.

What to do: With your fingers interlocked behind your head and your elbows out, slightly move your hands away from your head and hold for five deep inhalations. Do this a few times each day. Look straight ahead during this stretch.

If you play a racket sport or enjoy another sport in which one side is dominant, incorporate strengthening moves for the opposite side when you're not playing.

Also helpful: Consider taking up a new activity that uses muscles on both sides more equally, such as swimming, yoga or tai chi.

*It's always wise to consult a doctor before doing any new exercises.

Yoga—It Can Change Your Life!

Mary Louise Stefanic, a certified yoga and qigong instructor with a focus on therapeutic yoga. Ms. Stefanic was a staff member at the Loyola Center for Fitness and Loyola University Health System, both in Maywood, Illinois. She has been teaching yoga since 1969.

Not that long ago, yoga was viewed primarily as an activity for "youngish" health nuts who wanted to round out their exercise regimens. Now: Older adults—meaning people in their 60s, 70s, 80s and beyond—are among the most enthusiastic practitioners of this ancient healing system of exercise and controlled breathing.

Mary Louise Stefanic, a yoga instructor who has taught the practice for more than 40 years, reveals the unique benefits you can derive from yoga...

YOGA GOES MAINSTREAM

Virtually everyone can benefit from yoga. Unfortunately, many people are reluctant to try it because they assume that it's too unconventional and requires extreme flexibility. Neither belief is true.

What's more, its varied health benefits are largely what's making the practice so popular now with older adults. More than 1,000 scientific studies have shown that yoga can improve conditions ranging from arthritis, asthma, insomnia and depression to heart disease, diabetes and cancer.

You look better, too: Yoga is quite useful in helping to prevent rounding (or hunching) of the back, which occurs so often in older adults. This condition can lead to back pain and breathing problems as the rib cage presses against the lungs.

My experience: After teaching yoga to thousands of students, I'm continually amazed at how many tell me that it has literally changed their lives by helping them feel so much better physically and mentally.

GETTING STARTED

If you want to see whether you could benefit from yoga, ask your doctor about trying the following poses, which address common physical complaints. These poses are a good first step before taking a yoga class.* Yoga is best performed in loose, comfortable clothing and in your bare feet, so your feet won't slip. *Poses to try...*

●**Knees to chest pose.** For low back pain and painful, tight hips.

What to do: Lie on your back (on carpet or a yoga mat, available at sports-equipment stores for about $25). With your arms, hug both knees in to your chest. Keep your knees together and your elbows pointing out to each side of your body. Slowly rock from elbow to elbow to massage your back and shoulders. Take deep, abdominal breaths while holding your thighs close to your chest and hold for six complete inhales and exhales.

●**Mecca pose.** This pose also relieves back pain.

What to do: Begin by kneeling on the floor with your knees together. For added comfort, place a small towel behind your knees. Sit back on your feet, and lean forward from your waist so that your chest and stomach rest atop your thighs. Reach your arms out in front of you, resting your forehead to the floor while stretching your tailbone to your heels. Hold for six complete inhales and exhales.

●**Leg rotation.** For sciatica, a cause of back, pelvic and leg pain.

What to do: Lie on your back with both legs extended. Slowly bring your right knee to your chest and inhale. Rest your right ankle on the front of your left thigh, and exhale as you slowly slide it down along your left knee, shin and ankle to toes. This helps "screw" the top of your right thighbone into the hip socket, easing lower back and leg pain. Repeat on other side. Do three times on each side.

To conclude your session: While in a sitting position, press your palms together. Bring your thumbs into your breastbone. Tuck your elbows in and down, press your breastbone to your thumbs, lifting and opening your chest. Hold for six breaths.

Important: Even when you're not doing yoga, don't forget your breath. Slow, thoughtful, deep

*To find a yoga class near you, check your local community center and/or consult the International Association of Yoga Therapists, IAYT.org.

breathing is most effective, but don't perform it too quickly. I find the technique to be most effective when you hold the inhalation and exhalation for a certain number of counts.

What to do: Lie on your back, resting your hands on your belly so that your middle fingers touch across your navel. Inhale through your nose for a count of six, pushing your navel out so that your fingertips separate. Pause, then exhale for a count of nine, pulling your navel back in. Perform these steps two more times (more may make you dizzy). Do this in the morning and at night (deep breathing improves mental focus and can be energizing in the morning and calming at night).

Yoga Exercises Anyone Can Do

Susan Winter Ward, a Pagosa Springs, Colorado–based yoga instructor and the author of *Yoga for the Young at Heart: Accessible Yoga for Every Body.* She has taught yoga for 14 years and is the creator of the Yoga for the Young at Heart video series, which can be ordered on her website, YogaHeart.com.

Many people assume that they could never practice yoga because it requires so much flexibility. The truth is, inflexibility is actually one of the best reasons to do yoga.

Traditional yoga can be more challenging for people who suffer joint stiffness due to osteoarthritis or inactivity—the stretching as well as getting up and down from the floor, where some yoga poses are performed, can be difficult. But there is an alternative.

I've created a series of yoga exercises designed to be performed while seated in a chair.* These poses are accessible for people with physical limitations, due to multiple sclerosis or other conditions. Chair yoga also can be done at your desk, or while traveling on a plane or a train.

The following series of exercises require little space and no equipment other than a firm, steady chair. When combined with cardiovascular ex-

*Check with your doctor before beginning this or any exercise program.

ercise, such as brisk walking, and strength training, such as weight-lifting, chair yoga helps create a well-balanced exercise program. All inhalations and exhalations for these exercises should be done through the nose for a count of five.

For maximum benefits, practice the following exercises daily...

•**Breathing for relaxation.** Deep breathing brings extra oxygen into the lungs and bloodstream, both relaxing and energizing the body, and calming the mind.

What to do: Sit up straight. Place your right hand over your heart and your left hand over your stomach. Close your eyes and breathe in deeply. Exhale, then breathe in again, while focusing on lifting your chest and expanding your ribs. Inhale, then exhale while maintaining a straight spine. Repeat five to 10 times.

•**Butterfly curls.** These stretch the back of the neck, the spine, rib cage and arms.

What to do: Sitting toward the front of your chair, straighten your back and clasp your hands behind your head. Breathe in deeply and lengthen your spine while pulling your elbows back and letting your rib cage expand. Keeping your back flat, exhale and curl your head forward, pulling your elbows gently toward each other. Take a few deep breaths, lifting your chest toward your chin as you inhale and dropping your chin toward your chest as you exhale. Repeat five times.

•**Windmill.** This relaxes the shoulders, neck and arms.

What to do: Sitting up straight, inhale as you raise your right arm overhead. Bend your right elbow so that it points upward and your fingers touch your upper spine or neck. Exhale, then inhale again.

Next, stretch your left arm out to your left side and bend your elbow, bringing the back of your left hand to your spine. Exhale, pressing your hands gently toward each other while keeping your back and shoulder blades flat. Inhale, lifting your chest and gently pressing your hands toward each other as you exhale. If you like, you can hold a belt or strap between your hands. Repeat three to five times.

•**Expand your heart.** This pose relaxes the back, shoulders and chest, and aids breathing by creating space in the rib cage for the lungs to expand.

What to do: Sitting toward the front of your chair, clasp your hands behind you at the waist. With your elbows bent, press your shoulder blades together, lifting your chest. Inhale, drawing your elbows toward each other. Lengthen your spine as you inhale and lift your ribs away from your hips. Exhale as you press your knuckles down toward the chair seat. Repeat three to five times, taking long, deep breaths.

•**Seated push-ups.** This exercise strengthens the arms, back and shoulders.

What to do: Sit near the front of your chair and put your hands on the front corners of the seat. Inhaling deeply, with your elbows in toward your sides, straighten your elbows and lift yourself off the seat of the chair. Keep your legs and shoulders relaxed and avoid pushing with your feet. Exhale as you slowly lower yourself. Repeat at least five times.

•**Spinal twist.** This stretches the rib cage and spine and eases back strain. It also aids digestion by massaging the stomach and intestines.

What to do: Sitting up straight, cross your right leg over your left and place your left hand on the inside of your left knee. Inhale deeply as you twist to the right, pulling your right elbow and shoulder around toward the back of the chair. Keeping your back straight, take three to five deep breaths as you hold the pose. Lengthen your spine by lifting through the top of your head with each inhalation, and twist a bit farther to the right with each exhalation. Return to center, then repeat on the opposite side.

•**Cervical stretch.** This pose stretches and relaxes the arms, wrists, hands, shoulders, back and chest. It counteracts the effects of typing and eases headaches due to shoulder tension.

What to do: Sitting near the front of your chair, inhale deeply and raise your arms overhead. Interlace your fingers, palms facing the ceiling. Exhale, pressing through the heels of your hands. Inhale again, tucking your chin in toward your throat. While holding this position, exhale and let your chin drop toward your chest. Breathe deeply three to five times, feeling the stretch down to your shoulder blades with each exhalation.

•**Hamstring stretch.** This stretches the backs of the thighs, releases low back tension, strengthens the back and abdomen, and improves digestion.

What to do: Sitting toward the front of your chair, place both feet flat on the floor. While keeping your back flat and chest lifted, clasp your left knee just below the kneecap with both hands and pull your thigh toward your rib cage. Hold for three to five breaths. Switch legs and repeat.

Two-Minute Yoga Practice

Annie Carpenter, yoga instructor, Exhale Center for Sacred Movement, Los Angeles, quoted in *Yoga Journal*. Yoga Journal.com

Two-minute yoga practice is an effective overall stretch. Doing the Downward Dog pose everyday uses the strength of your arms and legs to stretch your spine, hips, hamstrings and calves. It also strengthens your quadriceps and ankles…and tones your arms and abdominals.

5-Minute Yoga Wake-Up

Carol Krucoff, C-IAYT, E-RYT, a yoga therapist and codirector of the Integrated Yoga for Seniors Professional Training at Duke Integrative Medicine, Durham, North Carolina. She is the coauthor of *Relax into Yoga for Seniors: A Six-Week Program for Strength, Balance, Flexibility and Pain Relief.* HealingMoves.com

To start your day off right, indulge in a five-minute ritual of simple yoga moves, beginning while you're still in bed and gradually building in intensity. Do these moves in the order given, repeating each exercise three to five times, and always breathing slowly and deeply.

LYING IN BED

•**Belly breathing.** Lie on your back, eyes closed, palms resting on your abdomen just below your navel. Focusing on your breath, relax your belly and inhale deeply for a count of four, feeling your hands rise. Exhale fully, drawing your belly in toward your spine. Open eyes and repeat.

•**Knee hug.** Lie on your back, knees bent and feet flat on the mattress. Raise your left leg and clasp your hands behind the thigh. Draw the leg toward your chest and hold for five slow breaths, feeling a stretch in your low back and hip joint. Repeat with the right leg.

•**Whole-body stretch.** Lie flat on your back, legs straight, arms extended overhead and reaching toward the headboard. (Move toward the foot of the bed to allow arms to extend more fully.) Stretch your whole body, taking several deep breaths. Alternately flex and point your feet…flex and circle your wrists.

SITTING UP

•**Neck stretch.** Sit tall on the edge of the bed, feet flat on the floor (or a footstool, if necessary). Inhaling, drape your right arm over the top of your head so that your right hand rests gently on the left side of your head, near your left ear. Exhaling, tilt your head to bring your right ear toward your right shoulder…then drop your left shoulder down, away from your left ear…and let the weight of your right hand gently enhance the stretch along the left side of your neck. Repeat on the other side, using your left hand.

•**Seated twist.** With feet flat on the floor, place your right hand on the outside of your left knee… place your left hand on the bed a few inches behind you. Inhale and lengthen your spine…then exhale as you turn your upper body gently to the left, bringing your chin toward your left shoulder. To encourage the twist, press your right hand against your left knee, keeping your legs still. Hold for several breaths. Repeat on the other side.

STANDING

•**Mountain pose.** Rise to standing, feet shoulder-width apart, weight evenly distributed. Stand erect, chin parallel to the ground, shoulders down. Inhale as you raise your arms overhead…exhale as you return your arms to your sides.

•**Dresser stretch.** Place your palms on top of a dresser, so hands are slightly above waist height. Step back until your arms are fully extended in front of you, and stand with feet shoulder-width apart. Using your hands for balance, with legs straight and head in line with your spine, slowly hinge forward at the hips until your torso is parallel to the floor. Hold for several breaths, feeling the stretch through your back and legs. Return to standing.

How to Find the Best Yoga Teacher

Carol Krucoff, C-IAYT, E-RYT, a yoga therapist and co-director of the Integrative Yoga for Seniors Professional Training at Duke Integrative Medicine in Durham, North Carolina. She is coauthor of *Relax into Yoga for Seniors: A Six-Week Program for Strength, Balance, Flexibility and Pain Relief.* HealingMoves.com

There's hardly a town or city in the US that doesn't offer one or more yoga classes these days.

But to get the most benefit from such a class, you need a well-qualified instructor—especially if you think that yoga isn't an option for you because of a chronic medical condition, such as arthritis or osteoporosis.

Instructors with the right training can provide you with modifications to help you avoid injuries. That way, you can get the full range of benefits from this ancient practice, which include improved strength, balance and flexibility…pain reduction… and relief of anxiety and depression.

Here's what everyone should look for to ensure that his/her yoga instructor is well-qualified…

•**Experience.** Finding an experienced yoga teacher is important for anyone taking a yoga class. But if you're an older adult and/or have a chronic health condition, be sure that the instructor has experience teaching such individuals for at least two to three years and has personally practiced yoga for at least five years.

•**Credentials.** Look for E-RYT and/or C-IAYT after the instructor's name. The former stands for Experienced Registered Yoga Teacher, which is earned through the Yoga Alliance (YA) and indicates at least two years' experience and 1,000 hours of teaching beyond a basic 200-hour teacher training. The latter, earned through the International Association of Yoga Therapists (IAYT), indicates 800 hours or more of specialized training beyond the 200-hour basic yoga teacher training. Someone who earns a C-IAYT will likely have taught for many years.

Good resources: Many hospital wellness centers and integrative medicine facilities offer yoga classes created specifically for people with arthritis, osteoporosis and other chronic medical conditions. The IAYT…Yoga Alliance (YogaAlliance. org)…and Silver Age Yoga (SilverAgeYoga.org) can help you locate an experienced local instructor. You can also click on "Find a Member" on the IAYT site, IAYT.org.

Yoga May Improve Sex Life

Lori Brotto, PhD, assistant professor of obstetrics and gynecology, and director, Sexual Health Laboratory, University of British Columbia, Vancouver, Canada, and leader of an article published in *The Journal of Sexual Medicine.*

Yoga may improve sex for women. Some women have trouble focusing when making love. In yoga, you are encouraged to concentrate on how the body responds to each pose. This can make it easier to tune in to sexual sensations as well. Most types of yoga can provide this benefit.

Yoga Can Be Dangerous: Avoid These Common Mistakes

Timothy McCall, MD, a board-certified internist and medical editor at *Yoga Journal*…coeditor of the 2016 medical textbook *The Principles and Practice of Yoga in Health Care*…and author of the best-selling *Yoga as Medicine.* DrMcCall.com

Yoga is good for you, right? Not always.

Troubling recent finding: For one year, researchers tracked more than 350 people who took yoga classes. Nearly 11% of the participants developed a new pain problem, often lasting a few months. And 21% reported that yoga had aggravated existing injuries.

What I tell my patients and clients: As a medical doctor and yoga instructor for more than 20 years, I know that the risk for injury from practicing yoga can be much lower than from many other forms of exercise such as running or tennis—if you avoid making common mistakes. And by staying injury-free, you will enjoy the many benefits of regular yoga practice—relaxation and stress relief…pain relief…a stronger, more flexible body…and a more peaceful mind.

Here's how to bypass the injury-causing errors people often make when they practice yoga…

WRONG TYPE OF CLASS

There are many different styles and types of yoga—from the gentle and restorative to the intense and aerobic. Some of the styles investigated in the study mentoined above were intense types in which participants move quickly from pose to pose without stopping. (*Examples:* Vinyasa Flow, Power Yoga and Ashtanga Yoga.)

In my experience, most yoga injuries happen to people doing more vigorous and acrobatic styles of yoga. Vigorous, flowing styles of yoga such as Vinyasa can be challenging and invigorating and therefore appealing. But it is not always a safe choice for anyone middle-aged or older because it's too fast and demanding, making injury more likely. Also, because the sequence of poses is quick, participants often do the poses incorrectly, with muscles and bones improperly aligned, increasing the risk for injury. The teacher may not notice these mistakes in alignment because students move so quickly from pose to pose.

My advice: If you are fit and under age 50, more athletically demanding yoga may be fine for you. If you are over age 50 and already practice flowing yoga without problems, you may be fine to continue, but the older you get, the riskier it becomes. If you are not fit or if you have a chronic health problem such as rheumatoid arthritis, poorly controlled high blood pressure or a degenerative disease of the nervous system such as Parkinson's, choose a gentler style of yoga. Examples may be called gentle yoga, restorative yoga or yoga for seniors. Other good choices include Yin Yoga and beginning Iyengar Yoga classes.

Helpful: If you want to practice a fast-paced Vinyasa-style yoga, first take a few classes in which you learn to do the poses slowly and correctly—and then speed up.

Red flag: Anyone who is pregnant, has multiple sclerosis or a chronic inflammatory condition such as lupus or inflammatory bowel disease should avoid hot yoga, including a type of hot yoga called Bikram Yoga—in which the room may be heated to 105°F. The intense heat can aggravate inflammatory conditions or harm a growing fetus.

UNDERTRAINED TEACHER

All the yoga teachers in the recent study had at least 200 hours of training—the amount required by the Yoga Alliance, a nonprofit association of yoga teachers and schools.

That might sound like a lot of training, but it's nowhere near enough to ensure quality instruction. In some instances, much of that training happens online without direct supervision by a qualified teacher.

Bottom line: You are more likely to be injured in a class conducted by a teacher who is undertrained.

My advice: If possible, find a teacher who has more training, say, 500 hours, or one who has many years of experience. To check the teacher's qualifications, you can call a yoga studio, check online or ask the teacher directly.

If you have a serious medical condition, consider consulting a yoga therapist, a yoga teacher trained to work with students with a wide variety of illnesses. To be certified in yoga therapy by the International Association of Yoga Therapists (IAYT), a teacher needs at least 1,000 hours of training. The IAYT website (IAYT.org) has a search function for finding IAYT members in a growing number of locations.

STRAINED BREATHING

In a good yoga class, you are taught to pay attention to your breath. And if you do that, the breath becomes an indicator of whether you are about to make a mistake and hurt yourself.

Often the first sign of an imminent mistake is strained breathing—gasping or holding your breath. If you maintain a discipline of breathing slowly and deeply, it's much less likely that you will hurt yourself. Added benefits of attending to your breathing include a greater sense of calm and mindfulness (steady focus in the present).

My advice: Tune into the breath throughout your yoga practice. If it becomes strained or uneven, make an adjustment that corrects the problem or come out of the pose.

TRYING TOO HARD

A common cause of injury in yoga is what I call "over-efforting"—trying to stretch more deeply into a pose when your breath and body are telling you that the extra stretch is not a good idea. Sharp pain and/or strained breathing are sure signs that the deeper stretch is a mistake. Over-efforting often happens because of peer pressure—almost everyone else in class is doing the pose in a certain way, so you want to keep up, too.

My advice: A yoga pose should be a balance of effort and ease. If the pose is more effort than ease—get out of it. If you get a sharp pain, particularly one in a joint such as the knee—get out of it. Even if the rest of the class is doing the pose...and even if the yoga teacher is telling the class to stay in the pose...if your body is telling you to get out of the pose, get out of it.

RISKIER POSES

There are several common yoga poses that are the most likely to cause injury, and they should be avoided by beginners and many people with chronic medical conditions. *These poses include…*

●**Headstands, which can damage the neck.** When I attend a general yoga class, it often is the case that about half the class should not be doing a headstand—ever. While doing the pose, their faces are red and strained, and they obviously can't wait for the teacher to tell them to come out of the pose. Upside-down poses also can be risky for those with eye problems caused by glaucoma, retinal disease or diabetes.

●**Shoulder stands and Plow pose.** These poses can overstretch the back of the neck. If your neck feels tight or uncomfortable, you probably should not be doing the pose.

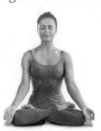

My advice: It may help to put folded blankets under your shoulders (but not under your head and neck) to take the strain off your neck.

●**Lotus pose,** a sitting pose in which you put the right foot over the top of the left thigh and vice

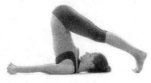

versa. This pose is only for people with flexible hips. If you use your hands to force your legs into this position, you create tremendous torque on your knee joint and you could rip or otherwise injure a knee ligament.

●**Chaturanga (yoga push-ups),** pictured here. In many athletic yoga classes, students cycle through a series of 12 poses known as a sun salutation. One element is Chaturanga, where you lower your body from Plank pose to a low push-up position. Doing this repeatedly can be murder on your shoulder—particularly if you

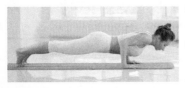

allow the top of your upper-arm bones to jut forward in the shoulder joint.

My advice: If you can't maintain good shoulder alignment, drop both knees to the ground in Plank pose, which takes some weight off, then descend the upper body to Chaturanga.

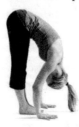

●**Deep back bends,** twists or forward bends. When in doubt, favor less extreme versions of these poses.

Surprising: Less demanding versions of poses confer most or all the health benefits of the deeper versions.

AGGRESSIVE ADJUSTMENT

Another potential cause of serious yoga injuries is when a teacher aggressively pushes on your body to take you more deeply into a pose (light touching to indicate how or where to move is fine).

My advice: Do not allow an instructor to manually force your body into any yoga position. If you are in a class with an instructor who does that, find a new instructor.

How to Make Yoga Safe If You Have Arthritis or Osteoporosis

Carol Krucoff, C-IAYT, E-RYT, a yoga therapist and co-director of the Integrative Yoga for Seniors Professional Training at Duke Integrative Medicine, Durham, North Carolina. She is coauthor of *Relax into Yoga for Seniors: A Six-Week Program for Strength, Balance, Flexibility and Pain Relief.* HealingMoves.com

I'd love to try yoga, but… It's a common lament of people with arthritis, osteoporosis or other chronic health problems. But yoga doesn't have to be off-limits if you have one of these conditions.

With a few precautions and a tailored approach, yoga is a wonderfully effective, research-backed method of improving strength, balance and flexibility…easing pain…and relieving the anxiety and depression that are often associated with chronic health complaints.

For anyone with one or more painful and/or limiting chronic conditions, the relaxation breathing and mindfulness that are central to yoga also can be exceptionally helpful.

Note: Older adults and people with health challenges should look for a class called "Gentle Yoga" or one geared to their needs, such as "Yoga Over 50" or "Yoga for Creaky Bodies." *Follow these steps to ensure that you stay safe if you have…*

ARTHRITIS

Decades ago, people with osteoarthritis and rheumatoid arthritis were advised to rest and "save their joints." Now we know that inactivity can actually cause stiff joints. Yoga relieves pain and stiffness, improves range of motion and sleep, and boosts energy levels and overall mood. *If you have arthritis, be sure to…*

•**Avoid putting excessive pressure on arthritic joints.** Arthritis in your left knee? Keep the toes of your right foot on the ground in single-leg balance poses like Tree Pose. If you have arthritis in both knees, you can relieve the load on your joints by lightly touching a wall or chair.

•**Understand the meaning of different types of pain.** Sharp, immediate pain—especially in a joint—is a sign to ease up. If you have dull pain in your muscles the day after a yoga session, that's likely delayed-onset muscle soreness after using your muscles in new ways—a sign that you're getting stronger! It generally goes away in a few days.

•**Don't overstretch.** This is especially true for people with rheumatoid arthritis, which can render joints loose and unstable.

To tell whether it's a good or risky stretch: Check your breath. If your breath is compromised in any way, back off.

•**Avoid chin-to-chest poses that place pressure on your head.** Poses, such as Plow, place undue pressure on vulnerable cervical spine joints.

•**Turn certain poses around to "take a load" off.** If a pose is bothering an affected joint, try turning it upside down or sideways, taking weight off the joint and letting gravity do the work for you. Happy Baby Pose, for example, can be done while lying on your back in bed.

Caution: Hot, red and/or swollen joints indicate active inflammation. Stick with rest or gentle range-of-motion activities for that joint. Talk with your health-care provider about appropriate treatment.

OSTEOPOROSIS

Yoga is an effective way to improve strength, balance and flexibility in people with osteoporosis. And because yoga improves your balance and strengthens bone, it may help lower your risk of falling and breaking a bone. *If you have osteoporosis, be sure to…*

•**Avoid rounding your spine when sitting or standing, since this position increases the risk for vertebral fracture.** In yoga poses—and in daily life—keep your spine long and hinge forward at your hips, rather than bending at your waist.

•**Don't twist your spine to its end range of rotation.** Instructors may encourage their students to twist as far as possible, using their hands to move even deeper into the twist. This is called end-range rotation and can increase fracture risk in people with osteoporosis. Keep any twists in the midrange, as you would when turning to look over your shoulder while driving. Move slowly, don't round your back and keep your spine elongated.

•**Avoid loading body weight on your neck and/or shoulders as occurs during such poses as Shoulder Stand and Plow.**

•**Keep your head on the ground during supine (face-up) poses.** Lifting your head when lying on the ground creates the forward-flexing, "abdominal crunch" action that can be dangerous because it places excess pressure on vertebral bodies and can lead to compression fractures. Yoga poses that can create this "crunch" are not necessarily supine—they include Standing Forward Bend and Seated Forward Bend. To perform these poses safely, hinge at the hips and keep your spine in neutral (don't round your back).

Yoga for Men: The Secret to a Flat Stomach, Healthy Heart and Better Sex

Timothy McCall, MD, a board-certified internist and medical editor at *Yoga Journal*...coeditor of the 2016 medical textbook *The Principles and Practice of Yoga in Health Care*...and author of the best-selling *Yoga as Medicine*. DrMcCall.com

About 36 million Americans regularly practice yoga for health and healing—but three out of four of them are women.

What few people realize: Despite its reputation as a "soft" exercise that's more suited to women, yoga can provide special health benefits for men—even helping to slow the growth of prostate cancer.

What all men need to know...*

BENEFITS FOR MEN

Hundreds of scientific studies on yoga have shown that it can improve health conditions ranging from sleep problems and sinusitis to high blood pressure and schizophrenia. Many of these benefits are particularly relevant for men. *For example, yoga has been shown to...*

•**Slow prostate cancer.** In a study published in *The Journal of Urology*, some men with prostate cancer did 60 minutes daily of gentle yoga (stretching, breathing, meditation, guided imagery and relaxation) for one year while others did not. Those who didn't do yoga had eight times more growth of cancer cells than those who performed yoga daily.

•**Reduce abdominal fat.** Stress is behind many "spare tires," because it triggers high levels of the hormone *cortisol*, which stimulates appetite and overeating and then plays a key role in turning extra calories into extra belly fat. For unknown reasons, visceral fat, which releases disease-causing

*Before starting yoga, check with your doctor if you have severe osteoporosis, problems with your spine or artificial joints—you may be at greater risk for injury. Also consult your doctor if you have any chronic health conditions or recent injuries. If you develop pain, dizziness or other symptoms while doing yoga, stop the pose and tell your teacher immediately..

inflammatory chemicals, is more prevalent in men than in women.

Good news: Yoga reduces cortisol, which helps control abdominal fat.

•**Help prevent a heart attack.** Each year more than 900,000 Americans have heart attacks, and the majority of them are men.

Recent research: Yoga can reduce many of the heart attack risk factors in people who have heart disease, including high blood pressure, elevated total and LDL "bad" cholesterol and high triglycerides.

•**Improve sexual performance and satisfaction.** In a study of 65 men reported in *The Journal of Sexual Medicine*, practicing yoga an hour a day for three months improved every dimension of sexual functioning—libido...erections...ejaculatory control...satisfaction with performance, intercourse and orgasm...and sexual confidence.

HOW TO START

Many middle-aged men make the mistake of thinking that because yoga looks easy, it is easy. While there are some easy versions that anyone can do, faster, more vigorous yoga styles require a fair degree of fitness and strength to even start. Even though yoga is generally safe for most people of all ages, if you're middle-aged or older and have never practiced yoga, it's best to start with a slower, less vigorous style. *My advice...*

•**Start with a yoga class, not with a book or DVD.** Taking a class led by a skilled yoga teacher is invaluable because the teacher can look at you, review what you're doing and guide you to the best injury-free experience. Expert instruction, mindfulness and not pushing too hard during practice can prevent most injuries, such as muscle spasms and ligament strains.

Helpful: If you do use a book or DVD to learn yoga, have a skilled yoga teacher look over your routine now and then to help you correct any mistakes.

•**Find a good class for men.** Ask a male family member, friend or colleague who practices yoga for his recommendation. If you don't know any men who practice yoga, ask a woman, or visit the website of the International Association of Yoga Therapists, IAYT.org.

● **Don't rush results.** Men are often achievement-oriented and want fast results. That's a mistake. Yoga is not about performance or competition—it's about how the poses help you.

● **Just do it!** This is the secret to success with yoga—simply doing a yoga routine, 15 to 20 minutes a day, every day.

For overall fitness, yoga is a good complement to cardio exercise and strength training. But remember, yoga also provides stress reduction, flexibility and mental focus.

WHAT YOGA ISN'T...

Misconceptions about yoga can keep some men from trying it. *Yoga is not…*

● **A religion.** It is practiced by Christians, Jews, Muslims and atheists.

● **Just stretching.** Yoga includes stretching poses (asanas), as well as many other techniques, such as breathing exercises and meditation.

● **A single style of exercise.** There are many styles of yoga, from slow and gentle (such as Ananda or Kripalu) to fast and vigorous (such as Power Yoga or Vinyasa Flow).

Simple Yoga Can Help You Beat the Post-Lunch Slump

Jennifer Mielke, a certified holistic health coach in New York City. She is a graduate of the Institute for Integrative Nutrition and a certified yoga teacher who regularly works with patients seeking remedies for fatigue.

For most of us, afternoon fatigue sets in around 3 pm. You might want to down a large latte (or worse, a soda). But don't repeat a cycle of buzzing and crashing! *Use this 24-hour plan to ensure energy during the afternoon slowdown and all day long…*

● *Breakfast:* **Eat avocado at breakfast.** It's rich in healthful fats, fiber and potassium, which will help energize you for hours to come. Blend it into a smoothie, or eat it with a drizzle of olive oil and tomato. If you don't like avocado, try soft-boiled eggs, which also are quick and energizing.

● *Midmorning:* **Talk with a friendly coworker, or call a friend for a quick chat.** Communicating with people you enjoy can be energizing. Also sneak in a revitalizing yoga stretch.

What to do: While sitting on the edge of your chair, extend your legs out straight with your heels touching the floor. Inhale and lengthen your spine. As you exhale, fold forward over your legs. In this position, take a few deep breaths. As you exhale, go deeper into the stretch. When you're ready, inhale and sit up.

● *Lunchtime:* **Take a 10-minute walk after lunch.** This can lead to increased energy for up to two hours afterward, according to recent research. Or try an energizing yoga pose.

What to do: While standing, inhale and reach your arms and hands toward the sky. Exhale and then touch your toes. Take a few deep breaths, then come back up to a standing position. Repeat several times. Avoid eating refined carbohydrates or sugar at lunch—these can cause blood sugar to spike, then crash, reducing energy.

● *Midafternoon:* **Splash cold water on your face.** It can be invigorating!

● *Before bed:* **Set the stage for a restful night's sleep.** Turn off all computer screens (your cell phone and TV, too!) an hour before bed. Melatonin, a hormone that induces sleep, is secreted in the dark. Screens can fool the body into thinking it's daytime, reducing melatonin.

Calming bedtime stretch: Lie on your back, and raise your legs up against a wall so your body forms a right angle. Breathe slowly and easily. Stay in this position for as long as is comfortable for you.

What Yoga Style Is Right for You?

Timothy McCall, MD, board-certified internist, medical editor of Yoga Journal and author of *Yoga as Medicine: The Yogic Prescription for Health and Healing.* DrMcCall.com

More than a dozen styles of yoga are practiced in the US. *Among the most common…*

●**Anusara.** This playful, warm-hearted and physically challenging style emphasizes body alignment (often with hands-on adjustments from the teacher) and a positive mindset that looks for the good in all people.

Best for: Physically fit people who want to be part of a like-minded community.

●**Integral.** Beginning classes include gentle poses, breathing techniques, meditation and discussions of ancient yoga texts. The principle of selfless service (such as volunteer work) is emphasized. Some centers offer special classes for students with physical limitations or health problems (such as heart disease or cancer).

Best for: People interested in traditional Indian yoga that includes more than just poses.

●**Iyengar.** Emphasizing meticulous body alignment, this style makes use of blocks, straps and other props so students with limited flexibility can safely and comfortably assume poses. Teacher training requirements are among the strictest.

Best for: Anyone new to yoga or especially in need of better body alignment, such as people with arthritis or back pain.

●**Viniyoga.** Gentle flowing poses are held only briefly. Safety and breath work are emphasized. Teachers often focus on private one-on-one sessions rather than group classes.

Best for: People who are new to yoga or out of shape or who are looking to use yoga to help alleviate any of a variety of chronic ailments.

To find a class: Yoga Alliance (888-921-9642, YogaAlliance.org) registers teachers who complete a certain number of hours of training in specific styles. If you have a medical condition, contact the teacher to see if a particular class is appropriate for you or to ask about private lessons. Yoga therapy has been shown in studies to be effective for a wide range of conditions, from diabetes and arthritis to cancer and chronic lung disease.

The Sleep-Better Yoga Plan

Carol Krucoff, C-IAYT, E-RYT, a yoga therapist and co-director of the Integrative Yoga for Seniors Professional Training at Duke Integrative Medicine in Durham, North Carolina. She is coauthor of, most recently, *Relax into Yoga for Seniors: A Six-Week Program for Strength, Balance, Flexibility and Pain Relief.* HealingMoves.com

The day is waning, your warm bed beckons… and yet your mind continues to race, making peaceful slumber a far-off dream. What's the best way to bring on the z's?

Many Americans opt for a powerful sleeping pill or even a nightcap to help drift off at bedtime. Even though these so-called sleep "aids" may help you doze off, they leave you vulnerable to wee-hour awakenings…or pose dangerous side effects such as dizziness that make you prone to falls.

An under-recognized solution: Yoga is a safe approach that can easily be added to your sleep-hygiene toolbox. *Here's how…*

THE YOGA SOLUTION

Yoga is a perfect sleep inducer because it is designed to quiet the mind—targeting the racing thoughts that can keep us from drifting off. Yoga is also a proven pain-fighter, easing backaches, arthritis and other common sleep saboteurs.

When adults over age 60 who had insomnia took three months of twice-weekly classes incorporating yoga poses, meditation and daily home practice, they reported significant improvements in their sleep, according to a study in *Alternative Therapies in Health and Medicine.*

HOW TO BREATHE RIGHT

When we are drifting off to sleep, the pace of our breathing naturally slows. But when our racing mind keeps us awake, turning our attention to our breath and deliberately slowing and deepening the breath can trigger a cascade of relaxing physiological changes—the heart rate slows, blood pressure decreases, muscles relax, anxiety eases and the mind calms.

Surprisingly, many people do not know the basics of correct deep breathing.

What to do: Put yourself in a comfortable position—lying on your back, for example—and place one of your palms on your belly. Relax your abdomen, and invite your breath to completely fill your lungs. You might notice that when you inhale fully this way, your belly rounds and your hand rises. With the exhale, your belly gently drops inward and your hand falls.

To get the most from abdominal breathing: Go a step further by making the exhale a bit longer. This type of breathing sends a clear signal to your central nervous system that everything is fine... just let go.

THE SLEEP-INDUCING POSES

Once you have become comfortable with the relaxed breathing described above, here are some sleep-better yoga poses to do right before bed. For each pose below, start by lying on the floor (on a yoga mat or carpet for comfort) or on your bed with your knees bent and your arms at your sides. If your chin juts up, place a small pillow or folded towel under your head so that your chin is at the same level or slightly lower than your forehead.

●**Knees to chest.**

What to do: Do the relaxed abdominal breathing described above for several minutes.

Once you're feeling relaxed, bring both knees toward your chest, holding onto your thighs or using a yoga strap (or a bathrobe tie) to catch your thighs and bring them toward your chest. Notice where you feel the sensation of stretch, and use your breath to help relax any tension. On the exhalation, draw your thighs in toward your body...on the inhalation, allow your thighs to drift away from your body. If it's uncomfortable to hug both legs, hug one leg at a time. Continue for six to 10 cycles of breath—each inhalation and exhalation is one breath cycle.

● **Neck release.**

What to do: Take an easy, full breath in, then as you exhale, rotate your head to the right. Your eyes can be open or closed, whichever feels better.

Inhale as you bring your head back to center, then exhale as you turn your head to the left. Continue for six to 10 breaths, moving with your breath. Next, turn your head as far as it will comfortably go to the right and relax your left shoulder toward the ground. Linger here for three to five easy breaths, then bring your head back to the center and repeat to the left.

●**Arms overhead.**

What to do: With your arms alongside your body and your palms facing down, tune in to your breath. As you inhale, extend your arms up and back so that the backs of your hands move toward the surface behind you. If your hands don't reach the surface behind you, that's fine. As you exhale, return your arms to their starting position along your sides. Repeat six to 10 times, moving with your breath—inhale your arms up and over...exhale them back down to your sides. Sleep tight...

Strong, Calm and Confident with Tai Chi

Roger Jahnke, OMD, a board-certified doctor of oriental medicine, lecturer and author of two books, including *The Healer Within*. He is director of the Institute of Integral Qigong and Tai Chi in Santa Barbara, California. IIQTC.org

Why do millions of people around the world practice tai chi? Because it's a wonderful way to integrate and nurture mind, body and spirit—to hone mental focus, build muscles and bones, and elevate self-confidence. To practice the meditative movements below, repeat each sequence for five minutes daily. Stand with feet shoulder-width apart, knees slightly bent, toes slightly angled out, posture erect (or sit in a sturdy chair). Move slowly and gracefully...match the rhythm of your deep breaths to your movements.*

Demonstrations: YouTube.com/iiqtc.

*Check with your doctor before beginning any new exercise routine.

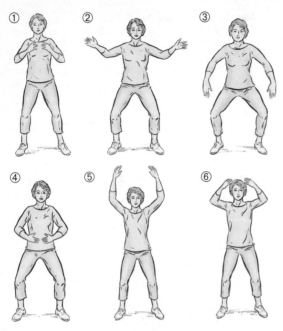

**GATHERING OF HEAVEN
AND EARTH**

In Chinese medicine, earth and sky represent yin and yang, powerful healing energies.

1. Start with hands in front of chest at heart level, several inches apart.

2. Open arms wide….begin to bend knees out to sides.

3. Sink into knees as far as is comfortable while reaching down and bringing hands toward each other, as if arms were encircling and gathering up earth energy.

4. Straightening legs, bring hands up toward heart.

5. Now, open arms wide…reach up and bring hands toward each other, as if encircling and gathering sky energy.

6. Lower hands, bringing them past face to heart level. Repeat sequence.

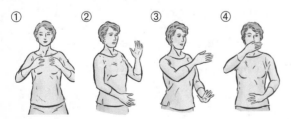

HANDS LIKE CLOUDS

In this movement, each time your hand drifts past your face, follow it with your gaze, imagining it as a tranquil, billowy cloud. Relax your shoulders…rest your mind.

1. Start with hands in front of heart, several inches apart.

2. Turning torso slightly to the left, lower your right hand to waist level…move both hands to left side of body.

3. Raise right hand and lower the left hand, so hands pass each other.

4. Turning torso to the center, bring right hand past face like a drifting cloud…bring left hand past center of body at waist level.

5. Repeat on other side. Turn torso and move hands to the right, left hand at waist level. Raise left hand and lower right hand. Turn torso to center…let left hand drift past face as right hand passes at waist level. Repeat sequence.

Illustrations: Shawn Banner

Are You Tough Enough for Tai Chi?—It Gives Benefits You'd Never Imagine

Peter M. Wayne, PhD, an associate professor of medicine at Harvard Medical School and director of the Osher Center for Integrative Medicine, jointly based at Harvard Medical School and Brigham and Women's Hospital, both in Boston. He has trained in tai chi for more than 35 years and is the author, with Mark L. Fuerst, of *The Harvard Medical School Guide to Tai Chi.*

Perhaps you've seen people performing the graceful, seemingly slow-motion movements of tai chi in a nearby park. If you've never tried it before, you may think that this form of exercise is easy to do and provides little more than a mild workout.

The truth: Even though tai chi consists of slow, gentle movements, this exercise is no pushover. Long known for its stress-reducing benefits, it also gives you an aerobic workout that's as intense as walking at a moderate pace…increases muscle strength and flexibility…improves breathing…improves posture and balance (to help prevent falls)…and focuses the mind.

What's new: Tai chi, which was developed centuries ago in China as a means of self-defense, is now linked to a number of health benefits, including improved cardiovascular health and bone density…and reduced back and neck pain.

Even better: Tai chi is safer than many forms of exercise because of its 70% rule: You never move your joints or exert yourself beyond 70% of your maximum potential.

Recently discovered benefits…

BETTER BREATHING

Many Eastern-based practices, including yoga, meditation and tai chi, emphasize diaphragmatic breathing, in which the muscles of the diaphragm (rather than the chest) are used to take in more oxygen. This style of breathing not only helps the lungs to move with less effort but also allows more oxygen to pass into the bloodstream.

Efficient breathing is more important than you might think. Multiple studies indicate that healthy breathing—as measured by "forced expiratory volume," the amount of air that you can exhale in one second—may help you live longer.

LOWER BLOOD PRESSURE

The stress relief that can come from tai chi, along with improved breathing and other factors, make it an ideal exercise for lowering blood pressure. In fact, research suggests that tai chi is at least as effective for lowering blood pressure as lifestyle changes that are usually recommended, such as losing weight and cutting back on sodium.

A Johns Hopkins study found that light-intensity tai chi improved blood pressure almost as much as moderate-intensity aerobic exercise.

PERIPHERAL NEUROPATHY

Millions of people with diabetes and other conditions have peripheral neuropathy, nerve damage in the hands and/or feet that causes numbness, tingling or pain. The condition is particularly troublesome because reduced sensations in the feet can impair balance and increase the risk of falling.

Research has found that people with peripheral neuropathy who practiced tai chi had improved sensitivity in the soles of the feet. They also had better balance and walking speed.

STRONGER BONES

You don't need to lift weights to increase bone strength and reduce risk for osteoporosis. Researchers in Hong Kong found that women who did tai chi three times per week had increased bone density within 12 months.

IT'S EASY TO GET STARTED

Tai chi classes are commonly offered at health clubs, YMCAs and even some hospitals. Classes are particularly useful because of the feedback given by the instructor and the group support, which helps keep you motivated.

Good goal: Two one-hour tai chi classes a week—plus at-home practice for at least 30 minutes, three times a week.

You can find a tai chi expert in your area at AmericanTaiChi.net.

A TASTE OF TAI CHI

Tai chi consists of dozens of different moves. *Here's one called "Tai Chi Pouring"…*

What to do: Stand with your feet shoulder-width apart. Slightly bend one knee and allow your weight to shift to that side. Briefly pause, and then gently bend your other knee and shift your weight in that direction. Pause again. "Pour" your weight back and forth for a few minutes while breathing deeply and feeling a relaxed flow connecting your whole body.

Qigong for Beginners

Roger Jahnke, OMD, board-certified doctor of oriental medicine, author of *The Healer Within* and director of the Institute of Integral Qigong and Tai Chi in Santa Barbara, California. IIQTC.org

The Chinese wellness system qigong (chee-GONG) combines four ancient practices, all meant to harness the body's self-healing powers. The basics are easy to learn and easy on the body, and they can be done at home. Here are samples of qigong movements and methods. Practice each daily to generate vitality and promote healing.

BODY MOVEMENT

Slow, gentle exercises build awareness of posture…increase strength, endurance and flexibility…and unlike vigorous exercises, do not cause injury or consume internal resources (such as energy) to fuel muscles.

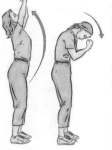

• **Gentle bending of the spine.** Stand with feet shoulder-width apart, knees slightly bent. Inhaling, raise arms above head, elbows slightly bent and palms facing skyward …tip head back and tilt the pelvis, arching back slightly. On the exhalation, bend elbows and bring arms down in front of you, hands fisted and pressed together…tuck chin to chest, tilt the pelvis under and round your back. Repeat five to 10 times.

BREATH PRACTICE

Deep breathing sends more oxygen-rich blood toward tissues…and "pumps" lymph fluid through the lymphatic system, a major part of the immune system.

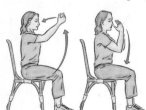

• **Gathering breath.** Sit with hands in your lap. Inhaling through the nose, move hands outward and upward, scooping up healing energy, until hands are just above face level, palms toward you and elbows slightly bent. Exhaling slowly, bring hands toward you, then downward past the chest and navel. Repeat five to 10 times.

MASSAGE

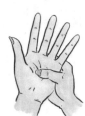

Reflexes refer to areas of the body that are separated physically, yet linked via acupuncture and energy channels. Self-massage of points on the hands, ears and feet has a healing effect on the organs, joints or tissues to which these reflexes connect.

• **Healing hand massage.** Grasp your left hand with your right hand, thumb against the palm and fingers on the back of the hand. Starting gently and gradually increasing the pressure, knead your left hand, including fingers and wrist. Spend extra time on any sore points—these areas are linked to body functions and organs that are not operating optimally. Continue for three to five minutes, then switch hands.

MEDITATION

Stress overstimulates the nervous system and exhausts the adrenal glands (which secrete stress hormones). Meditation counteracts stress, enhancing healing brain chemicals and hormones.

• **Qigong meditation.** Stand, sit or lie comfortably. Inhale fully, imagining you are drawing in qi (vitality) from the universe through hundreds of energy gates (acupuncture points) all over your body's surface. Exhale slowly, visualizing healing resources circulating inside you. Continue for five to 15 minutes, mentally directing the healing flow to wherever your body needs it most.

Illustrations by Shawn Banner.

3

No Time to Exercise

Get One Hour of Fitness in 5 Minutes

Tom Holland, exercise physiologist and certified strength and conditioning specialist based in Darien, Connecticut. He is author of *Beat the Gym: Personal Trainer Secrets—Without the Personal Trainer Price Tag.* TeamHolland.com

If you're like most people, finding the time for exercise can be as challenging as the exercise itself. But you don't have to carve an hour out of your schedule—a five-minute workout one or more times per day can lead to noticeable improvements in your physical strength and cardiovascular fitness. (For a tougher, "fast" workout, see page 39.)

You don't need fancy equipment. *These very basic and well-known moves will work all the major muscle groups…*

1. Do a one-minute warm-up. You can jog in place or do jumping jacks to increase your heart rate and blood flow, raise your body temperature and improve your muscle elasticity. This will prepare your body for more vigorous exercise.

2. Do 30 seconds of squats. From a standing start, bend your knees, as if you're about to sit on an imaginary chair. Do not go any lower than a 90-degree angle where your thighs are parallel with the floor and your heels are down. Then return to a full standing posture. Hold your arms out in front of you for balance as needed. Repeat as many times as possible.

Beginner strategy: If you can't do deep squats, do more shallow squats—lower your body only a few inches. Then increase this depth as the days pass and you get stronger.

3. Do 30 seconds of push-ups. You probably already know how to do push-ups—with your hands positioned slightly more than shoulder width apart.

Beware of pitfalls: Keep your body straight, butt in line, and your neck in a neutral position. Repeat this exercise as many times as possible in 30 seconds.

Beginner strategy: If you are not yet strong enough for a traditional push-up, do "knee push-ups," where your knees are on the ground instead of your toes.

4. Do a 30-second plank. Position yourself in the push-up position—body perfectly straight, supported by your toes and hands with arms extended, hands below your shoulders. Contract your abs, and hold this position for 30 seconds.

Beginner strategy: Support yourself on your toes and forearms rather than on your toes and hands…and/or try to hold the plank for less than 30 seconds.

5. **Repeat steps two through four.** Perform a second round of the three exercises above.

6. **Do a one-minute cool-down.** Jog in place for 30 seconds, then do 30 seconds of stretches. Stretch your quads by holding one foot up behind your backside for a few seconds (grasp a chair for balance if necessary), then repeat with the other foot. Stretch your shoulders by grasping your right elbow with your left hand and pulling your right arm across your body (keep your right shoulder down), then repeat on the left arm. If any other parts of your body feel tight, go ahead and stretch those, too.

10 Easy Ways to Sneak Exercise Into Your Day

Carol Krucoff, C-IAYT, E-RYT, a yoga therapist and co-director of the Integrative Yoga for Seniors Professional Training at Duke Integrative Medicine in Durham, North Carolina. She is coauthor of, most recently, *Relax into Yoga for Seniors: A Six-Week Program for Strength, Balance, Flexibility and Pain Relief.* HealingMoves.com

Getting the recommended 30 minutes of exercise a day can be challenging. But the good news is that you don't have to work out for a half-hour straight to boost your health. Guidelines from the American Heart Association and the American College of Sports Medicine state that three 10-minute bouts of moderate-intensity physical activity (such as a brisk walk) can be just as effective as exercising for 30 minutes straight. And other evidence suggests that even shorter periods of activity—in fact, every step you take—adds up to better health.

Don't let bad weather or a busy schedule ruin your exercise plans. *Try these simple strategies to slip exercise into your day…*

1. Break the elevator/escalator habit. Climbing stairs is a great way to strengthen your heart, muscles and bones. The Harvard Alumni Health Study, which followed 11,130 men (mean age 58 at the beginning of the study) for about 20 years, found that those who climbed 20 to 34 floors per week had about a 30% lower risk of stroke. Take the stairs at every opportunity and even look for ways to add extra flights, such as using the bathroom on a different floor. If you must take an elevator up a tall building, get off a few flights early and walk.

2. Use muscle, not machines. In our push-button world, we expend about 300 to 700 fewer calories per day than did our grandparents, who had to do things like chop wood and fetch water. Drop the "labor saving" mentality, and embrace opportunities to activate your life. Use a rake instead of a leaf blower…wash your car by hand…get up and change the TV channel.

3. Walk to a coworker's office instead of sending an e-mail. William Haskell, PhD, calculated, in *The Journal of the American Medical Association*, that the energy expenditure lost by writing e-mails for two minutes every hour for eight hours per day five days a week—instead of two minutes of slow walking around the office to deliver messages—adds up to the equivalent of 1.1 pounds of fat in one year and 11 pounds of fat in 10 years.

4. Take exercise breaks. Energize your body with movement instead of caffeine by turning your coffee break into a "walk break." Every hour or two, get up and walk around or stretch.

5. Wait actively. If you're forced to wait for an airplane, hairdresser, dentist, doctor, restaurant table, etc., take a walk. To boost the calorie burn of your walk, move purposefully—as if you're late for a meeting—rather than just strolling along.

6. Do the housework boogie. Play lively music when you're doing household chores, and dance off extra calories by moving to the beat.

7. Try aerobic shopping. Take a lap or two around the mall or grocery store before you go into a store or put anything in your cart.

8. Socialize actively. Instead of sitting and talking (or eating) with friends and/or family, do something active, such as bowling, playing Ping-Pong, shooting baskets or dancing.

9. Install a chin-up bar in a convenient doorway. Whenever you walk through, do a pull-up or simply "hang out" and stretch. Chin-up bars are available at sporting-goods stores and online for less than $20.

10. Practice "phone fitness." Stretch, walk or climb stairs while you're talking on your cell phone or cordless phone.

This 7-Minute Workout Really Works

Chris Jordan, MS, CSCS, director of exercise physiology at Human Performance Institute in Orlando, Florida. He designed the exercise programming portion of the Corporate Athlete Course, which was described in an article—which he coauthored with Brett Klika—in *American College of Sports Medicine's Health and Fitness Journal.* HPInstitute.com

D on't have the time to exercise? Then here's the workout for you! It is a series of 12 resistance and aerobic exercises that can be completed in seven minutes. It's a tough seven minutes. The exercises are easy to learn, but they will push your body to the limit.

HOW IT WORKS

We designed the following workout for "corporate athletes"—busy adults without a lot of free time or access to a health club. The exercises can be done at home or in a hotel room because the only "equipment" that's required is the weight of your body and a sturdy chair.

This approach, known as high-intensity circuit training, is effective for weight loss as well as metabolic and cardiovascular health. Workouts that are done at high intensity—during which the heart will beat at up to 80% to 90% of its maximum rate—cause changes in the muscles that are comparable to the changes produced by lengthier workouts at moderate intensity.

You don't need a heart monitor to determine exercise intensity. I recommend the talk test. If you can speak an entire sentence while exercising, you're not pushing hard enough. If you can't speak at all, you're working too hard. You're in the right zone when you can speak a few words before pausing for breath.

On an exertion scale of one to 10—with one being at rest, and 10 being almost impossible—the

workout should be an eight or a nine. This can be a very tough workout. No one should do it without getting a physical and the go-ahead from a doctor.

EASE INTO IT

If you're not already an athlete, start slowly. While you're learning and getting in shape, you might take a little longer than seven minutes to complete all 12 of the exercises. Your goal is to get the time down to seven minutes using correct form and technique for each exercise. Do the seven-minute workout every other day.

You may need to go to your local fitness center and get guidance from a certified fitness professional. When you get stronger, you can do the seven-minute workout two or three times in a row if you wish for the ultimate 15-to-20-minute workout.

It's important to do the exercises in the order listed.

Reason: The workout includes total-body exercises, which are more aerobic in nature, and exercises that give the lower- and upper-body muscles some time to recover. When you're doing a leg exercise, the muscles in the upper body have a chance to rest. When you're working the upper body, the legs have the opportunity to rest. These intervals of exertion and rest help make the workout so effective.

THE EXERCISES

Aim to perform 15 to 20 repetitions of each exercise over a period of 30 seconds, but don't compromise form and technique for repetitions. When you finish one exercise, don't rest. Immediately start the next one.

Caution: If you have high blood pressure or heart disease, skip the isometric exercises (wall-sit, plank and side plank). These movements involve extended muscle contractions that can impede blood flow. A trainer can suggest safer alternatives.

•**Jumping Jacks.** Start the routine with a classic jumping jack—with your feet shoulder-width apart, arms at your sides, jump slightly and spread your legs while bringing your arms together over your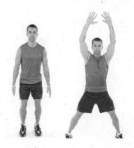

head until your hands almost touch. Jump again as you bring your feet back to the starting position while lowering your hands to your sides.

Helpful: If you're uncomfortable doing jumping jacks, you can run or walk in place.

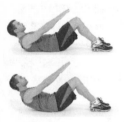

●**Wall-sit.** Start out standing with your back against a wall. Bend your knees, and slide down until your thighs are parallel to the floor. Hold the position for 30 seconds.

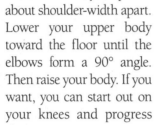

●**Push-up.** Support your body on your hands and toes, your palms about shoulder-width apart. Lower your upper body toward the floor until the elbows form a 90° angle. Then raise your body. If you want, you can start out on your knees and progress to a full push-up as you become stronger.

●**Abdominal crunch.** Lie on your back, with your knees bent, your feet flat on the floor and your arms extended toward your knees. Using the abdominal muscles, lift your head and shoulders a few inches off the floor. Then lower your head/shoulders back down.

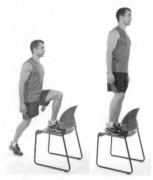

●**Step-up.** Leading with your left leg, step onto a sturdy chair. (If you aren't sure of your strength or balance, you can substitute something that's lower than a chair, such as a step or a low bench.) Use the strength of your left leg to bring your other foot onto the chair. Then step off the chair, leading with your left leg. Repeat, alternating legs each time.

●**Squat.** Stand with your feet shoulder-width apart and your arms at your sides. Bend your knees, and squat until your thighs are parallel to the floor.

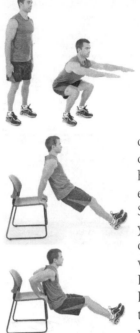

While lowering your body, extend your arms in front of your body. Keep your knees over your toes. Then rise to the starting position.

●**Triceps dip on chair.** Sit on the edge of a sturdy chair (or step or low bench), with the heels of your hands on either side of your butt. Slide off the seat so that your weight is supported on your hands. Your legs will be extended forward. Bend your elbows, and lower your butt toward the floor. When your waist is a few inches lower than the seat of the chair, push up with your arms until your elbows are straight. Keep your shoulders flat, not shrugged.

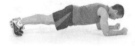

●**Plank.** Lie facedown on the floor while supporting your weight on your toes and forearms. Hold the position, keeping your body straight for 30 seconds.

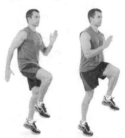

●**High knees/running in place.** This exercise combines a running motion with exaggerated knee lifts. While "running," raise your knees as high as you comfortably can, without compromising your rhythm or balance. Stay on your toes, not your heels.

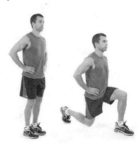

●**Lunge.** While keeping your upper body straight, step forward with one leg. Lower your hips until both knees are bent at a 90° angle. Push back with the leading leg until your body returns to the

40

starting position. Then step forward with the other leg and repeat.

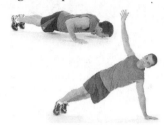

●**Push-up and rotation.** Assume the normal push-up position. As you come up, rotate your body so that your right arm rises overhead. Return to the starting position, and lower yourself. Do another push-up, this time extending the other arm. Do this for 30 seconds, alternating sides.

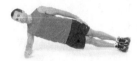

●**Side plank.** Lie on your side, with one forearm under your shoulder. Your upper leg will be directly on top of the lower leg, with your knees straight. Raise your hips until your body forms a straight line from the ankles to the shoulders. Hold the position for 30 seconds, then repeat on the other side.

The Ultimate Workout: Two Exercises Keep You Fit!

Michael J. Joyner, MD, physician-researcher and leading expert on human performance and exercise physiology at the Mayo Clinic, Rochester, Minnesota. His research has focused on how humans respond to various forms of physical and mental stress. DrMichaelJoyner.com

If you're like most efficiency-minded Americans, you may be on the lookout for the exercise that's going to whip you into shape, keep you fit and slow down aging—with the least amount of time and fuss. For those of us looking to streamline our workouts to just the essentials, two simple exercises can do the job. They are challenging but worth the effort…and can be easily modified to suit your individual fitness level.

THE DYNAMIC DUO

Burpees and jumping rope are the dynamic duo, in my opinion. Why burpees and jumping rope? Of all the exercise choices, these maintain high vigor while promoting strength, endurance, balance and coordination all at once—precisely the capabilities that tend to deteriorate as we age, increasing our risk for falls and other mishaps. *These exercises are also…*

●**Compact.** Both can be done almost anywhere —whether you're in a hotel room…in your family room…or in your backyard.

Note: If you're indoors, you need adequate ceiling height to jump rope.

●**Quick.** The regimen can be compressed into a tidy five minutes if you're starting out and extended to a 10-, 20- or 30-minute workout when you're ready to up your game.

PERFECTING YOUR TECHNIQUE

To get the maximum benefits and reduce your risk for injuries, it's important to do both of these exercises properly…

●**Burpees.** Unless this exercise is already part of your workout, start slowly to make sure you've got the right technique. Ready?

●Stand straight with your arms at your sides.

●Squat down until you can put your hands on the ground in front of your feet.

●Kick your legs back into the plank position, straight behind you.

●Do a push-up on your toes or on your knees.

●Pull your legs back into the squat position.

●Jump up as high as you can with your arms overhead.

For a somewhat easier version: Do the same exercise without the push-up and jump. If the plank position is too difficult, modify it by kicking your legs back only halfway.

●**Jumping rope.** Maybe you haven't jumped rope since you were a kid, but it will come back to you. Keep the jump low to minimize the impact on your ankles and knees. When you feel ready, try using a weighted jump rope (which incorporates 1-, 3- or 5-pound weights) to rev up your heart rate and build upper-body strength. Skip the added weight if you have existing shoulder, arm or wrist problems. Use a jump rope that feels right to you—whether it has anti-slip handles or plastic beads strung on a nylon cord.

WARMING UP

Jumping jacks and running in place are great ways to warm up. These exercises are also good substitutes for burpees and jumping rope if you haven't been physically active in a while and/or want a gentler way to ease into your routine.

If jumping jacks and running in place don't appeal to you or you are concerned about your risk for falling or joint pain, there are other ways to modify the burpee–jump rope regimen while you increase your fitness.

Instead of burpees, try: Knee bends (also known as "squats"). If you're worried about your knees, skip the knee bends and simply stand with your back against a wall and lift up one leg with your knee bent as high as you feel comfortable. Repeat with the other leg.

Or try push-ups, either on the floor or against a counter.

Instead of jumping rope, try: Brisk walking— set a pace that puts you at the edge of being short of breath.

THE WORKOUT

To begin a burpee–jump rope regimen, do five burpees alternating with 30 seconds of jumping rope. Do each set three to five times (for a total of 15 burpees and a minute and a half of jumping rope…or 25 burpees and two and a half minutes of jumping rope). Then work up to sets of 10 burpees alternating with one minute of jumping rope. As your stamina builds, continue to alternate exercises until you work up to longer sets of up to two minutes of each. Try to do the burpee–jump rope workout two to three days a week with brisk walking or cycling on the other days.

Important: If you have any chronic medical conditions, consult your doctor before trying this workout. Stop immediately if either activity causes pain. It will take time to build up your stamina. Scale up according to your age and ability.

The Quick, Powerful Workout You're Probably Not Getting

Wayne L. Westcott, PhD, a professor of exercise science and chair of the exercise program at Quincy College in Quincy, Massachusetts. He is coauthor of several books, including *Strength Training Past 50.*

Until recently, fitness gurus have advised people to "take the stairs" mainly as a substitute for do-nothing elevator rides.

Now: Stair-climbing is becoming increasingly popular as a workout that's readily accessible (stairs are everywhere)…often climate-controlled (indoor stairs)…and free.

It burns more calories than walking…strengthens every muscle in the legs…and is good for your bones as well as your cardiovascular system. It may even extend your life span.

Compelling research: A study found that participants who averaged eight flights of stairs a day had a death rate over a 16-year period that was about one-third lower than those who didn't exercise—and more than 20% lower than that of people who merely walked.

A CONCENTRATED CLIMB

Walking is mainly a horizontal movement, with an assist from forward momentum. Stair-climbing is a vertical exercise. Your body weight is lifted straight up, against gravity. Climbing stairs also involves more muscles—in the calves, buttocks and the fronts and backs of the thighs—than walking. Even the arms get a workout. Canadian researchers found that it required double the exertion of walking on level ground—and 50% more than walking up an incline.

As a weight-loss tool, stair-climbing is hard to beat. An hour of climbing (for a 160-pound person) will burn about 650 calories. That compares with 400 calories an hour for a 15-minute-mile "power walk"…and 204 calories for a leisurely stroll.

IT'S EASY TO START

Inconvenience is one of the biggest barriers to exercise. It sometimes feels like a hassle to change into workout clothes and drive to a health club...or even exercise at home. But you can always find a set of stairs—in your neighborhood, at work, at the mall or at home.

You don't need fancy workout gear to climb stairs (uncarpeted stairs are preferred). Because it doesn't involve side-to-side movements, you don't necessarily need to invest in specialized shoes. You can do it in any pair of athletic shoes or even work shoes, as long as they don't have high heels.

HOW TO CLIMB

When getting started, begin with a single flight of stairs. When that feels easy, take additional flights or increase the intensity by going a little faster. Work up to five minutes, then slowly increase that to 10, 15 and 20 minutes, if possible, three times a week. *Other tips…*

•**Keep your upper body straight.** There's a natural tendency to lean forward when you climb stairs, particularly because a forward-leaning position feels easier. Remind yourself to stand straight when you're climbing and descending. It will give your legs a better workout...strengthen your abdominal and other core muscles...and help improve your balance.

•**Swing your arms.** You don't need an exaggerated swing, but keep your arms moving—it helps with balance and provides exercise for your arms and shoulders. You'll often see stair-climbers with their hands or arms on the rails. It's OK to use the rails if you need the support, but it reduces the intensity of the exercise. It also causes the stooped posture that you want to avoid.

•**One step at a time.** Unless you're a competitive stair-climber, you'll probably do best by taking just one step at a time. Ascending stairs is a concentric exercise that increases muscle power...it's also the part of the workout that gives most of the cardiovascular benefit.

Coming down the stairs is an eccentric (also called "negative") movement that puts more stress on the muscles and increases strength.

Important: Descend the stairs slowly, and keep "jolts" to a minimum. It sounds counterintuitive, but the descents cause more muscle soreness than the climbs.

You can take two steps at a time on the ascent—if your balance is good and you're bored with single-step plodding. The faster pace will increase the intensity of your workout, particularly when you give your arms a more exaggerated swing. To minimize jolts and maximize safety, however, stick to single steps on the descent.

TO END YOUR WORKOUT

The "Figure 4" stretch is a great way to conclude a stair-climbing workout. It stretches the calves, hamstrings, gluteals, low back and upper back.

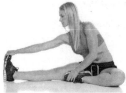

Photo: iStock.com

What to do: While sitting on the floor with your right leg straight, bend your left leg so that your left foot touches your right thigh. Slowly reach your right hand toward your right foot. Then grasp your foot, ankle or lower leg, and hold for 20 seconds. Repeat on the other side.

Caution: Stair-climbing should be avoided if you have serious arthritis or other joint problems. It's less jarring than jogging, but it's still a weight-bearing exercise that can stress the joints. People with joint issues might do better with supported exercises, such as cycling, rowing or swimming.

Before taking up stair-climbing as a form of exercise, check with your doctor if you're middle-aged or older, have arthritis, a history of heart or lung disease or if you've been mainly sedentary and aren't confident of your muscle strength—or your sense of balance.

Too Busy to Go to the Gym? Get Fit in Just a Few Minutes

Joan Price, a certified fitness instructor and motivational speaker based in Sebastopol, California, and author of several books, including *The Anytime, Anywhere Exercise Book.* She credits her commitment to exercise for her success in twice regaining the ability to walk and dance after two head-on car crashes. JoanPrice.com

Lack of time is a primary reason people give for failing to get the recommended 30 to 60 minutes of moderate-intensity exercise most days of the week. Admittedly, it can be tough to find such a big chunk of time in your busy schedule.

What helps: Instead of feeling compelled to cram an entire day's worth of exercise into a single block of time, commit to fitting in little bursts of physical activity—two minutes, five minutes, 10 minutes—throughout the day. The more these "fitness minutes" add up, the more you reap the benefits of exercise, including improved health, better weight control, increased energy and a sense of well-being.

IN THE MORNING

• **When your alarm clock rings**—instead of pressing the snooze button, get up and use those extra minutes to do some gentle yoga poses.

• **While brushing your teeth**—do calf raises. Standing, slowly rise onto the balls of your feet… hold for several seconds…return to the starting position. Repeat, continuing for two minutes.

• **In the shower**—give your upper back muscles a workout. Squeeze your shoulder blades together…hold for five to 10 seconds…rest for a moment. Repeat 10 to 15 times.

• **While you style your hair**—squeeze your buttocks muscles as hard as you can for 10 seconds…rest for several seconds…repeat five to 10 times.

• **When going down stairs**—turn around at the bottom of the stairs and go back up, making one or more extra up-and-down trips.

• **As the coffee is brewing**—hop on your right foot 10 times…then hop on the left foot. Repeat twice.

• **When letting the dog out**—go with him for a short walk.

OUT AND ABOUT

• **At the gas station**—walk inside to pay rather than swiping a credit card at the pump. Instead of sitting in your car as the gas flows, clean all your windows, alternating the hand that holds the squeegee.

• **At every red light**—do shoulder shrugs and roll your shoulders…repeatedly tighten and release your thigh muscles…rotate one wrist, then the other wrist.

• **When parking**—instead of finding a spot close to your destination, get one a few blocks away.

• **Upon entering a store**—if all the items you need will fit in a shopping basket, choose a basket instead of a cart.

• **As you shop**—if you need a cart, do 10 bicep curls with weightier items—soup cans, juice jugs—before placing them in your cart. (If you feel silly doing this in public, do your bicep curls at home as you put the items in the pantry.)

• **While waiting in line**—work your abdominal muscles. Suck in your belly and tighten your abs… hold for 10 seconds…relax. Repeat five to 10 times.

• **On a long car trip**—stop every 50 miles or so, and take a walk around a rest stop or scenic area.

• **When traveling by bus, plane or train**—walk up and down the aisle for at least five minutes every hour.

AT YOUR DESK

• **While on the phone**—march in place or pace around your office.

• **As you read e-mail**—lift your right foot several inches off the floor…rotate your ankle clockwise several times, then counterclockwise…lower the foot. Repeat on the left side.

• **If you need to talk with a coworker**—walk over to her office instead of phoning. When you get back to your own desk, before sitting down, hold your arms out to the side and circle them forward 15 times, then backward.

• **Each time you finish a task**—do "chair dips." With feet flat on the floor, place your hands on the armrests and push your body up (so your rear end hovers above the seat)…hold for several seconds… lower yourself back into the chair. Repeat 10 times. (Skip this if your chair has wheels.)

• **During your lunch break**—take a walk through the office complex.

• **In the restroom**—stand and reach for the sky for 30 seconds…then do 10 jumping jacks.

• **If you drop a pencil (or at least once a day)**— do a variation on toe touches. Stand up, bend down, pick up the pencil, straighten up…drop the pencil again. Repeat 10 times.

IN THE EVENING

●**Before starting dinner**—take a quick ride around the neighborhood on your bicycle.

●**At the dinner table**—do leg lifts. Sit with feet flat on the floor. Straighten your right leg to hold your right foot out in front of you…lift your right thigh a few inches off the chair and hold for several seconds…lower the foot. Repeat 10 times, then switch to the left leg.

●**Doing laundry**—when you grab a basket of clothes, tighten abdominal muscles and, with your back straight, lift the basket from hip height to chest height five times.

●**Listening to the radio or a CD**—dance around the room for one entire song. Repeat several times.

●**While watching TV**—pop an exercise video or DVD in your player. Every time the TV show cuts to a commercial break, turn on the player and follow along with the workout for several minutes.

●**Climbing the stairs**—take the steps two at a time. (Do not do this if you have balance problems.)

●**After washing your face**—tilt your head slowly from side to side, feeling a good stretch along your neck…try to touch your chin to your chest to stretch the back of your neck.

●**Before climbing into bed**—raise your arms overhead…tilt gently to the right, feeling the stretch along the left side of your torso…then tilt to the left. Repeat five times.

●**When you lie down**—do knee hugs. Lie on your back with your knees bent, feet flat on the mattress. Raise one leg, place your hands behind the thigh and draw the leg toward your chest. Hold for 30 seconds…return to starting position. Repeat with the other leg.

●**Closing your eyes**—breathe in and out deeply 10 times, feeling grateful for all that your body was capable of doing during the day.

One-Minute Workouts? Yes—Because Every Brisk Minute Counts

Jessie X. Fan, PhD, professor of family and consumer studies, University of Utah, Salt Lake City. Her study was published in *American Journal of Health Promotion.*

This is great news—really great news—for everyone.

Remember when we all first started talking about "aerobic" exercise (this goes back decades), and we were told that our heart rates had to remain elevated for at least 20 consecutive minutes to get any benefit? That's why we exercised our patooties off in so many long Jazzercise classes back in the '70s and '80s. And that's why some people who thought they didn't have the time or stamina to work out for 20 minutes felt that there was no point in exercising at all.

Fast-forward to the first decade of the new millennium, when experts discovered that shorter bouts of exercise—just 10 minutes rather than 20—were enough to confer benefits, so long as a person reached a weekly total of 75 minutes of vigorous exercise or 150 minutes of moderate-intensity exercise.

The problem is, fewer than 4% of American adults do reach that goal.

Now the great news: A recent study reveals an easier way to hit that target, providing a motivational boost for exercisers and nonexercisers alike. What's the secret? Every single minute of brisk activity counts when it comes to better health, even if you don't clump those minutes together in bunches of 10. In other words, even a one-minute workout does a body good! *Here's why…*

GETTING INTENSE

After the 20-minute-minimum mandate gave way to the 10-minute-minimum recommendation, researchers started wondering whether even shorter bursts of activity might be beneficial. They also wanted to know just how intense the activity had to be to show a benefit.

They used data from the ongoing National Health and Nutrition Examination Survey, in which participants undergo in-depth interviews and full physical exams. The analysis for the new exercise study also included data gathered when, for seven days straight, 4,511 participants wore accelerometers, devices that track the duration and intensity of movement measured in counts per minute (cpm).

Based on the accelerometer data, researchers created four categories of physical activity...

• **Higher-intensity long bouts**—10 or more minutes at 2,020 cpm or higher.

• **Higher-intensity short bouts**—less than 10 minutes at 2,020 cpm or higher.

• **Lower-intensity long bouts**—10 or more minutes at 760 to 2,019 cpm.

• **Lower-intensity short bouts**—less than 10 minutes at 760 to 2,019 cpm.

The higher-intensity long bouts correspond to the Centers for Disease Control and Prevention's current recommendations, while allowing for the brief interruptions that may come when incorporating physical activity into normal living (such as pausing during a brisk walk before being able to cross the street and continue). Also, because there's some controversy on exactly what constitutes moderate versus vigorous activity, the researchers looked at two commonly used thresholds of 760 cpm and 2,020 cpm. (Activity level is translated into real-life terms below.)

RESULTS: EVERY MINUTE HELPS

Most participants logged the majority of their activity in lower-intensity long bouts, while higher-intensity activity was primarily logged in very short bouts of one or two minutes.

Looking only at higher-intensity long bouts, women logged an average of just 46 minutes of high-intensity long-bout physical activity per week, while men logged 61 minutes...so both genders fell short of the recommended target.

But: When shorter bouts of higher-intensity activity were factored in, women averaged 144 minutes per week and men averaged 246 minutes per week...a much more encouraging showing.

Then came the real test—determining whether those minute-long mini-bouts of activity actually did a body good. To that end, researchers looked at the participants' body mass index (BMI) data. Of course, BMI isn't the only measure of health and well-being, but a great many health risks are reduced when BMI is kept down within the normal range.

After adjusting for other factors that affect BMI (age, calorie intake, smoking status, etc.), the researchers found that lower-intensity activity was not associated with any differences in BMI. *But higher-intensity activity was another story...*

For women: Each minute of higher-intensity activity—whether from a short or long bout of activity—was associated with a better BMI. For example, for a typical 5-foot, 5-inch woman, each daily minute of higher-intensity activity had the equivalent calorie offset of 0.41 pounds for short bouts and 0.26 pounds for longer bouts. So if you were to compare two such women who followed the same diet, the woman who engaged in just one more minute per day of higher-intensity short-bout activity would weigh 0.41 pounds less than the other woman. Do the math and this can add up. If one woman typically gave that quick one-minute burst of activity just 10 times in the course of her day, she would weigh four pounds less than the other—which is the difference between having pants that fit and pants that don't.

For men: Each minute of higher-intensity activity per day had the equivalent calorie offset of 0.27 pounds for short bouts and 0.20 pounds for longer bouts—again showing that short bouts of activity did have an impact. Analyzed another way, the researchers said, each extra minute per day of higher-intensity short-bout activity was associated with a 2% drop in a man's likelihood of being obese.

The researchers were not sure why lower-intensity activity was not associated with lower BMI. It could be that only higher-intensity activity triggers the secretion of hormones that cause more calories to be burned even after a bout of exercise ends.

Why this is good news: For many people, short bouts of activity are much easier to accrue than long bouts—so a little extra effort can have an important health payback in terms of weight. Remind yourself, for instance, that it really is worthwhile to pick up your walking pace and to take the stairs instead of the escalator. Working such short little bursts of higher-intensity activity into your day absolutely adds up to better health!

Here are the cpm ratings (according to an earlier study from the University of Massachusetts, Amherst) for some everyday activities that qualify as "higher-intensity"...

- **Walking at 3 mph on a flat surface**—2,970 cpm
- **Walking at 3 mph on a modest incline**—3,137 cpm
- **Climbing stairs**—2,770 cpm
- **Descending stairs**—3,157 cpm
- **Moving an object (less than 25 pounds)**—2,156 cpm
- **Organizing a room/putting away household items**—3,384 cpm

Add a Mini-Workout to Your Workday

James A. Levine, MD, PhD, professor of medicine in the division of endocrinology and director of the Non-Exercise Activity Thermogenesis Laboratory, both at the Mayo Clinic in Rochester, Minnesota. He is also the coauthor of *Move a Little, Lose a Lot.*

Catrine Tudor-Locke, PhD, associate professor and director of the Walking Behavior Laboratory at Pennington Biomedical Research Center in Baton Rouge.

Given that more than 80% of jobs in the US are now sedentary (compared with just 50% five decades ago), day-in-day-out sitting represents a huge and growing health problem. But there's good news—because breaking up sedentary time with spurts of activity has been shown to help offset the health risks of sitting. So, even when we're stuck at the office, we can protect ourselves with some creative get-up-and-go strategies and a few nifty gadgets sold at sporting-goods stores and/or online.

Here are some specific moves...

- **Stand up when you can.** Using the muscles necessary to stand activates substances that have good effects on how the body uses and stores sugars and fats. Plus, standing burns three times as many calories as sitting.

- Automatically get to your feet whenever a co-worker stops by to talk.

- When on the phone, stand and rise up onto your toes, then lower your heels back to the ground...repeat these heel lifts as many times as you can.

- **Get an adjustable-height computer workstation.** Raise it so you can see the screen and reach your keyboard while standing...lower it when you want to sit down. (Avoid prolonged standing if you have back problems.)

- **Step on it.** Standing is better than sitting, but walking is even better than standing.

- Walk fast to the restroom (and take the stairs to one on a different floor), then do an extra lap around the office before heading back to your desk.

Helpful: Drink plenty of water throughout the day—this forces you to take more frequent bathroom breaks (as well as promoting good hydration).

- Rather than meeting with a colleague or two in your office or a conference room, have a "walking meeting" in the corridor.

- If you have enough space and the whir of a machine won't bother coworkers, try a treadmill desk (a treadmill with a flat surface at the front). You don't have to use it all day or even go fast—walking for one hour at a leisurely pace burns 100 to 200 calories more than sitting for the same period of time. Or use a mini-stepper—a small device with two footpads that lets you step in place against resistance—when standing at your adjustable-height workstation.

- **When you must sit, move some muscles.** You're not trying to "feel the burn" with an intense workout—the idea is just to move as much as you can.

- Sit on a stability ball (a large inflatable plastic ball). The continuous tiny adjustments necessary to stay upright on the ball will engage many more muscles (especially the abs, back and pelvis) than sitting on a chair. An average-height woman needs a 21-inch-diameter ball…use a 17-inch ball if you are shorter than five feet…use a 25-inch ball if taller than five feet, seven inches.

•**When waiting for a report to print, do some seated biceps curls or shoulder presses with five-pound hand weights.** Or use a resistance band (a three-foot-long strip of latex) for some seated chest presses or triceps toners.

•**March in place as you read your e-mail, raising your knees as high as you can without hitting the underside of your desk.**

•**Put a portable mini-cycle (a diminutive version of a stationary bicycle) beneath your desk and pedal while you work.**

Helpful: Encourage your coworkers—especially your boss—to join in your "deskercise" movement. If workday physical activities are frowned upon or laughed at, they fail quickly. But when everyone is into them, you get a sense of merriment in the workplace—and then people are quite happy to get moving.

You Can Exercise Less and Be Just as Healthy

Barry A. Franklin, PhD, director of preventive cardiology/cardiac rehabilitation at William Beaumont Hospital in Royal Oak, Michigan. He is a past president of the American Association of Cardiovascular and Pulmonary Rehabilitation and the American College of Sports Medicine. He is also coauthor, with Joseph C. Piscatella, of *109 Things You Can Do to Prevent, Halt & Reverse Heart Disease.*

D o you struggle to fit the recommended amount of exercise into your busy schedule? Well, what if we told you that the amount of exercise needed to reap health benefits might be less than you think? Maybe you could free up some of your workout time for other activities that are important to you and beneficial to your health—like playing with your kids or grandkids, volunteering for a favorite charity or cooking healthful meals.

THE LATEST IN EXERCISE RESEARCH

A recent study published in the *Journal of the American College of Cardiology* found that people lived longest when they ran, on average, for 30 minutes or more, five days a week. Surprisingly, that research also showed that people who jogged at an easy pace for as little as five to 10 minutes a day had virtually the same survival benefits as those who pushed themselves harder or longer.

Also surprising: A study recently done at Oregon State University found that one- and two-minute bouts of activity that add up to 30 minutes or more per day, such as pacing while talking on the telephone, doing housework or doing sit-ups during TV commercials, may reduce blood pressure and cholesterol and improve health as effectively as a structured exercise program.

HOW TO EXERCISE SMARTER, NOT HARDER

Here are four strategies to help you exercise more efficiently…

•**Recognize that some exercise is always better than none.** Even though exercise guidelines from the Centers for Disease Control and Prevention call for at least 150 minutes of moderate exercise each week, you'll do well even at lower levels.

A study in the *Lancet* found that people who walked for just 15 minutes a day had a 14% reduction in death over an average of eight years. Good daily exercises include not only walking but working in the yard, swimming, riding a bike, etc.

If you're among the multitudes of Americans who have been sedentary in recent years, you'll actually gain the most. Simply making the transition from horrible fitness to below average can reduce your overall risk for premature death by 20% to 40%.

•**Go for a run instead of a walk.** The intensity, or associated energy cost, of running is greater than walking. Therefore, running (or walking up a grade or incline) is better for the heart than walking—and it's easier to work into a busy day because you can get equal benefits in less time.

For cardiovascular health, a five-minute run (5.5 mph to 8 mph) is equal to a 15-minute walk (2 mph to 3.5 mph)…and a 25-minute run equals a 105-minute walk.

A study of runners found that their risk of dying from heart disease was 45% lower than nonrunners over a 15-year follow-up. In fact, running can add, on average, three extra years to your life.

Caution: If you take running seriously, you still should limit your daily workouts to 60 minutes or less, no more than five days a week. (See below for the dangers of overdoing it.) People with heart symptoms or severely compromised heart function should avoid running. If you have joint problems, check with your doctor.

•**Ease into running.** Don't launch into a running program until you're used to exercise. Make it progressive. Start by walking slowly—say, at about 2 mph. Gradually increase it to 3 mph…then to 3.5 mph, etc. After two or three months, if you are symptom-free during fast walking, you can start to run (slowly at first).

•**Aim for the "upper-middle."** I do not recommend high-intensity workouts for most adults. Strive to exercise at a level you would rate between "fairly light" and "somewhat hard."

How to tell: Check your breathing. It will be slightly labored when you're at a good level of exertion. Nevertheless, you should still be able to carry on a conversation.

Important: Get your doctor's OK before starting vigorous exercise—and don't ignore potential warning symptoms. It's normal to be somewhat winded or to have a little leg discomfort. However, you should never feel dizzy, experience chest pain or have extreme shortness of breath. If you have any of these symptoms, stop exercise immediately, and see your doctor before resuming activity.

TOO MUCH OF A GOOD THING?

Most people who run for more than an hour a day, five days a week, are in very good shape. Would they be healthier if they doubled the distance—or pushed themselves even harder? *Not necessarily. Risks linked to distance running include…*

•**Acute right-heart overload.** Researchers at William Beaumont Hospital who looked at distance runners before and immediately after marathon running found that they often had transient decreases in the pumping ability of the right ventricle and elevations of the same enzymes (such as *troponin*) that increase during a heart attack.

•**Atrial fibrillation.** People who exercise intensely for more than five hours a week may be more likely to develop atrial fibrillation, a heart-rhythm disturbance that can trigger a stroke.

•**Coronary plaque.** Despite their favorable coronary risk factor profiles, distance runners can have increased amounts of coronary artery calcium and plaque as compared with their less active counterparts.

Watch out: Many hard-core runners love marathons, triathlons and other competitive events. Be careful. The emotional rush from competition increases levels of epinephrine and other "stress" hormones. These hormones, combined with hard exertion, can transiently increase heart risks.

Of course, all this doesn't mean that you shouldn't enjoy a daily run…or a few long ones—just don't overdo it!

A Faster, Smarter Way to Get Fit

Martin Gibala, PhD, a professor and chair of the kinesiology department at McMaster University in Hamilton, Ontario, Canada. He has published more than 100 peer-reviewed articles and is coauthor of *The One Minute Workout: Science Shows a Way to Get Fit That's Smarter, Faster, Shorter.*

Very few of us can say that we have "extra" time. If something on our to-do list has to be eliminated, it's usually that hour spent at the gym.

But what if you could significantly pare down your exercise time?

You've probably heard of high-intensity interval training (HIIT). With HIIT, you intersperse bouts of intense exercise—say, 30 seconds of all-out pedaling on a bike—with equal or longer periods of recovery (complete rest or low-intensity exercise). Repeat that a few times, and you're done for the day.

What's new: Researchers have discovered that with HIIT, you can get significant health benefits even faster than previously thought.

HOW HIIT HELPS

Traditional aerobic workouts, involving continuous low-to-moderate intensity exercise, strengthen the heart…improve metabolism…and reduce the risk for heart disease, high blood pressure, diabetes and other chronic diseases. What's exciting about HIIT is that it offers the same health benefits as a traditional workout—but in a different way.

Here's why: Each time you push yourself into high action, you create a disturbance in your body's *homeostasis*, which is how the body behaves at rest. Each disturbance forces the heart to beat faster, the lungs to process more oxygen and the muscles to consume more fuel.

Very quickly, your body adapts to these changes. Muscles grow more *mitochondria*—your cells' powerhouses—making them more efficient at producing energy. The heart pumps more blood with each beat. You become fitter, and your cardiovascular disease risk goes down.

High-intensity workouts with frequent intervals cause more disturbances in homeostasis than traditional workouts, which push the body into a more constant state of physical exertion.

FASTER, BUT EQUAL

In a 2016 study, researchers at McMaster University compared two training protocols in sedentary men. One group followed standard exercise guidelines—they rode exercise bikes at a moderate pace for 45 minutes, three days a week.

The second group did a special HIIT workout—a 20-second all-out, hard sprint…followed by two minutes of slow cycling…repeated twice for a total of three sprint-rest cycles. Add in a few minutes for a warm-up and cooldown, and that's a sweet workout of just about 10 minutes.

Results: After 12 weeks, men in both exercise groups showed similar improvements in insulin sensitivity (the body's mechanism for regulating blood sugar) and cardiorespiratory fitness. All men also developed stronger muscles.

Bottom line: Men who followed the 10-minute HIIT workout three times weekly had the same health benefits as men who did traditional exercise for 45 minutes three times weekly.

ALMOST ANYONE CAN DO IT

You may assume that high-intensity workouts are riskier than easy ones, especially for people who are out of shape or have a high risk for heart disease. The truth is, any form of exercise, including HIIT, slightly increases cardiovascular risks during workouts…but your overall heart disease risk goes down. In fact, a wide variety of HIIT protocols have been applied to people with many different conditions, including cardiovascular disease, diabetes and metabolic syndrome.

To play it safe: If you have health problems or heart disease risk factors—smoking, high blood pressure, a sedentary lifestyle, etc.—check with your doctor before starting any new exercise program.

GETTING STARTED

Even though an HIIT workout is designed to push exercisers out of their comfort zones, you can adapt it to suit your preferences in a less strenuous way. All that's required are bursts of exercise followed by lower-intensity activity.

Do you like walking? You can do 30-second fast walks. Start slowly, then push yourself to about 70% of your upper limit—breathing hard, but not gasping for air. Then slow down for a few minutes. Alternate fast/slow for up to 30 minutes (with a short cooldown at the end), three or more times a week.

Those who are healthy, fit and have the all-clear from their doctors, may want to try this 10-minute workout that incorporates just one minute of high-intensity exercise. First, warm up for three minutes with low-intensity exercise. *Then…*

•**Blast through 20 seconds of an all-out sprint (or bike, swim, etc.).**

•**Recover with light activity for two minutes.**

•**Repeat the cycle until you've done three sprints.** End with a two-minute cooldown of light activity.

4

Improve Your Workout: Exercise Smarter and Safer

Get More from Your Workouts!

Tom Holland, MS, CPT, an exercise physiologist, certified sports nutritionist and certified strength and conditioning coach. He is author of four fitness books, including *Beat the Gym: Personal Trainer Secrets—Without the Personal Trainer Price Tag* and hosts the podcast "Fitness Disrupted" on iHeartRadio.

Anyone who sticks to an exercise program knows that the commitment involves a lot of time and, in some cases, money if you belong to a gym or fitness center.

Trap: All too often, people follow ineffective routines that cause them to waste their time and money. Here are my secrets for getting the most from your workout…*

SECRET #1: **Do the right amount of cardio.** If you don't do enough cardiovascular exercise, you won't get the maximum benefits. But, if you do too much, you'll increase your risk for injury. So how much cardio should you do?

My advice: Follow this simple formula—for every pound you weigh, do one minute of cardio each week. For example, if you weigh 150 pounds,

*Consult your doctor before beginning or significantly changing an exercise regimen.

you should do 150 minutes of cardio (incorporating a variety of exercises) per week.

Because women in general will end up doing less cardio than men with this formula, it's wise for them to spend more time doing strength training (see below). Genetically, women have less muscle than men, and as a woman ages, the preservation of lean muscle becomes vital.

SECRET #2: **Understand what the programs on cardio machines really mean.** Let's say that you opt for a "fat-burning" program on a treadmill because you want to lose (or maintain) body weight. Based on the "calories burned from fat" percentages given with these programs, it appears that you will burn more fat if you work out at a lower intensity. But that's not true. Because these fat-burning calculations are based on percentages—not total calories burned—they are easily misunderstood. *For example…*

Workout #1: A 30-minute cardiovascular workout at an easy intensity burns 250 calories and 20 g of fat. With this workout, 72% of calories burned are from fat.

Workout #2: A 25-minute intense cardio workout burns 330 calories and 25 g of fat. That's the equivalent of 68% of calories burned from fat.

The easier workout burns a larger percentage of fat, but the more intense workout burns more fat and calories in total—and in less time. The more calories and fat burned, the more weight you will lose.

SECRET #3: Skip the heart-rate zone charts. The most widely used maximum heart-rate zones are calculated by subtracting the exerciser's age from 220. For example, if you are age 50, your maximum heart rate would be 170 (220 − 50 = 170). This is supposed to be the highest heart rate you should reach during a workout. However, research has found that in most cases the number is too low.

My advice: Whether you choose to use a treadmill, StairMaster, stationary bike, elliptical trainer, etc., simply focus on varying the intensity of your workout. Use a scale of one to 10, with 10 being the most intense. On some days do a lower intensity workout (around a five or six), and on other days bring it up to a seven or eight. Mix in short intervals (10 to 60 seconds) of high-intensity (nine to 10) exercise.

Important: Always get your doctor's approval before following any maximum heart-rate formulas.

SECRET #4: Don't slight your strength-training regimen. Many people complain that, as they age, they eat and exercise the same amount but still gain weight. One of the main causes of this is loss of muscle mass. The more muscle mass you have, the more calories you burn. Strength training preserves and even increases muscle mass, keeping metabolism at a high level.

Strength training also increases bone density and functional strength and preserves joint health.

My advice: As with cardio workouts, vary your strength-training routines. Some days use machines, others use dumbbells or stretch bands. You also could do squats, push-ups and lunges. If you have trouble incorporating separate strength-training sessions into your workout, an efficient method is to do circuit training. This approach involves strength exercises with short bursts of cardio in between.

Important: Don't spend too much time on ab crunches. The appearance of abs is largely due to diet. The best way to reduce abdominal fat is with healthful eating and cardio exercise. Spend only 10% of your strength-training sessions on ab exercises. This will define the abdomen once you have decreased abdominal fat.

SECRET #5: Start with an exercise you hate. Because you're less likely to perform exercises you hate, doing them will have a big impact on your body.

My advice: Do just one exercise you don't like at the beginning of a workout—if you put it off until the end of your exercise session, chances are you won't do it. Incorporate one exercise you hate for a few weeks, then switch to another you dislike. This prevents your body from getting used to the hated exercise.

See What's Missing from Your Workout…

Tom Holland, MS, CPT, an exercise physiologist, certified sports nutritionist and certified strength and conditioning coach. He is author of four fitness books, including *Beat the Gym: Personal Trainer Secrets—Without the Personal Trainer Price Tag* and hosts the podcast "Fitness Disrupted" on iHeartRadio.

First things first: If you exercise regularly, pat yourself on the back. But if you're like most people and do just one exercise over and over again, listen up.

By simply varying your exercise routine, you can greatly improve the health benefits of your workout…overcome any boredom that might creep in… and even reduce your risk for injury.

The good news is, you don't need a lot of fancy equipment to vary your workout. *Here's how to mix it up if your favorite exercise is…*

WALKING

If you are a walker, add high-intensity interval training (HIIT). Whether you frequent your local outdoor track or use a treadmill, walking is arguably one of the best forms of exercise there is.

But to maximize the benefits, you need to ramp up your speed (and/or perhaps incline or resistance if you're using a treadmill). The best way to do this is to up the ante on your workout with some HIIT, which intersperses short bursts of increased intensity.

While your regular walking routine may feel like a five on a scale of one to 10, during HIIT intervals, you should feel like you're exercising at a seven or an eight. The variety makes a low-intensity, steady exercise like walking more interesting and fun, and people who have fun when they exercise are more apt to stick with it.

If you're trying to lose weight: HIIT burns extra calories both during and after the workout.

To try it: Walk or use a treadmill at a comfortable warm-up pace for three minutes, then alternate 60 seconds at a normal pace with 60 seconds at a faster pace or higher incline for the remainder of the workout. (Pumping your arms helps. Be sure you know how to use the safety cord if you're on a treadmill.) Do a three-minute cooldown at a slower pace. Try adding HIIT to your walking routine one to three times per week.

TENNIS

If you love tennis, add some foam rolling. Pulled muscles and strains are ubiquitous among tennis players in their 50s, 60s and beyond, thanks to the quick, sudden movements and direction changes. But just a few minutes of pre-tennis self-massage with a foam roller could be enough to keep you on the court.

Why foam rolling? Because this technique, which involves moving a foam roller back and forth along different parts of the body, enhances blood flow to different muscles, performing it preworkout can improve flexibility and range of motion, reducing one's risk for injury, according to research published in *International Journal of Sports Physical Therapy.*

Also: Foam rolling lower-body muscles prior to exercise alters perception of fatigue, so you won't tire as quickly.

To start rolling: Target your calves, quadriceps and iliotibial bands, the thick connective tissue running down the outside of each hip to just below the knee.

For calves, sit on the floor and place the roller perpendicular underneath your outstretched legs. While supporting most of your weight with your hands, lift your hips and slowly move the roller up and down your calves for 10 to 30 seconds.

Flip over to roll out your quads...and turn on your side for the iliotibial bands—roll these areas for 10 to 30 seconds each. Try this rolling routine before tennis matches and a few times per week.

YOGA

If yoga is your thing, add cardio exercise. Yoga offers balance, flexibility, strength and stress relief. But unless you're practicing a fast-paced vinyasa yoga that has your heart working hard enough to make conversation difficult, it's probably not counting toward the standard recommendation of at least 150 minutes weekly of moderate cardiovascular exercise.

Mix things up with jogging or fast walking, biking, swimming or fast-paced aerobics classes. Just make sure that you're spending most of your time at your target heart rate for 30 minutes a day, five days a week. It's fine to do three 10-minute sessions to reach your goal.

Your target heart rate: Aim for 50% to 85% of your maximum heart rate, which is 220 minus your age. So if you're 55, your maximum heart rate is 165, and your target heart rate 83 to 140 beats per minute.

Exciting recent finding: Heart disease patients practicing yoga in addition to aerobic exercise had twice the reduction in blood pressure, cholesterol levels and body mass index compared with those who did either exercise alone.

Also: For all types of exercise, do strength training two days a week for a well-rounded regimen.

HIIT for Runners

Roundup of experts on exercise, reported at Shape.com.

Better way for runners to get started with high-intensity interval training...

Start with 15 seconds of an all-out sprint, and add 15 seconds each time you exercise until you hit the one-minute level. Use the right amount of recovery time—your recovery time should be four times as long as the high-intensity period.

Example: Four minutes of walking or jogging for every one-minute sprint. The body needs that long to get ready for the next intense push. After you finish your workout, keep moving for several hours. Walk, stretch your muscles, and stand up and move around every 30 to 60 minutes to help your muscles recover properly.

Smarter Not Harder Ways to Exercise

Edward J. Jackowski, PhD, founder and CEO of Exude Fitness, a New York City–based fitness company (Exude. com) that specializes in one-on-one fitness training. He is author of *Escape Your Shape: How to Work Out Smarter, Not Harder* and *Hold It! You're Exercising Wrong* and the DVD *Escape Your Shape: 21-Day Body Makeover.*

Want to feel better? Exercise. Lose weight? Exercise. Ward off disease, prevent injuries and recover from health problems faster? Exercise, exercise, exercise.

A true health panacea, exercise is an appropriate prescription for just about everything and everyone.*

Problem: Exercise is a vague term that many people (including doctors) think they understand—but about which they get little expert guidance. As a result, we often waste time and effort on fitness regimens that offer minimal benefit and may even lead to injury.

Here are eight common mistakes that are made concerning fitness…plus smart and simple solutions that will help you get the most from your workouts.

MISTAKE: **Confusing activity with exercise.** You can't get fit from an occasional play-till-you-

drop game of tennis or a nightly stroll around the block—yet many of us convince ourselves that sporadic bursts of effort or low-intensity activities fulfill their exercise needs. While it is true that some exercise is better than no exercise, true fitness comes from workouts that are consistent and challenging but not exhausting.

Smarter: Each exercise session should include all of the following…

•**A warm-up.**

•**Stretches to increase flexibility.**

•**Cardiovascular workout, such as walking fast enough to raise your heart rate for 10 minutes.**

•**Strengthening moves that build muscles in your upper body, core (torso) and lower body, such as biceps curls, sit-ups and lunges.**

•**A cooldown, such as relaxed walking, to gradually lower your heart rate.**

MISTAKE: **Working out for too long a period.** Your entire session should not exceed 60 to 75 minutes. Your body won't reap significant additional health benefits from exercising longer than this. What's more, if your body gets used to extended workouts and then you have to cut down—due to increased demands at home or at work, for instance—you'll gain weight if you don't also cut calories. This is because your body will no longer be expending as many calories as it is accustomed to burning.

Smarter: Schedule an hour or so of exercise into your calendar three or four times per week—then stick with it. The idea is to make exercise a consistent part of your life, not an ordeal that knocks you out so much on Tuesday that you can't face the gym again until Saturday.

MISTAKE: **Lifting weights that are too heavy.** Many weight-lifters believe that the heavier the weight, the better the effect on body shape. But if one of your reasons for working out is to slim down, heavy weights won't help—in fact, they'll make you bulk up.

Smarter: To reduce your size while still building strength, use lighter weights and increase the number of repetitions.

*Always check with your doctor before beginning any exercise program.

Example: Do 25 leg lifts with two-pound leg weights instead of 15 lifts with five-pound weights. The lighter weights will still challenge your muscles, but the muscles won't grow as big. If you do want to build muscle size, use heavier weights and do fewer repetitions.

MISTAKE: **Relying on classes to keep you fit.** A well-choreographed class with an excellent instructor is a good way to learn proper technique. But what will you do when you can't make it to class or the teacher is absent? You may end up skipping your workout altogether.

Smarter: Create an alternate routine for the days when you can't take a class—preferably one you can do alone, anywhere, anytime. Also create a mini version that you can do no matter what your time constraints may be.

MISTAKE: **Working through an injury.** Maintaining a consistent exercise schedule does not mean that you should keep working out when you're hurt. Doing so probably would worsen the injury and undermine your fitness goals.

Smarter: *To avoid paying the price for overworking an injury, remember the word PRICE...*

● **P is for PROTECTING your body from further injury by laying off until you feel better.**

● **R is for RESTING the part of your body that aches.**

● **I is for ICE**—apply to the painful area for 30 minutes twice daily for a few days to ease swelling and pain. Do not use heat on a new injury.

● **C is for COMPRESSION**—wrap the sore area with an Ace bandage (not too tight!) for a few days.

● **E is for ELEVATE**—to take pressure off the injured area, elevate it whenever possible.

When you are pain-free, return to your exercise regimen. If pain is severe or does not abate after several days, see your doctor.

MISTAKE: **Rushing to buy an exercise machine.** If you can afford it and know that you'll use it as one part of your overall routine, it's fine to buy a machine, such as a treadmill. However, most people end up stuffing that machine in a corner and forgetting about it—or overusing it and building up one particular body part while neglecting the rest.

Smarter: Use machines at a local gym...build a repertoire of exercises that need no equipment, such as running, jumping jacks and push-ups... buy only versatile, portable, low-cost gear, such as an elastic resistance band and a jump rope.

MISTAKE: **Extending your knees over your toes.** Lunges and squats are excellent exercises— but if you let your knees extend too far forward, you strain the knee joints and increase the risk for injury to the cartilage, tendons and ligaments.

Smarter: Keep an eye on your alignment. You always should be able to see your toes just beyond the tops of your knees.

Better: Perform these exercises in front of a mirror so that you can periodically check your form.

MISTAKE: **Believing that jump ropes are just for little girls.** If you haven't jumped rope since elementary school, you're missing out on one of the simplest and most effective exercises. Jumping rope is an aerobic activity, so it's good for your heart...improves all-over muscle strength by working the entire body at once...builds bones because it is weight-bearing...and is low-impact if done on a surface with natural give, such as a wood floor or a thin mat.

Smarter: To add jumping rope to your fitness routine, start slowly—try to do 20, then 50, then 100 jumps in a row. As your endurance builds, aim to jump rope for 10 minutes straight during the cardio portion of your workout two or three times per week. Even if you have problems with incontinence, keep jumping—my clients say that their symptoms improve within a few weeks, perhaps because the exercise strengthens pelvic area muscles.

Bonus: Jumping rope burns twice as many calories as playing singles tennis, but it places much less pressure on your joints.

7 Mistakes That Can Sabotage Your Walking Workout

Robert Sweetgall, who passed away in 2017, was president of Creative Walking, a Kirkwood, Missouri, company that designed walking and fitness programs for schools, corporations and other clients. He walked/ran across the US seven times. Sweetgall is coauthor, with Barry Franklin, PhD, of *One Heart, Two Feet: Enhancing Heart Health One Step at a Time.*

We all know that walking is very good for us. But what most people don't realize is just how powerful this simple exercise is. Studies have shown that walking promotes heart health, strengthens bones, spurs weight loss, boosts mood and even cuts risk for cancer and Alzheimer's.

Latest development: In recent studies involving patients with peripheral artery disease (PAD), plaque buildup in the arteries that can contribute to heart attack or stroke, walking improved their painful symptoms as much as medication and, in some cases, even more than bypass surgery or balloon angioplasty to treat the affected artery.

What's more, even a small amount of walking goes a long way toward improving health. Recent research has found that walking just a half-mile a day helps prevent diabetes, and another study has shown that walking for just two hours a week reduces breast cancer risk by 18%.

While many people take walking for granted, the majority of walkers could significantly improve the health benefits by tweaking their walking techniques and using the right equipment.

Common walking mistakes—and what to do instead…

MISTAKE #1: Tilting forward. Some walkers tilt their upper bodies forward, as though they're walking into the wind. They think that this position increases speed. It does not—and it greatly increases pressure on the lower back while straining the shins.

Better: Walk with your head high and still, shoulders relaxed and chest slightly out. In this position, you can rotate your eyes downward to survey the path and look ahead to view the scenery around you.

MISTAKE #2: **Swinging the arms inefficiently.** Many walkers waste energy by swinging their arms side to side or pumping their arms up and down. These exaggerated movements add little to cardiovascular fitness and make walking less efficient because arm energy is directed upward or sideways rather than straight ahead.

Better: For maximum efficiency, pump your arms straight ahead on a horizontal plane, like you're reeling in a string through your midsection. This motion improves balance, posture and walking speed.

MISTAKE #3: **Using hand and/or ankle weights.** While some people like to walk with weights to boost the intensity of a walking workout, the risk for injury far outweighs the benefits of using weights. The repetitive stress of swinging weights can cause microtears in the soft tissues of the arms and legs.

Better: To increase exertion, walk uphill or on an inclined treadmill.

Another good option: Try Nordic walking (see next article) for a total-body workout. With this type of walking, you use specially designed walking poles (one in each hand) to help propel your body forward.

Compared with regular walking, Nordic walking can increase your energy expenditure by 20%, according to a study from The Cooper Institute. It works the abdominal, arm and back muscles and reduces stress on the feet, ankles, knees and hips while improving endurance.

MISTAKE #4: **Not doing a warm-up.** You're inviting muscle soreness and potential injury if you hit your top speed at the start.

Better: Be sure to warm up. Start slowly, accelerating over the first five to 10 minutes…and end slowly, decelerating over the last five minutes. A slow start allows your muscles to warm up and become flexible, while enabling your cardiorespiratory system to get used to higher workloads. A proper cooldown helps eliminate the buildup of lactic acid, which can lead to muscle soreness.

***MISTAKE #5*: Doing the same walk every day.** It's best to alter your routine for maximum health benefits and to maintain motivation.

Better: Do shorter, faster-paced walks some days (cardiovascular conditioning) and longer, moderate-paced walks on other days (calorie burning). Also try walks on steeper terrains and walks that alternate faster intervals with slower intervals.

***MISTAKE #6*: Not keeping a walking log or journal.** Every day, indicate how far and fast you walked and any other observations you wish to record in a notebook or on your computer. Keeping a journal helps foster a sense of accomplishment and self-esteem and is the single most effective method for ensuring that you'll stick to a walking program.

***MISTAKE #7*: Choosing cushy shoes.** A study in *The American Journal of Sports Medicine* found that, on average, expensive, high-tech footwear caused twice the injuries as shoes costing half as much.

Some high-priced, cushiony shoes can make you feel as if you're walking on a foam mattress, but they have an inherent "wobble" that can cause your foot to move side to side, leading to potential foot, ankle, knee and hip injuries.

Better: Thin-soled shoes with minimal support. They force the muscles in the legs and feet to work harder, which improves strength and balance and helps prevent injuries.

When transitioning to thinner-soled shoes, make the switch gradually, breaking them in on shorter walks. They can feel awkward at first, so give your feet time to adjust.

Of course the right shoe is a very individual choice, but I like Karhu shoes, which promote forward momentum.

Cost: About $55 to $140, depending on the model. Other people like the so-called "barefoot" shoes, such as Vibram FiveFingers.

Helpful: Avoid cotton socks, which can lose their support and shape after a few washings. Try socks made from blends that include acrylic fibers, Coolmax and/or spandex/elastic. Soft wool socks also can work.

Tip: Powder your feet with cornstarch before a long walk to reduce friction, heat buildup and blisters.

TAKE THE LONGEVITY TEST

The more steps it takes you to walk the same distance each year, the weaker your core muscles are becoming.

Self-test: Each year on your birthday, go to a track and walk one lap, recording the number of steps on your pedometer. Aim to complete the lap in about the same number of steps each year. If it takes you more steps each year, you are regressing toward the "senior shuffle" and compromising your core-muscle strength and overall vitality.

What to do: In addition to walking regularly, start a core-muscle strengthening regimen (see exercises beginning on page 64) and a stretching program to tone your hip and leg muscles.

Power Up Your Walking: Nordic Walking...Boost Calorie Burn by 20% or More

Wayne Westcott, PhD, professor of exercise science, researcher and chair of the exercise science program at Quincy College in Quincy, Massachusetts. He has worked as a strength training consultant for numberous national organizations, such as the American Council on Exercise, the American Senior Fitness Association and the National Youth Sports Safety Foundation. He is the author or coauthor of several books, including *Building Strength and Stamina, Strength Training Past 50, Strength Training for Seniors, Complete Conditioning for Golf,* and *Strength and Power for Young Athletes.*

Nordic walking, popular in Finland, is coming into fashion in the US. The secret to its success is the rubber-tipped poles that work the upper body and core to burn more calories during a revved-up form of fitness walking. Also known as pole walking, this technique was first used for summer training by cross country skiers, but soon became popular with the Finnish walking public.

Nordic walking supplies a better workout overall than normal walking, and many people especially enjoy this form of vigorous outdoor exercise that enables them to breathe in fresh air as they trek over varied terrain.

MORE BANG FOR THE BUCK

In Nordic walking, you use two lightweight aluminum or fiberglass poles to push off each step, as if you were a cross-country skier. This technique reduces wear and tear on the knees and ankles, since you are requiring your triceps, pecs and forearm muscles to take some of the weight off your joints. As for energy consumption or weight loss, Nordic walking provides more bang for the buck, too. Most Nordic walkers report not feeling like they have to work harder, yet they burn an additional 20% to 40% more calories compared with normal walking—primarily because the upper body is more involved.

As with many forms of exercise, the right technique is essential. Nordic walking can be done on neighborhood streets (flat or hilly), or a more challenging hiking trail—your choice. The more challenging the terrain, the better the workout. The correct equipment is important, too. Poles must be proper length for your height or you risk back strain and diminished benefits. Most poles come with instructions, so read them carefully. You can learn more about Nordic walking at AmericanNordicWalking.com.

FREQUENCY, INTENSITY AND CONSISTENCY

To keep energy and interest levels high, many people like to vary their exercises, choosing Nordic walking one day, biking or fitness walking the next. *Whatever exercise regimen you choose, try to meet three key criteria...*

•**Frequency.** Try to get out there three or four days a week.

•**Intensity.** Activity should be vigorous enough to raise the heart rate 60% to 85% of maximum heart rate.

•**Consistency.** For your body to reap real benefits, workouts must be a minimum of 15 to 20 minutes long.

Walking for Exercise? Here's How to Find the Right Intensity

Study titled "Walking Cadence (Steps/Min) and Intensity in 21–40 Year Olds: CADENCE-Adults" by researchers at University of Massachusetts Amherst, published in *International Journal of Behavioral Nutrition and Physical Activity.*

You've probably heard the standard recommendations to get 150 minutes of aerobic exercise per week at moderate intensity...or 75 minutes at vigorous intensity. But what does "moderate" really mean? And how much harder is "vigorous"?

If walking is your thing—and it is one of the best possible forms of aerobic exercise—there are lots of electronic fitness trackers (not to mention good, old-fashioned pocket pedometers) that promise to give you the answers. The problem is, these devices are not always affordable or convenient to use. And some people don't like being "plugged in" all the time.

Now an ongoing study focusing on the health benefits of walking, which earlier research has pegged as everything from improved heart health to reduced risk for constipation, has uncovered an easy way to determine the intensity of your exercise—without using a pricey electronic device or a fancy pedometer.

Recent finding: In analyzing the first batch of results from their study-in-progress, researchers at the University of Massachusetts Amherst report that simply counting the number of steps you take per minute will determine your walking cadence—which is a surprisingly simple but reliable way to ensure that you're exercising hard enough.

Study details: In this initial report, published in *International Journal of Behavioral Nutrition and Physical Activity*, 80 study participants (all from the 21- to 40-year-old group) were asked to walk on a treadmill for five-minute intervals with two-minute periods of recovery between each session. The treadmill speed was bumped up by half a mile per hour for each five-minute effort until the participant was running...working at 75% of his/her maximum heart rate…or self-reported as exercising at a "somewhat hard" level.

The researchers counted the walkers' cadence, and their exercise intensity was verified by a portable device that calculates oxygen consumption. With these results in hand, the researchers found that walking cadence is a good indicator of exercise intensity.

The numbers you need to know: A walking speed of moderate intensity begins at approximately 100 steps per minute, according to this study, while a vigorous intensity kicks in at about 130 steps per minute.

To quickly calculate your own cadence on any given walk: Wear a watch with a second hand (or set the timer on your smartwatch) and go for a walk. Simply count the number of steps you take in 15 seconds, then multiply that number by four. Voila! That final number is your walking cadence.

To put a little groove into your step: If you hum "Stayin' Alive" by the Bee Gees to yourself while you walk, and match your steps to the beat, you'll be right at 100 steps per minute. Walking to the beat of Cyndi Lauper's "Girls Just Wanna Have Fun" or Billy Ray Cyrus's "Achy Breaky Heart" will put you at a cadence of 120. And to boost your effort up to 130, step out to Jennifer Lopez's "On the Floor" or Lady Gaga's "The Edge of Glory."

Reboot Your Workout!

Robert Hopper, PhD, exercise physiologist and author of *Stick with Exercise for a Lifetime*, with Rebecca Shannonhouse, editor-in-chief, health content, Bottom Line Inc.

Have your workouts started to feel…well, like work? You go to the gym, but not as often as you used to—or need to.

Sound familiar? Sooner or later, motivation vanishes from our exercise routines. But the "routine"—which inevitably leads to boredom—is actually part of the problem.

How to get on track, according to Robert Hopper, PhD, an exercise physiologist and author of *Stick with Exercise for a Lifetime*…

●**Pick an activity that you really enjoy.** Sounds obvious—but how many of us head straight for the treadmill or the same piece of equipment every time we go to the gym? Instead, think of a sport you really love to do. It might be biking, skiing, golf or racquetball. Think of it as your activity, and do it whenever you can.

●**Choose your workouts strategically.** This means opting for activities that support your favorite form of physical activity.

Example: If you're a skier, biking and lower-body weight training will help keep you in shape to hit the slopes.

●**Pay yourself.** A bit too extreme? It actually works for a lot of people.

Helpful: Try one of the motivational smartphone apps—such as Pact, which allows you to team up with friends so you can all get paid for working out…or StickK, which donates your contribution to a favorite charity when you meet your fitness goals—or to one you despise when you don't.

I'm excited to try these new approaches, so if you'll excuse me…I'm off to the gym!

Improve Your Treadmill Workout

Bruce Pechman, known as "Mr. Bicep." Based in San Diego, he has practiced fitness training for more than 30 years and has competed in more than 20 bodybuilding competitions. He appears regularly on such news programs as *Fox & Friends*, *KTLA Morning Show* and *Good Morning San Diego*. MrBicep.com

Using a treadmill is a great way to get the benefits of walking or running—while avoiding exposure to inclement weather and vehicle exhaust. A treadmill also offers a better workout than the other commonly used piece of exercise equipment, an exercise bike. A study at the Milwaukee Veterans Administration Hospital found that an average, medium-intensity treadmill workout burns 700 calories per hour—200 more than one hour on an exercise bike.

However, many people don't get the most from their treadmill workouts, because they make these mistakes…*

MISTAKE: Holding on. People hold the treadmill rails or walk with their arms close to their sides.

Problem: Holding the rails can reduce the total calories burned by one-third or more. Swinging your arms when you walk or run increases energy use. It also works the obliques, the muscles on both sides of the abdominal wall.

Solution: Unless you need to hold the rails—because of a disability or balance issues—let your arms swing naturally on a treadmill. Do this even if it requires you to walk or run at a slower speed.

MISTAKE: Standing too far forward. People tend to "hug" the control console at the front of a treadmill, either because they're reading something propped on top or because they want to be near the controls.

Problem: Walking too close to the front of the treadmill shortens your natural stride. This prevents muscles and joints from achieving a full range of motion and reduces workout efficiency.

Solution: Once you start the treadmill, take a step-and-a-half backward. This is enough to permit a normal stride—and to allow your arms to swing back and forth without hitting the console.

MISTAKE: Leaning forward. The forward momentum of treadmills encourages people to lean forward as they walk or run.

Problem: Leaning skews the body's biomechanics. It can cause neck and back pain and makes it more difficult to achieve a normal stride.

Solution: Stand upright…pull in your stomach…keep your shoulders back…and keep your head level.

MISTAKE: Not adjusting the incline. Most home treadmills can be adjusted to an incline of as much as 12%. Treadmills in health clubs go as

*Talk to your doctor before starting any exercise program.

high as 20%. Unfortunately, many people never use this feature.

Problem: Walking on a horizontal surface burns fewer calories than walking uphill. With an incline setting, you give your hamstring, gluteal and quadriceps muscles more of a workout.

Solution: Set the machine on horizontal for the first five minutes of your workout to warm up. Then choose a challenging incline, and keep it there for the duration of your workout. Using a 6%-to-7% incline will burn 20%-to-40% more calories than using only the horizontal position.

MISTAKE: Complacency. People who use treadmills tend to settle into a comfortable routine and stay there.

Problem: "Coasting"—sticking to the same speed or incline—leads to a workout plateau, where any improvement in strength and conditioning essentially stops.

Solution: Push past your comfort zone. When your usual routine starts feeling easy, increase the incline or speed.

OK to Lean Forward When Working Out on a Treadmill?

Edward J. Jackowski, PhD, founder and CEO of Exude Fitness, a New York City–based fitness company (Exude. com) that specializes in one-on-one fitness training. He is author of *Escape Your Shape: How to Work Out Smarter, Not Harder* and *Hold It! You're Exercising Wrong* and the DVD *Escape Your Shape: 21-Day Body Makeover.*

If you are hunched over while working out on a treadmill (or on an elliptical or other aerobic exercise machine), you will get less weight-bearing benefit (for osteoporosis prevention) and burn fewer calories than you would if standing upright. When leaning forward, you're distributing your body weight to your arms and upper body instead of placing your weight primarily on your legs, as you should. Leaning too far forward can lead to low-back and shoulder discomfort or even injury. Also, be sure not to grip the handrails. This position does not simulate the walking that you naturally do in everyday activities and will prevent you from developing better balance. If you need additional support while on the treadmill, hold the handrail just long enough to regain your balance, then release your hands and move your arms as you would while walking down the street. If you have balance problems, start at a slow enough pace so that you can comfortably walk hands-free, and stand upright for maximum results.

The Surprising Way to Get More from Your Exercise

Paul A. Estabrooks, PhD, behavioral scientist, professor and Harold M. Maurer Distinguished Chair of the department of health promotions at University of Nebraska Medical Center in Omaha. He is an author of "Group-Based Physical Activity for Older Adults Randomized Controlled Trial," recently published in *Health Psychology*.

We all want to get as many health benefits as possible from the exercise we do.

What you might not realize: Group workouts—especially those that have a few special features—offer an array of unexpected health benefits. *What you need to know to tap into this powerful exercise booster…*

If you're skeptical that group workouts could offer more than an intense solitary jog on your treadmill, there's a body of research that gives some convincing reasons why going solo may not be the best approach. *Compared with solo exercise, group workouts are linked to…*

•**Less pain.** When adults exercised for 45 minutes on rowing machines, those who had rowed in groups demonstrated a higher pain tolerance versus solitary rowers, according to research published in *International Journal of Sport and Exercise Psychology*. Researchers theorize that physically syncing up with others stimulates a release of feel-good endorphins.

•**Greater motivation to push harder.** A phenomenon called the Köhler effect motivates people to strive harder when working in a group. Research

conducted at Kansas State University found that this phenomenon really kicks into high gear when you exercise with people you perceive as stronger than yourself, inspiring exercisers to work out nearly 200% longer and harder than when working out alone.

Caveat: Simply being in a room with other people isn't enough to reap all of these great benefits. The key is finding what researchers call a "true group class."

THE MAGIC OF A TRUE GROUP CLASS

A true group class is one in which the instructor takes steps to promote bonding among participants and a collective goal. For example, your instructor might start class by saying, "Over the next 45 minutes, we are going to collectively walk the equivalent of three laps around the Parthenon."

Important: Typically, group-based fitness classes are more effective than solo workouts only when they use these types of group dynamic strategies. In a meta-analysis published in *Sport & Exercise Psychology Review,* researchers compared the benefits of home workouts, standard exercise classes and true group classes.

Result: True group classes were deemed the most beneficial—mainly because people stick with exercise longer when they are working out in these groups. Solo exercise at home ranked last.

The special ingredient seems to be the bonding that takes place in these classes. Feeling like you belong to a group is a very basic human need…one that research has linked with improved health and longevity—especially as one ages.

WHAT TO LOOK FOR

To find a class with this dynamic…

•**Find an instructor you love.** If you feel inspired and challenged by the instructor, the rest of the class likely feels the same way. This creates a sense of connection among participants and gives everyone something to chat about in the locker room.

•**Exercise with people your age.** A study of 627 adults published in *Health Psychology* found that being in a class with other people your own age improves the chances that you will stick with your exercise plan—more so than being among classmates of the same gender. Look for a class with members who are within about five years of your own age.

•**Look for a class with competition built in.** Boot camps and boutique fitness classes—such as those offered by Orangetheory Fitness, a nationwide fitness franchise, and Flywheel Sports, which offers cycling studios at 42 locations across the US and an app for on-demand cycling workouts you can do at home (with purchase of the Fly bike)—encourage friendly competition by allowing participants to compare their performance results.

•**Experiment with virtual group classes.** No class available? You can still reap the benefits of a collective workout with a virtual group class, such as those offered by Peloton, which provides cycling workouts you can do while streaming live and on-demand fitness classes with instructors and fellow participants.

Note: While on-demand classes offer the benefit of friendly competition, they do not provide the positive effects associated with bonding.

Work Out Better with a Buddy

Cedric X. Bryant, PhD, chief science officer, American Council on Exercise, San Diego. He has served on the exercise science faculties of Arizona State University, Pennsylvania State University and the US Military Academy at West Point and has authored or coauthored numerous books, including *Strength Training for Women.*

Whether you plan to walk briskly around the neighborhood each morning or train for a triathlon, an exercise partner may be just what you need. *Advantages of working out together…*

•**Exercising is more fun when you play,** chat or engage in friendly competition with another person.

•**You're less likely to skip a workout when someone is counting on you to show up.**

•**A partner minimizes your risk for injury—** spotting as you lift weights, correcting your body alignment in yoga poses.

•**You work muscle groups and deepen stretches in ways that are difficult to do on your own.**

•**You save money by sharing equipment,** swapping fitness DVDs or carpooling to the tennis court.

The key to success is to make a good match—so your best friend or nearest neighbor may not be the optimal choice. *Ask yourself if you and a potential partner are similar enough in these key areas…*

•**Fitness level.** Is she interested in a leisurely bike ride around the park, while you want to train for a cycling trip through France? That's not a fit.

•**Schedule.** If you're a morning exerciser and she's a night owl, can you find a compromise—such as lunch hour?

•**Temperament.** Do you both like to talk while you lift weights, or would one of you find the other's chatter distracting?

•**Commitment.** Is she game to jog in any weather, while you run for shelter when clouds roll in?

There are no right or wrong answers to the questions above—it's just a matter of compatibility. *If you have doubts, keep looking…*

•**Check the bulletin board at a local community center, spa or gym.**

•**Ask a personal trainer for a referral.** She even may offer you and your new partner a two-for-one discount.

•**Search** ExerciseFriends.com…or Craigslist.org (look under "community" for your city) for a match.

Important: Always check with your doctor before beginning a new exercise program.

STRENGTH TRAINING FOR TWO

Many strength-training moves can be adapted for partners. Here are examples of exercises for the upper, mid and lower body. For more techniques, experiment with your buddy or consult a trainer.

•**Medicine ball push.**

Equipment: A four- to 10-pound medicine ball (a weighted ball about the size of a basketball, sold at sporting-goods stores, about $20).

Partner 1: Stand facing your partner, about three feet apart. Hold the ball between your hands at chest level, a few inches in front of you, elbows bent and pointing out to the sides. Step forward with the right foot and gently throw the ball, using a pushing motion, so it arcs just above head height.

Partner 2: Extend arms to meet the ball, bending elbows as you catch it to bring the ball toward your chest.

Both partners: Take turns throwing and catching 10 to 15 times, alternating the foot that steps forward as you throw.

Modification: If you have bone loss or wrist problems, use a ball no heavier than six pounds.

●**Stability ball crunches.**

Equipment: A 21-inch-diameter inflatable stability ball (about $20 at sporting-goods stores). If you are shorter than five feet tall, use a 17-inch ball…if taller than five feet, seven inches, use a 25-inch ball.

Partner 1: Kneel and face your partner, one arm extended forward at chest height, palm facing away from you to create a "target" for your partner to clap. Between each of her "crunches," move your palm to a slightly different location—giving her a moving target.

Partner 2: Recline face-up, low to mid-back pressed against the ball, knees bent at a 90-degree angle, feet shoulder-width apart and close to where your partner is kneeling. Hold your hands a few inches in front of your chest, elbows bent. Using abdominal muscles, do a crunch by lifting your upper body up and away from the ball…at the top of your crunch, straighten one arm and clap your partner's palm…lower back down. Do 10 to 15 crunches, alternating the hand that claps.

Both partners: Switch positions.

Modification: If balance is a problem, lie on the floor instead of the ball to do crunches.

●**Squats.**

Both partners: Stand back-to-back, keeping your torso firmly pressed against your partner's from shoulder blade to hip throughout the exercise. Together, slowly bend knees and lower hips while moving feet forward until thighs are parallel to the floor (as if sitting on a chair) and knees are directly above ankles. Hold for about 30 seconds. Then slowly straighten knees and raise hips while walking backward until you are standing once again. Rest for about 15 seconds. Repeat five to 10 times.

Caution: If you have knee problems, limit the depth of your squat to your pain-free range.

TANDEM STRETCHING

For safety, always move slowly and gently, clearly communicating when your stretch has reached the desired level of intensity. Do the stretches below after your aerobic or strength-training workout, as part of your cooldown. Finish with the breathing exercise.

●**Chest-opening stretch.**

Partner 1: Stand erect, arms reaching behind you, elbows straight but not locked, palms facing each other.

Partner 2: Stand facing your partner's back, just beyond her outstretched hands. Grasping her wrists, pull gently and steadily toward yourself to open your partner's chest…hold for 15 to 30 seconds…rest…repeat two to four times.

Both partners: Switch positions.

●**Straddle stretch.**

Both partners: Sit on the floor facing each other. Holding hands, spread legs as wide as possible, knees straight, toes up, feet pressed against your partner's feet. As one partner slowly leans forward, the other leans back…then switch, continuing the forward-and-backward movements. After about 30 seconds, widen your straddle if possible. Repeat several times.

●**Yoga breathing.**

Both partners: Sit cross-legged on the floor, facing away from each other, backs touching, spines straight. Breathing through the nose, inhale deeply, pause for a few seconds, then exhale slowly. Continue for one minute, matching the rhythm of your partner's breathing. Then switch, so that one partner inhales as the other exhales, continuing for another minute. Use this meditative breathing technique to calm your mind and prepare for the rest of your day.

Core-Strengthening Moves You've Never Tried

Brad Schoenfeld, PhD, certified strength and conditioning specialist and an associate professor in exercise science at Lehman College in New York City where he directs the Human Performance Lab. He is the assistant editor-in-chief of the National Strength and Conditioning Association's *Strength and Conditioning Journal* and author of several fitness books, including *Science and Development of Muscle Hypertrophy* and *Strong & Sculpted*. LookGreatNaked.com

---

A re you tired of doing the same old crunches in an attempt to get a flatter stomach and stronger core? Especially since research shows that standard crunches don't really do the job that well because they target only a limited number of core muscles. Brad Schoenfeld, a certified strength and conditioning specialist and author of *Strong & Sculpted*, here recommends five unique, effective and fun-to-do exercises…and there's not a traditional crunch in the bunch.

Schoenfeld's core makeover works the abdomen and sides, as well as the mid-back, low-back and hip areas—muscles essential for maintaining good balance and posture and preventing back pain (not to mention looking good in form-fitting clothes). His exercises require no equipment and can be done at home on a mat. (As with any new exercise activity, get your doctor's OK before beginning.)

You can work your core muscles every day as an add-on to your regular exercise session or as a stand-alone mini-workout. Unless otherwise indicated, try to do 10 repetitions of each move…as you improve, increase to 15 or 20 reps.

●**Toe touches** target the abdominal muscles, especially the upper abs.

Start: Lie face-up, arms and legs extended straight up toward ceiling. Raise head several inches off floor…raise upper back slightly to maintain tension on target muscles.

Move: Contracting abs, curl torso up and forward as much as possible, reaching for toes, while keeping lower back on floor…hold for a count of one…slowly return to starting position.

●**Side jackknives** work the sides of the abdomen.

Start: Lie on left side, legs straight and together. Bend left arm and prop yourself up on left forearm, so left side of torso is several inches off floor. Bend right elbow and place right fist gently against right ear, so right elbow points toward ceiling.

Move: Raise right leg about 18 inches…at the same time, bend at right side of torso (without twisting) to raise torso as high as you comfortably can, bringing right elbow closer to right leg…hold for a count of one…slowly return to starting position. After one complete set, repeat on opposite side.

●**Superwoman (or man)** strengthens the lower back and buttocks area.

Start: Lie face-down with arms stretched out overhead and resting on floor…legs straight and together…and head and neck aligned with spine.

Move: Keeping front of torso on floor, tighten buttocks muscles and simultaneously lift arms and legs off floor as high as possible (as though flying like Superwoman)…hold for a count of one…slowly return to starting position.

●**Reverse curls** focus on the lower abs.

Start: Lie face-up on floor, arms at your sides. Bend knees and bring them toward chest until buttocks are lifted slightly off floor.

Move: Contracting abs, tilt pelvis toward chest and raise buttocks as high as possible while keeping mid-back and upper back pressed against floor…hold for a count of one…slowly return to starting position.

●**Bird dog** builds strength in the entire core.

Start: Get down on hands and knees, keeping back straight and head aligned with spine.

Move: Straightening left leg, simultaneously extend left leg and right arm until they are parallel to floor. Hold for as long as possible…slowly return to starting position. Repeat on opposite side.

Beyond Sit-Ups: 5 Key Exercises to Strengthen Your Core

Jim White, RD, ACSM EP-C, registered dietitian, certified fitness instructor and owner, Jim White Fitness and Nutrition Studios, Norfolk, Virginia. JimWhiteFit.com

Melanie Finnern, registered yoga teacher based in Maplewood, New Jersey. She teaches various classes at Baker Street Yoga. BakerStreetYoga.com

If you think sit-ups and crunches are all you need to do to keep your core toned, you're missing out. They're only strengthening your abs.

To protect your back from injury, improve your posture, enhance your balance and strengthen your ability to do everyday tasks with ease, you need to exercise all your core muscles, including the muscles in your pelvic area and your back.

These five movements, many culled from yoga poses, tone all your core muscles.

You don't need to do all of them each time you work out, but try incorporating all five over the course of your week. As with any exercise, if you feel pain, stop.

●Boat Pose (Paripurna Navasana)

Focuses on strengthening: Core stability muscles in your spine and pelvis.

Sit on the floor with your legs extended straight in front of you, and place your hands on the floor, slightly in front of your hips, fingers pointing to-

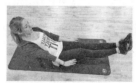

ward your feet. Lean back slightly while lifting your legs, keeping them as straight as possible, until your legs and back form a 45-degree angle. Now lift and extend your arms straight out in front of you—either alongside your legs and parallel to the floor, or grasping behind your knees or thighs. Hold for as long as you can, aiming for a goal of one minute as you get better at the exercise. To end, lower your legs and return to starting position.

●Crow Pose (Kakasana)

Focuses on strengthening: Abdominals and spine.

Begin by squatting on the floor like a frog—your feet hip-width apart, your hands on the floor,

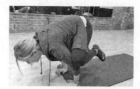

shoulder-width apart and fingers spread, with your arms inside your legs. Your knees should be against the backs of your upper arms. Lean forward slowly, pressing your arms into your knees, until you can balance with your feet off the floor. Avoid rocking into the pose—and keep your gaze forward. Hold for up to one minute before returning to your starting position.

●Side Plank (Vasisthasana)

Focuses on strengthening: Obliques (the muscles on the sides of your abdomen).

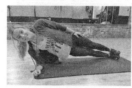

Begin with your feet and hands on the floor, back and legs straight in an inverted "V." Then turn, lowering the weight of your body onto your right forearm and your right foot. Stack your left foot on top of your right, and rest your left hand on your left thigh. Keep your body in a straight line by tightening your abdominals and thighs. For added challenge, extend your left arm up toward the ceiling. Hold the pose for up to 30 seconds. Then slowly return to starting position and repeat on the left side.

●Mason Twists

Focuses on strengthening: Obliques and center abdominals.

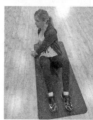

Sit on the floor with your knees bent, your feet flat on the floor and your hands flat on the floor next to your hips. Tighten your abdominals and, keeping your back straight, lean back about 45 degrees while you lift your feet until your calves are parallel to the floor—so you're balancing on your gluteal muscles (buttocks). Clasp your hands together and hold them in front of your stomach. Moving only your upper body, twist to each side, bringing your clasped hands as close to the floor on each side as you can. Continue alternating side to side for 15 to 30 seconds. Rest and repeat. (An easier version of this exercise is to keep your feet flat on the floor, knees bent.)

●**Flutter Kicks.**

Focuses on strengthening: Lower abdominals.

Lie on your back with your arms by your sides and your legs fully extended. Lift your head and feet a few inches off the floor, slightly bending your knees.

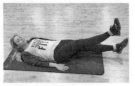

Keeping your abdominals taut, move your legs up and down in a scissor-like motion (or like a basic swimming kick) in small, fast movements without letting your feet touch the ground. Kick for 10 to 15 seconds. Rest and repeat.

Photo credit: Jim White, RD, ACSM EP-C, Jim White Fitness and Nutrition Studios.

Forget Sit-Ups: Here's a Better Core Workout

Vik Khanna, PA, MHS, clinical exercise specialist, health educator and chief exercise officer of Galileo Health Partners, based in Ellicot City, Maryland. He is coauthor of *Ten Commandments of Faith and Fitness: A Practical Guide for Health and Wellness.*

There are few exercises as quintessential as the sit-up. Virtually all of us did them in gym classes when we were growing up. Many people still regularly perform sit-ups in an effort to strengthen the muscles of the core (abdomen, sides and lower back). But conventional sit-ups may cause more harm than good.

Recent development: In a report in *The United States Army Medical Department Journal,* more than half the injuries caused by the Army's standard fitness test were linked to sit-ups. Various branches of the US Armed Forces are now evaluating the use of sit-ups. So what does that mean for people who need core conditioning in their fitness regimens? *Here's the latest thinking…*

TOO HARD ON THE SPINE

Sit-ups not only target mainly the rectus abdominis, the wall of abdominal muscles that bridges the area between the rib cage and the hips but also make excessive use of the hip flexors to raise the torso up toward the knees. The side oblique mus-

cles and lower back, which are crucial for everyday activities, are left out.

But suppose that you are moving a heavy piece of furniture. Strong abdominals will help, but so will strength and stability in the back, sides and legs—areas that are not helped by sit-ups. You'll move better—with more balance and power and less risk for injury—when you exercise all the core muscles as an integrated unit.

A real downside: The most common way people do sit-ups leads them to curl their upper body into a "C shape" as they rise from the floor, which puts tremendous stress on the spinal column. This increases risk for disk herniation, back or nerve pain and muscle strain in the lower back.

A BETTER CORE WORKOUT

Based on my research and work as a conditioning coach for athletes, I believe the following exercises are superior to sit-ups because multiple muscle groups are worked together. In general, a healthy adult can do these exercises three or more times a week.

●**Forearm plank.** Known in yoga as the dolphin plank, it is a whole-body exercise that works the core as well as the shoulder girdle, buttocks and legs. A straight-arm plank puts more emphasis on the triceps (muscles on the back of the upper arm) and the shoulders, while the forearm plank also works the core and hips. The forearm plank is a better choice for people with limited shoulder stability or arm strength or who have carpal tunnel syndrome or other wrist problems.

What to do: Once you're in position (imagine the upper position of a push-up, except that

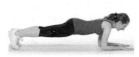

your forearms are on the floor and your upper arms are perpendicular to the floor), focus on keeping your body and head in one straight line looking at a spot on the floor just in front of your hands.

Tighten your abdominal muscles—this will help you hold the position and keep your back straight. It's harder than it looks, especially as the seconds pass and you realize how thoroughly you must engage your muscles from your toes to your shoulders to keep from collapsing to the floor. Keep your jaw relaxed, and breathe deeply throughout the exercise.

I try to hold the position for two or more minutes. For beginners, 10 to 15 seconds is about the limit. If you can hold the position with good form for 30 to 60 seconds, you are probably strong enough to try some variations. *For example…*

While holding the plank, lift one leg a few inches off the floor…flex the foot toward your knee or point the toes backward. Hold for a few seconds. Repeat with the other leg.

●**Side plank.** This variation of the forearm plank is challenging because you support your weight on just one arm, using the oblique muscles in your sides, the deep transverse abdominal muscles and many muscles in the hips, low back and thighs.

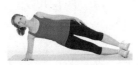

What to do: Lie on your right side while resting on your forearm. Contract your abdominal, side and hip muscles, and raise your hips off the floor until your body is in a straight line. Hold the position for at least 30 seconds, then lower yourself back down and switch sides. Alternate sides until you have done three on each side.

●**The McGill curl-up.** Developed by the spine researcher Stuart McGill, this movement is an abdominal crunch with a surprisingly small range of motion that works multiple core muscles. In this exercise, you barely come off the floor, and you never force your spinal column into that hazardous "C" shape.

What to do: Lie on your back, with one foot planted flat on the floor and the other leg straight out. Place one hand on top of the other under the

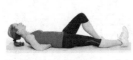

arch in your lower back. This preserves the natural curve and reduces spine pressure.

Keeping your neck in a neutral position, contract your abdominal and oblique muscles so that your upper body just comes up off the floor. You may feel your shoulder blades lose contact with the ground, but your back should remain straight, while your hands support the curve in your lower back. Hold the position for a few seconds, then lower back

down. Do three to five reps with your left leg bent and then three to five with the right leg bent. Try to work up to three to five reps held for about 10 seconds each on each side.

Also: Don't tuck your chin into your chest during the rising motion, and don't curl your back or round your shoulders. Keep your upper body in a straight line by activating only the abdominal and oblique muscles. This keeps your spinal column in a safe and supported position, reducing the risk for muscle strain and spinal disk damage.

You Can Work Out Like an Olympic Athlete

Timothy Miller, MD, director of the endurance medicine program, which specializes in treating endurance athletes, and associate professor of clinical orthopaedics at The Ohio State University Wexner Medical Center in Columbus. Dr. Miller is also a volunteer team physician for the US Olympic Track and Field Team.

Watching Olympic athletes perform their incredible feats can be awe-inspiring… and humbling. But don't despair.

Even if you're not an Olympic athlete, you can still perform at your highest potential by adding highly effective Olympic training routines to your own workout.

Helpful: You can add all—or just a few—of the exercises below to your current fitness routine to increase your endurance, gain strength and boost bone density…*

FARTLEK WORKOUT

●**Which Olympic athletes do this? Cyclists and distance runners.**

Good for: Anyone who wants to add speed and endurance to a walking, running or cycling routine.

What is it? Short bursts of high-intensity movement—a few seconds to a minute—that take place within a longer aerobic routine. Many people refer

*If you have a chronic medical condition or a recent injury, or are at increased risk of falling, consult your doctor before trying these exercises.

to this workout method as Fartlek (which means "speed play" in Swedish), but it is also known as interval training.

How can I do this? Do a 30-minute walk or jog in your neighborhood. Begin with a 10-minute warm-up of a slower-paced run or walk (use a stopwatch to keep track of your time). Once you're warmed up, sprint (or walk fast) between two mailboxes (or telephone poles or any other regularly spaced marker)…then return to your regular pace for the distance of three mailboxes. Sprint or walk fast again, continuing the same interval pattern for 10 minutes. Afterward, return to your regular pace for 10 minutes. Then cool down for a few minutes with a slower run or walk.

For a 30-minute cycling routine, pedal slowly for a 10-minute warmup. Then do 30-second sprints pedaling as fast as you can followed by one minute of slow pedaling for a total of 10 minutes. Then cycle for 10 minutes at a comfortable pace and end with a cooldown.

ECCENTRIC EXERCISES

• **Which Olympic athletes do this? Power lifters and gymnasts.**

Good for: Anyone who wants to strengthen his/her calves, Achilles tendons and biceps.

What is it? These exercises, which are the most efficient way to build strength, focus on working the muscle when it lengthens. In this phase, you consciously slow the descent of a weight (or gravity). This means that you use resistance twice—once while lifting the weight and once while lowering it.

How can I do this? Biceps curls and heel drops.

Biceps curl: To begin, choose a light hand weight (about three to five pounds)…or use small soup cans. Stand with your feet shoulder-width apart, elbows at your sides and forearms at 90-degree angles from your body, with your palms and weights facing up. Hold your left arm steady. Lift your right arm toward your shoulder for a count of two to three seconds, keeping your elbow at your side.

Lower the weight slowly and with control for a count of three to four seconds, keeping your mus-

cles contracted. This is the eccentric phase of the exercise. Alternate arms for a total of 12 to 15 repetitions on each arm. Perform the whole set two to three times. When you can perform 10 reps easily, increase the weight.

Heel drop: Stand with the balls of your feet on the edge of a stair. Drop your heels as low as you can in a slow, controlled motion, taking about three to four seconds to completely lower them. Then push your heels back up for a count of two to three seconds. Repeat 12 to 15 times. Do two to three sets.

PLYOMETRIC TRAINING

• **Which Olympic athletes do this? High jumpers, gymnasts, sprinters and basketball players.**

Good for: Anyone who wants to build leg strength.

What is it? Also known as "jump training," these exercises require your muscles to exert maximum force in short intervals.

How can I do this? Box jumps. Most gyms have jump boxes of varying heights (six inches, 18 inches, etc.), or you can buy one at a sporting-goods store or online. Pick a height you can jump onto so that both feet land squarely on the box.

Stand with feet slightly wider than shoulder-width apart, knees bent. Using your arms to help generate power, jump on the box landing softly on two feet, knees flexed. Keep your hands in front of you for balance. Then jump back down to the starting position. Repeat 10 times for a total of three sets.

Best Time of Day for Exercise

Liz Neporent, MS, CSCS, exercise physiologist based in New York City and author of *Fitness for Dummies* and *Weight Training for Dummies.* She is a contributor to ABC National News and serves emeritus on the executive board of the American Council on Exercise.

Are you a person who likes to roll out of bed and hit the gym…or the pool, the track or the tennis court—or do you prefer an afternoon or evening workout? Exercise however you like, but according to a recent study, you might want to put some planning into when you work out. Belgian researchers found that exercising before eating—on an empty stomach, something most people have only first thing in the morning or late afternoon—has several beneficial effects, including preventing weight gain and warding off a truly serious disease.

AN UNUSUAL STUDY—THEY ATE JUNK FOOD

In the study, 27 healthy young men ate a horrible diet high in sugar, fat and calories—chosen because it was just about guaranteed to create both weight gain and a reduction in the body's ability to process blood sugar effectively.

The Belgian men were divided into three groups. The control group had to eat the awful diet and avoid exercising. Men in the second and third groups—in addition to eating the same unhealthful diet—both exercised, performing the same workout. But the second group did it soon after breakfast and the third group did it before breakfast, exercising on an empty stomach.

HOW DID THAT WORK FOR THEM?

The results were surprising and dramatic. As one might expect, the control group (the one that simply pigged out) gained a lot of weight and also saw their ability to control blood sugar (insulin sensitivity) plunge. The "exercise after eating" group also gained weight, but not nearly as much as the control group. Their insulin sensitivity also went down, just as it did in the control group.

But the "exercise before eating" group was a whole different story. Despite eating the terrible diet, this group did not gain weight…not only that, their insulin sensitivity didn't fall, so even their bad diet did not make them insulin resistant. A breakthrough finding? You bet. As the authors said, "This study for the first time shows that fasted (empty stomach) training is more potent than 'fed training' to facilitate adaptations in muscle and to improve glucose tolerance and insulin sensitivity…"

SO DON'T EAT FIRST?

Should you forgo eating before working out? Not necessarily—it depends on your goals. People whose interest is in heightening their performance—who are, for instance, training for an upcoming event or beginning interval training—might do better to eat first, since they'll need energy to push themselves harder and harder. But if it's weight loss or maintaining general fitness that you are after, evidence does seem to be trending toward not eating before working out. The benefit of the before-breakfast interval is that most of the food consumed the day before is well through the small intestine and thus the inflow of nutrients is at its ebb.

One caveat—if you find that exercising on an empty stomach makes you feel dizzy or faint, this may not be a good approach for a vigorous workout. Or you may need to have a small, healthful snack that includes protein before you do any exercising. While you won't get the same benefits as exercising on an empty stomach, the fact that you're exercising is still a good thing!

How to Stay Injury-Free from a Lifelong Triathlete

Tom Holland, MS, CPT, an exercise physiologist, certified sports nutritionist and certified strength and conditioning coach. He is author of four fitness books, including *Beat the Gym: Personal Trainer Secrets—Without the Personal Trainer Price Tag* and hosts the podcast "Fitness Disrupted" on iHeartRadio.

During the past 30 years, exercise physiologist Tom Holland has completed more than 60 marathons, 25 triathlons and several ultramarathons stretching as far as 50 miles. Although the 50-year-old has asked a lot of his body, he has not endured a single significant injury since he separated his shoulder playing football in high school. Avoiding injury is vital to staying active and independent as we age—and even to avoiding physical therapy, which could easily cost $100 per session. *So we asked Holland to share his secrets for remaining injury-free despite being extremely active…*

•**I listen to my body.** I don't subscribe to the saying "No pain, no gain." If I feel an unusual twinge or tweak while I'm exercising, I stop what I'm doing. If I felt something was really wrong in the middle of a marathon, I'd take myself out (thankfully, it has never happened). Pushing through pain is how small issues become major injuries.

That doesn't mean I get to skip my workout whenever something seems off. It just means that I switch my focus to a different part of my body. If the twinge was in my knee, for example, I do upper-body exercises that day instead.

•**I do a little of many things rather than a lot of one thing.** I love running. I could happily run every day. I'm less a fan of swimming and biking, but I took up triathlons anyway—because excessive focus on one activity puts great stress on certain body parts while leaving others underdeveloped, increasing the odds of injury.

A balanced fitness plan includes upper- and lower-body work and addresses all five components of fitness…

Cardiovascular endurance: Activities that get the heart rate up and keep it up for at least several minutes, such as jogging, swimming and biking.

Muscle endurance: Using a muscle continuously over an extended period, such as holding a plank position or ascending long staircases without pausing.

Muscle strength: Such as lifting weights.

Body composition: Making sure, through diet and exercise, that you develop and maintain a healthy balance of fat and muscle.

Flexibility: Such as from stretching, yoga or Pilates.

You can incorporate all of the above without spending hours a day exercising—just don't do the same thing every day!

•**I begin very slowly with unfamiliar exercises and activities.** The risk for injury is greatest when we try new things. We don't yet know the proper forms and techniques…and our bodies aren't yet used to performing the necessary actions.

The first few times I try something, I set aside my ego and keep the reps slow and the difficulty low. There have been times when I've lifted so little weight at the gym that people have asked me if something is wrong. Better that my pride gets hurt than my body.

•**I'm extremely cautious about group fitness classes.** Fitness classes tend to be designed to be challenging for the strongest people in the class—which can leave novices at risk for injury as they struggle to keep up. Many instructors do not closely monitor participants' technique, either—they just shout encouragement from the front of the room. Even yoga can be dangerous for novices. I have a number of friends who sustained injuries in yoga class that could have been avoided with better oversight from the instructor.

Fitness classes can be socially fun and great motivators—I myself take some. But before trying any new class, I confirm that it's appropriate for someone at my level…and I ask the instructor to keep a close eye on my form. If I find that I can't keep up during the class, I don't try to—in fitness classes, ego gets people injured.

•**I'm always working on my balance.** Falls cause injuries. Preventing falls requires maintaining your ability to keep your balance, which naturally declines with age from loss of muscle strength and joint flexibility and changes in the inner ear.

Incorporating balance exercises into your day is as simple as standing on one foot while you brush your teeth, put on your socks or ride an elevator.

For even better balance, add to your workouts an exercise called a *single-leg floor touch.* Stand with your feet hip-width apart. Lift your right foot off the floor, raising the leg behind you, and hinge forward at the waist until your torso is parallel with the floor. As you do so, lightly touch the floor with your right hand. (You should bend your left leg as you do this—this is not a stretching exercise.) Balance for a few seconds in that position, return to start, then repeat for a total of 10 reps. If needed for balance, hold your left arm out to the side or grasp something sturdy. Then switch sides, and do 10 reps with your left leg raised and left hand touching the floor.

●**I don't do exercises that often cause injuries.** I don't do straight-leg lifts—an exercise where you lie flat on your back and lift your fully extended legs. These put too much strain on the lower back. I don't do upright rows, where a barbell (or pair of dumbbells) is lifted repeatedly from waist height to collarbone height with the hands facing inward toward the body in an overhand grip. These put too much stress on the shoulders. And I don't do behind-the-neck lat pull-downs, where a bar attached to weights by a cable is pulled down until it is behind the neck. This also puts excessive stress on the shoulders. (Lat pull-downs are safe when the bar is pulled down to a position in front of the head.)

●**I do lateral training.** The most common exercise equipment includes treadmills, ellipticals, stationary bikes and stair climbers. The most common outdoor exercises include jogging and bik-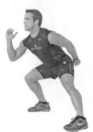ing. What do all of these have in common? They all feature forward-only or forward-and-back movement, not side to side. That's one reason why seemingly fit people often get hurt when they play basketball, tennis or touch football for the first time in a while—these sports require rapid side-to-side movement, which their exercise routines have not prepared them to do.

I include side-to-side, or "lateral," exercises in my workouts. A lateral elliptical machine, which many gyms now have, is one way to do this. You also can train laterally with simple lateral lunges—stand with your feet shoulder width apart…take a big side step to your right, leaving your left foot where it is…bend your right knee until your right thigh is almost parallel with the floor, keeping your left leg straight, your right knee approximately above your right foot, and both feet pointed forward. Return to standing without repositioning your left foot, then repeat to the left, and do 10 lunges on each side.

Photos courtesy of Tom Holland.

Even Simple Home Exercise Equipment Can Be Tricky When It Comes to Safety

Barbara Bushman, PhD, professor in the department of kinesiology at Missouri State University in Springfield, a fellow of the American College of Sports Medicine (ACSM) and editor of *ACSM's Complete Guide to Fitness & Health.*

Exercising at home is convenient and economical. Yet even with simple equipment, such as weights, resistance bands, balance boards and balls, there's a risk for injury if appropriate safety precautions are not taken. At a good gym, professional trainers are on hand to help, and equipment is regularly checked for damage (and puppy teeth aren't a factor)—but at home, you're on your own. *Here's how to stay safe when using…*

●**Hand weights or barbells with weight plates…**

●Wear weight-lifting gloves to help you maintain your grip—otherwise a barbell or dumbbell can easily slip out of sweaty hands.

●Always wear shoes to help protect your feet in case you do drop a weight.

●If you have a weight bench, check regularly to assure that all nuts and bolts are tight—these can loosen over time and make the bench unstable.

●Never try to lift more weight than you can comfortably handle unless another person is right there to spot you.

●**Elastic resistance bands or tubes…**

●These are economical, portable and versatile alternatives to weights, but they do wear out—so before each use, check for tiny tears. If you spot a rip or weak area, it's time to replace your band or tube.

●If the equipment has a handle (as many tubes do), be sure the elastic tubing is properly secured in the handle.

●Avoid abruptly letting go of the band or tube while it is stretched—otherwise, it may snap back and hit you. This can be particularly serious if it hits you in the eye.

●When anchoring the band or tube to another object, choose something stationary, such as a door hinge. Do not anchor to a lightweight piece of furniture or a doorknob—if the furniture suddenly moves or the door flies open, you could lose your balance and fall.

- **Balance boards…**

- Typically a flat board atop an inflated base shaped like an upside-down dome, these also are called wobble boards because they challenge your balance—so the primary safety concern is to prevent falls.

Best: Do your workout next to a bar or other stable surface (choose one with no sharp edges) that you can grab if you start to lose your balance.

- Opt for a balance board with a textured top surface rather than a smooth one. This helps keep feet from slipping.

- Master simple stationary exercises (such as just standing on the balance board) before challenging yourself with exercises involving movement or the addition of hand weights.

- **Inflatable fitness balls…**

- If a ball explodes while you're sitting or lying on it, the sudden fall to the floor could leave you with an injury to the back, neck, head or other area. Pay a few extra dollars for a ball labeled "burst-resistant," which is designed to deflate relatively slowly if punctured.

- Also check the product label for inflation instructions. Overinflating may cause the ball to pop while you're pumping it up, potentially hurling pieces of plastic into your eye.

- If possible, do your ball workout on a floor that is carpeted or padded with rubber tile so you won't land as hard in the event of a sudden fall.

- Be sure the floor is free of sharp objects… stay away from furniture…and keep pets out of the area.

- **Treadmill.** The treadmill causes more injuries than any other type of exercise equipment, according to the Consumer Product Safety Commission.

- If your treadmill has a safety cord that clips to your clothing, be sure to use it (and if your unit does not have this feature, consider upgrading to one that does). At one end of the cord is a key that plugs into the treadmill. If you lose your footing and fall, the cord disengages from the machine, shutting off the treadmill automatically. Without this safety feature, you could wind up having your face sandpapered by the treadmill's moving belt.

- Familiarize yourself with your treadmill's speed and grade options. Incorrectly manipulating the controls could cause the treadmill to speed up or raise its incline when you were expecting to go slower or lower, and that could send you flying.

- Use caution when placing towels, magazines, water bottles or other objects on the console at the front of the treadmill. An object that drops onto the treadmill could wind up underfoot, causing you to trip.

- **Multistation Home-Gym Machine.** These combination units are designed to provide a full-body workout—which means they have many moving parts that can cause injury if the equipment is improperly assembled or maintained.

- It is worth paying extra to have a professional set up your unit. If you're buying a new multistation, ask the store manager whether professional assembly is included in the purchase price—and confirm that the job won't be done by an untrained deliveryman. For help putting together a used unit or to make sure that yours has been assembled correctly, check with a local store that sells similar equipment.

- Even with all the nuts and bolts in the right places, inattention can lead to accidents—so stay alert and keep hands and other body parts well clear of the multistation's moving weight stacks, leverage arms, pulleys and cables.

- Examine your unit's pulleys, connections and other moving parts at least once a month for signs of wear, including fraying or other damage. Follow the manufacturer's directions for lubricating and tightening the unit's components and replacing worn parts promptly.

- **Stationary Bicycle.** These are relatively safe, but you'll still want to exercise caution.

- Avoid wearing pants that flare at the ankle—depending on your bike's style, the fabric could get trapped in the spinning mechanism and wrench your leg. The same goes for untied or unnecessarily long shoelaces.

•A seat that is too low puts strain on your knees.

Best: Adjust the seat height so that there's a slight bend in the knee when your foot is at the far reach of the pedal stroke.

•A recent study in *The Journal of Sexual Medicine* found that using a bike on which the handlebars were positioned lower than the saddle was linked with decreased genital sensation in women.

Best: To lessen the pressure, raise your handlebars higher than your seat. Also, consider using a cushioned seat cover or wearing padded shorts to increase comfort—so you'll be eager to get back on your bike when it's time to work out again.

For added safety: No matter what type of equipment you choose, if you are not familiar with it, it's a good idea to take a few lessons from a qualified fitness professional…or buy a how-to DVD featuring a credentialed instructor, not a celebrity.

4 Dangerous Fitness Myths—Don't Turn Your Exercise Regimen into an Injury Trap

Wayne Westcott, PhD, professor of exercise science, researcher and chair of the exercise science program at Quincy College in Quincy, Massachusetts. He has worked as a strength training consultant for numberous national organizations, such as the American Council on Exercise, the American Senior Fitness Association and the National Youth Sports Safety Foundation. He is the author or coauthor of several books, including *Building Strength and Stamina, Strength Training Past 50, Strength Training for Seniors, Complete Conditioning for Golf,* and *Strength and Power for Young Athletes.*

D on't believe everything you hear when you are trying to get in shape or stay in shape. There are plenty of myths and half-truths.

Among the most dangerous fitness myths to avoid…

FITNESS MYTH #1: **A little pain means you're getting maximum benefit from your workout.** Despite the popular cliché "no pain, no gain," you should never feel prolonged, stabbing or sharp pain during a workout or continue to exercise when something hurts.

The risk: Pain means damage. It could be a warning sign that you have overstressed or overstretched a muscle, tendon or ligament. It also can indicate joint damage. People who continue to exercise when they hurt risk more serious injuries, such as torn muscles or tendinitis (inflammation of a tendon).

Exception: A little soreness after exercise means that you have had a good workout. When you exercise hard, the muscles develop microscopic tears that lead to rebuilding of tissue and an increase in strength. If you are very sore, however, you have overworked your muscles.

Warning: Don't believe the myth that you can exercise longer and harder if you take an anti-inflammatory pain reliever, such as *ibuprofen* (Motrin), before going to the gym. Taking a pre-workout anti-inflammatory may reduce muscle performance and prevent you from feeling an injury while working out.

Important: If you have arthritis or another painful condition that requires daily treatment with aspirin, ibuprofen or another anti-inflammatory medication, ask your doctor if it's safe to take the drug prior to workouts. The combination of exercise and anti-inflammatories might increase the risk for damage to the gastrointestinal lining, according to recent research.

FITNESS MYTH #2: **You should stretch before exercising.** Trainers used to advise everyone to stretch before lifting weights, going for a run, etc. Do not do it.

The risk: Tendons and ligaments take longer to warm up than muscles. People who stretch when they're "cold" are more likely to suffer from muscle and tendon strains and other injuries than those who begin their workouts with a progressive warm-up. Static stretches, in which you stretch a muscle to a point of tension and hold the stretch for a certain period of time, can be particularly harmful before a workout.

Recent finding: New research also has shown that people who do static stretches before working out can't exercise as long and may have reduced muscle strength.

Exception: You can start a workout with dynamic stretches, slow movements that mimic the exercise patterns you're about to do. Before taking a run, for example, you could do some fast walking and slow jogging. This type of stretching is safe and prepares the muscles for exercise.

Also: Stretch *after* vigorous activity. That's when muscles and tendons have the best blood flow and elasticity, and you're less likely to get injured. *Good postworkout stretches…*

• **Figure Four.** Sit on the floor with both legs out in front of you. Bend your left leg, placing the sole of your left foot against your right inner thigh. With your right hand, reach for your right ankle and hold for 30 seconds. Perform twice on each side to stretch your hamstrings and calves.

• **Letter T.** Lie faceup on the floor with your arms in a T-position. Slowly cross your left leg over your body, allowing your torso to rotate so that your left foot is near your right hand. Keep your leg as straight as possible. Hold for 20 seconds. Perform twice on each side to stretch your hips and lower back.

FITNESS MYTH #3: Do not rest during workouts. You have probably heard that the best strength-training workouts involve nonstop action, with no rest (or very little rest) between exercises.

The risk: Failing to rest will cause muscle fatigue and poor form, a common cause of injuries. Also, you won't fully train the muscles because they need time to recover.

When you're working the same muscles, you need to rest 30 to 90 seconds between sets.

Example: Do eight to 12 biceps curls…take a 30- to 90-second break…then curl the weight again.

Exception: With circuit training, you move quickly from one exercise to the next. You might do a biceps exercise, then a leg exercise, then return to the biceps. Even though you're constantly moving (and getting a good cardiovascular workout), you're allowing one group of muscles to rest while you work a different part of the body.

FITNESS MYTH #4: High-heat exercise works the muscles more. Some people believe that high-temperature workouts—including "hot" yoga, spinning and others in which the room temperature may be 90°F or even hotter—make the muscles more limber and improve the body's ability to remove toxins.

The risk: It forces the heart to do double-duty—not only to bring oxygen to the muscles and remove wastes that accumulate during exercise, but also to pump more blood to the skin to dissipate the extra heat. If you're tempted to try high-heat workouts, ask your doctor first.

Does "Running the Stairs" Hurt the Knees?

Wayne Westcott, PhD, professor of exercise science, researcher and chair of the exercise science program at Quincy College in Quincy, Massachusetts. He has worked as a strength training consultant for numberous national organizations, such as the American Council on Exercise, the American Senior Fitness Association and the National Youth Sports Safety Foundation. He is the author or coauthor of several books, including *Building Strength and Stamina, Strength Training Past 50, Strength Training for Seniors, Complete Conditioning for Golf,* and *Strength and Power for Young Athletes.*

If you like to "run the stairs" in your exercise regimen, you may be able to modify your workout to reduce your chance of knee (and hip, lower back and muscular) injuries.

Your best bet is to jog up the stairs, then walk back down.

Here's why: When you're running, the fraction of time your feet are in contact with the ground and supporting your weight decreases. Add the impact of bouncing, and the average "landing force" absorbed by your ankles, knees and hips is about three times your body weight. (Walking reduces the landing force absorption by about half.) Jogging up those stairs reduces this force because your foot does not drop as far as it would on level ground. Jogging down the stairs increases the landing force because your foot has to fall farther. Walking, of course, is a lower-impact exercise and less risky.

Post-Workout, Pain-Free

Men's Journal. MensJournal.com

After your workout, take a hot shower for five minutes, then turn the water as cold as you can stand for one minute. Repeat this for at least three cycles, and end with cold water. Alternating between hot and cold water dilates your blood vessels and helps facilitate circulation, reducing inflammation and pain, which helps you recover faster.

When to Stop Exercising

Gabe Mirkin, MD, a sports-medicine physician and former associate clinical professor at the Georgetown University School of Medicine in Washington, DC. A former marathon runner, he now bikes, at age 85, seven days a week for a total of 150 to 180 miles. Dr. Mirkin is the author of more than 20 books, including *The Healthy Heart Miracle: Your Roadmap to Lifelong Health.*

Increasing your physical fitness through vigorous exercise is one of the best things you can do for your health. But a successful exercise program also depends on knowing when to stop exercising.

People who try to push themselves extremely hard—or who fail to recognize subtle red flags that they're overdoing it—risk experiencing muscle strain, serious injury or even death from a heart attack or stroke.

The eight most critical signs that you should ease up—or perhaps even take a break from your workout routine…

•**Sudden dizziness, an irregular heartbeat, chest pain or unusual shortness of breath.** These are signs that there's not enough blood getting to your brain (resulting in dizziness)… to your heart (leading to irregular heartbeat or chest pain)… or to your body tissues in general (triggering unusual shortness of breath). Any of these scenarios could indicate a potentially serious cardiovascular problem, such as heart attack.

If you experience any of these symptoms, stop exercising and immediately seek medical help in a hospital emergency department. Your doctor will perform tests to diagnose whether your symptoms are caused by a serious medical condition or are harmless. (In some cases, healthy people can experience temporary irregular heartbeats, chest pains caused by a muscle cramp, or shortness of breath caused by sudden pain.)

•**Wheezing or a feeling that your lungs are so full that you can't get more air into them while exercising.** These can be signs of asthma, but shortness of breath also can be caused by the inability of your heart to pump enough blood to your muscles. If you have these symptoms, consult your doctor. Though asthma attacks while working out are often due to "exercise-induced asthma," the attack is caused not by exercise itself, but by breathing cold, dry air.

The problem often can be avoided by exercising in a room with an air humidifier during the winter or by tying a kerchief around your head to cover your mouth while working out in cool, dry conditions—this lets you rebreathe some of the moist air that you exhale. If the problem persists, you may need a prescription bronchodilator medication (an inhaled substance that dilates the bronchial airways to facilitate airflow) before cold-weather workouts.

•**Chills, headache, severe muscle burning or aching, dizziness or blurred vision.** If these occur in hot weather or inside a hot building, stop exercising immediately. You could be having a heat stroke—a potentially fatal condition. If you don't feel better right after stopping your workout, get medical help immediately in a hospital emergency department. Your body temperature could be so high that you will need to be cooled right away to prevent brain damage.

• **"Feeling the burn" as you exercise.** This means that lactic acid (a compound that is produced when the body breaks down carbohydrates to use for energy) is making your muscles acidic, which is necessary to increase muscle strength and endurance. However, the longer you stay in the burn, the longer it will take for your muscles to recover for your next workout.

As soon as you feel the burning sensation, begin exercising at a very low intensity until the burn disappears, then gradually increase the intensity again. Repeat this process throughout your workout.

• **Sore, stiff muscles the day after a workout session.** This syndrome, known as delayed-onset muscle soreness (DOMS), typically occurs eight to 24 hours after intense exercise that puts too much force on your muscles.

If this happens, exercise at an easy level for as many days as it takes the soreness to disappear, then resume your harder workouts. Just be sure to follow the "backing off the burn" method described above.

Important: Easy exercise, such as slow walking or cycling, is better than full rest when recovering from muscle soreness because it makes your muscles fibrous and tougher. In contrast, complete rest does not make your muscles as strong or your body as healthy as daily exercise does.

• **Pain or tenderness that doesn't go away.** If you feel even the slightest pain or tenderness in a specific spot while exercising, stop for the day to protect yourself from getting an overuse injury to a bone, tendon or ligament. Such injuries are always preceded by localized tenderness on one side of the body—unlike DOMS, which usually is felt on both sides of the body and does not worsen with easy exercise. Don't resume exercising until the pain or tenderness is completely gone.

If the problem persists, see a podiatrist (for foot pain) or an orthopedist trained in sports medicine—you may have inflamed tissue or a biomechanical problem that's overstressing a certain part of your body.

• **An elevated heart rate upon awakening.** A good way to check your fitness level is to take your resting heart rate (the number of times your heart beats per minute while you're sitting or lying still) immediately after waking up in the morning. Your resting heart rate generally should be under 75 beats per minute. As your fitness level improves, this rate will gradually drop—a sign that your heart and muscles are working more efficiently.

If your resting heart rate suddenly increases by 10 beats or more per minute, you may have been pushing yourself too hard—a syndrome known as overtraining—or you could be coming down with a cold or other type of infection, which causes your heart to beat faster as your body tries to fight off an infection. In either case, you should avoid intense workouts in favor of easy daily exercise sessions until your heart rate returns to normal.

• **Tired, cramping muscles.** If you've been exercising regularly (in warm or cold weather) and your muscles start cramping or feeling unusually tired, you may have perspired so much that your body is dehydrated or has low sodium levels. If this occurs, stop exercising for a few days. Drink at least a full glass of water with every meal, add extra salt to your food and eat some salted foods, such as nuts or canned soup. If you have high blood pressure, discuss this approach first with your doctor.

5

Everyday Ways to Stay Fit

5 Exercises That Make Everyday Life Better…and Keep Your Body Younger

Beth and Lee Jordan, both certified American Council on Exercise (ACE) health coaches and personal trainers based in Jacksonville Beach, Florida.

What are your fitness goals? Amazing endurance? Extraordinary strength? Lightning speed? If so, more power to you—literally. But many of us just want to stay healthy so we can keep doing the activities we need to do…and activities we love to do…for a good long time.

Try this test: Can you put your socks on standing up? Can you stand up from a chair without using your arms, sit back down, and repeat another 11 times within 30 seconds? Can you stand on one foot for 30 seconds? These are tests of functional fitness, sometimes called neuromotor or neuromuscular fitness.

The good news is that you can improve your functional fitness level with simple exercises. The goal is to increase your ability to do the activities that you need to do every day at home, at work and during recreational fun…such as lifting work files or children or grandchildren…carrying the laun-

dry down to the basement and back…bending down to garden…keeping your balance getting in and out of the tub and when you're out for a nice hike. It's a combination of balance and power.

Functional fitness exercises combine upper- and lower-body movements into what are known as compound exercises, while emphasizing core stability. They often mimic real everyday movements.

These exercises are especially important as you age, when your muscles weaken and simple activities can feel more difficult. All the things you used to barely give a thought to can become challenging if you don't give those muscles some extra attention.

Get started with these five functional exercises designed to help you keep living the active life you enjoy…for a long, long time.

BENT-OVER DUMBBELL ROW

What it helps you do: Bend over to reach things…and pick up an object such as a laundry basket, package of mulch or bag of groceries.

How to do it: Use a dumbbell with a weight that challenges you but that you can lift repeatedly. Stand next to a bench or chair and, holding the dumbbell in your right hand, bend at a 90-degree angle so that your back is parallel to the floor. Brace your left hand and left knee on the bench or chair. Your weight will be on your right foot, and your right hand should hang down directly under

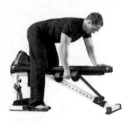

your shoulder, holding the weight. Keeping your back straight, head in line with your spine and abdominal muscles taut, pull the dumbbell up toward your shoulder as far as you can. Your elbow should remain higher than the dumbbell. Then lower the weight by straightening your arm toward the floor. Repeat several reps and then switch sides.

SINGLE-LEG SQUAT

What it helps you do: Control and balance your own weight when walking on unstable ground, going up and down stairs, getting out of bed and getting up out of a chair.

How to do it: Start by standing with your feet hip-width apart, one foot several inches in front of 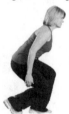 the other, with feet parallel. Slowly squat down as far as you're able to, without losing balance and keeping your bent knee of the leg in front behind your toes. Your hands can be on your hips or your arms can be extended straight out in front of you. Rise to your starting position. Perform several reps and then switch legs.

FORWARD LUNGE

What it helps you do: Move with ease during activities such as yard work, vacuuming and putting groceries in your cupboard.

How to do it: Start in a standing position. Keeping one leg in place, step your other foot out in front of you and bend your knees—your ultimate goal is for them to both reach 90-degree angles. 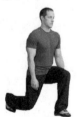 (Once you get good at this, your front thigh and back shin should be parallel to the floor). Push off with your front leg to return to your starting position. Maintain a straight spine and taut abdominals throughout the movement, keeping your arms at your sides or your hands on your hips. Perform several reps, alternating legs with

each lunge. (Once you're comfortable with the forward lunge, try side lunges and walking lunges with twists.)

SUPERMANS

What it helps you do: Maintain a healthy posture while sitting, standing and walking.

How to do it: Lie on your stomach, facing straight down, with your head in line with your spine, legs 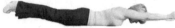 extended straight, toes pointing, and your arms extended straight out in front of you, palms facing each other. Simultaneously, lift both your arms and your legs a few inches off the floor. Make sure your head stays aligned with your spine during the entire movement, and avoid arching your back or lifting your head. Hold the lift for a few seconds, and then gently return your arms and legs to the starting position. Perform several reps.

FARMER'S WALK

What it helps you do: Increase your grip strength and improve coordination when walking and carrying items at the same time.

How to do it: You'll need to walk during this exercise. Don't worry if you don't have much space—this is fun if you have a lawn, driveway or walkway to use, but you can also just go in circles inside. Start in 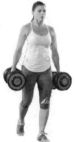 a standing position with a dumbbell beside each foot. (Choose a weight that's challenging for you but not so heavy that you can't lift it.) Keeping your back straight, squat down and grip the handles of the weights, lifting them as you stand back up, keeping your weight on your heels. Then take short, quick steps as you walk for up to 100 feet. Remember to breathe throughout the walk. Set the weights back down on the floor. Rest and repeat.

GETTING STARTED WITH A FUNCTIONAL FITNESS ROUTINE

How often should you do these exercises? The American College of Sports Medicine recommends about two or three 20-to-30-minute sessions each week. You'll still want to keep up a regular routine of aerobics, strength training and flexibility exercises, too.

As with any new exercise routine, it's always a good idea to check with your doctor before getting started...and that's especially true if you have any joint problems or other physical challenges. And as with any physical activity, if it starts to hurt, stop.

Are these five exercises the only way to improve functional fitness? Of course not. Yoga and tai chi are also great, and they "count" toward the recommendations. You can even do functional exercises with a paper towel tube.

But if you're looking for a streamlined routine, the five exercises above all work together to improve your ability to do the things that matter every day.

Note: The images in this story that demonstrate each exercise are used with permission, courtesy of the American Council on Exercise. You can see more in their Exercise Library by visiting AceFitness.org. Search "exercise library."

The Definitive Antidote to Sitting All Day

Bernard Duvivier, MD, PhD, a postdoctoral researcher at Maastricht University Medical Center, the Netherlands, and lead researcher of the study titled "Reducing sitting time versus adding exercise: differential effects on biomarkers of endothelial dysfunction and metabolic risk" published in *Scientific Reports.*

One thing we know for sure: Sitting for most of the day is terrible for your health, raising your risk for diabetes, obesity, high cholesterol and high blood pressure. But the remedy has been confusing. First, we thought that getting 30 minutes of cardio exercise every day was the answer because it benefits heart health and overall health. Then the "marching orders" were to get up from our desks every hour to stand, walk or stretch because incremental amounts of movement seemed to help undo the negative effects of sitting. There were even reports (widely misinterpreted) that sitting a lot wasn't bad for you after all. (It is.) So, which is it? Research done at Maastricht University in the

Netherlands may have found the definitive fitness prescription for people who, because of their jobs or another reason, sit a lot.

The study: The researchers wanted to identify the specific health effects of both cardio exercise and informal movement. To do this, they recruited 61 adults with different health profiles. About one-third were of normal weight and generally healthy, another third were overweight and the final third were overweight and had diabetes. The one thing that all participants had in common was that none exercised regularly.

Each participant was first tested for markers of heart and metabolic health, including cholesterol levels and insulin resistance, and then they completed three different four-day sessions, spaced 10 days apart to avoid skewing results, representing markedly different lifestyles...

• **"Sit" sessions.** Participants sat for 14 hours straight each day and got up only to use the bathroom.

• **"Exercise" sessions.** Participants sat for 13 hours and spent one hour pedaling a stationary bike each day.

• **"Sit Less" sessions.** Participants sat for eight to nine hours and spent seven to eight hours standing or casually walking around each day.

After each four-day session, the researchers repeated the health tests and compared the results to the original ones. *Here's what they found...*

• **"Sit" session.** No surprise here—nonstop sitting does not do a body good. The participants showed increased insulin resistance and higher cholesterol levels. Blood tests also showed unfavorable changes to endothelial cells...those that line the inside of blood vessels. When these cells don't work well, there is a greater risk for blood fats accumulating in the arteries and for arterial stiffness, two risk factors for high blood pressure and hardening of the arteries, precursors to cardiovascular disease.

• **"Exercise" session.** The endothelial health of the participants improved compared with where it was after the sit sessions, but cholesterol and insulin sensitivity didn't budge.

●**"Sit Less" session.** The light but frequent physical activity of these sessions was associated with improved cholesterol and insulin sensitivity, but endothelial health did not budge.

What this means for you: The results show that exercise and light activities benefit your heart and metabolic health in different ways—and that you need to do both.

Exercise improves endothelial health by "training" blood vessels—increasing blood flow temporarily stresses them, and as a result, they become healthier, in much the same way that muscles become stronger and healthier from the stress of strength training. Exercise helps reduce blood pressure by increasing nitric oxide levels.

Light activity—standing, walking, stretching—improves what's called insulin signaling. Your cells become more sensitive to insulin, and glucose is more easily cleared from the blood. It's also possible that simply walking and standing throughout the day keeps insulin levels steady because the muscles you engage use blood glucose for fuel. Light activity might help improve cholesterol, in part due to an increase in an enzyme that boosts levels of HDL, the good cholesterol, and helps your body break down triglycerides (blood fats).

WAYS TO SIT LESS

More studies are needed to better pinpoint the ideal dose of light activities, but recent guidelines from countries including Australia and Belgium suggest that you get up every 30 minutes. *But you can build that rather robotic regime into activities that more naturally match your lifestyle, for example…*

●**Hold walking meetings** (get outside when the weather's nice) and walk to colleagues' desks instead of sending e-mails.

●**Walk around the field during your child's sports games and practices rather than sitting in the bleachers.**

●**When watching TV, do chores during the commercials.**

●**Drink more water**—besides keeping you hydrated, you'll have to get up to visit the bathroom more often (choose the farthest one you have access to).

●**Set an alarm on your phone to remind you to move every half-hour.**

Move Your Trunk for Better Health

Karen Erickson, DC, chiropractor, Erickson Healing Arts, an integrative chiropractic practice in New York City. She is a fellow of the American College of Chiropractic, and on the inaugural leadership team for the American Chiropractic Association's Council on Women's Health.

Twist and shout…work it on out! Remember the 1960s dance called the Twist? All the millions of people twisting to Chubby Checker and The Beatles' version of "Twist & Shout" very likely weren't focused on improving their health. But it turns out that moving your trunk, as the gyrations of the Twist did so well, actually is very good for you. So come on, come on, come on—let's do some trunk twisting!

Your trunk, the part of your body from your shoulders to your hips, doesn't get much of a workout doing daily activities. For one thing, we spend a lot of time sitting—12 hours a day, on average. But even if you're one of the 33% of Americans who have a gym membership and actually use it, most exercises don't involve moving your trunk either. When your trunk stays mostly static, it reduces the ability of your rib cage, diaphragm and lungs to expand. This can diminish lymph and blood circulation to the muscles and organs of the trunk. Lack of trunk movement also weakens core muscles, leading to poor posture and raising risk for tension and injury to the back, shoulders and hips.

You can reverse all that by stretching your trunk and strengthening your core muscles. It's not difficult, and doing it daily pays off big. Right away, you'll notice improved posture and increased flexibility. You may even feel less winded, because your diaphragm, the principle breathing muscle, will work better, too.

SIMPLE TRUNK-TONING MOVES

One of the easiest ways to get some trunk movement into your day is to walk while swinging your arms. Do this empty-handed so that your arms can swing freely. Try for 20 to 30 minutes daily.

Three more easy moves that do wonders for flexibility, circulation and general well-being…

PLANK

There are many variations on the Plank, which engages your abdominal muscles and helps build core strength. For basic Plank, get into a push-up position, with hands directly below the shoulders and arms straight. Hold the position for 10 to 30 seconds to start, building up to one minute. Do once a day.

Variation: Once you can hold the position for one minute, try a three-legged plank—lift one foot slightly off the floor for 30 seconds, then lower it back to the floor. Switch feet and repeat.

BRIDGE

The Bridge exercise engages your glutes and tones your entire torso. Start by lying on your back, arms at your sides, with your knees bent and your feet flat and close to your buttocks. (You should be able to touch your heels with your fingertips.) Next, raise your hips as high as you can, resting your weight on your head and upper back. Ideally, your body will be in a straight line from your shoulders to your knees. Hold the position for 15 seconds, working up to one minute. Then slowly lower your hips back to the floor. Repeat four times.

Tip: Remember to breathe naturally during the exercise—don't hold your breath.

TRUNK TWIST SERIES

This three-part exercise stretches your entire core and helps counteract leaning forward to read, text, etc.—plus it feels great!

Step 1: Stand with your legs shoulder-width apart. Place your hands on your shoulders, and slowly twist to your right…then to your left. Repeat the left-to-right twist two times.

Step 2: With your hands still on your shoulders, bend your torso sideways as far as comfortable without straining your low back and hold for several seconds…then bend to the opposite side and hold for several seconds. Repeat two times.

Step 3.: With your hands clasped behind your head, slowly bend backward by lifting your chest toward the ceiling. Hold the stretch for a few seconds, then slowly straighten up. Repeat two times.

Caution: Only bend as far as is comfortable, keep your chin tucked and don't let your head flop back. Stop if you feel a strain in your neck or lower back.

Finish: End by gently bending your head and upper torso forward to balance the stretches you just did.

One Strong Workout Hikes Metabolism for Days

Study by researchers at UT Southwestern Medical Center, Dallas, reported in *Molecular Metabolism*.

A recent study showed that metabolism-influencing brain neurons stay active for up to two days after a single workout. This means that taking a day or two off from exercise does not harm long-term fitness routines, as long as the workout before the time off is sufficiently intensive.

Exercises That Help With Everything You Do

Larkin Barnett, personal fitness trainer, Pilates and yoga instructor, and past professor of dance and exercise science at Florida Atlantic University in Boca Raton, and the author of *Functional Fitness: The Ultimate Fitness Program for Life on the Run.*

Functional training is a form of exercise that strengthens the muscles that we use in everyday activities, such as standing, walking, sitting, doing chores and carrying packages.

How it works: Functional training helps integrate the limbs and the trunk muscles for fluid, powerful movements…puts your body into proper alignment…improves posture and balance…and promotes deep breathing for relaxation.

A functional fitness routine can be incorporated into cardiovascular and strength-training workouts. *The exercises described below are designed for people of all fitness levels and should be performed daily…*

SIT UP AND TAKE NOTICE

Benefits: Corrects trunk alignment, including weak abdominal muscles that don't provide sufficient support for the lower back…and enhances stamina and endurance.

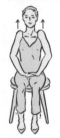

Good for: Carrying objects…walking and running…and relieving muscle tension caused by working at a desk or a computer.

What to do: While sitting in a straight-backed chair, scrunch your shoulders up toward your ears, then relax them. Inhale slowly while you raise your shoulders, then exhale slowly as you lower them. Do this three to five times, feeling tension drain out of your shoulders and neck.

Next, sit tall, perched on your sit-bones (you can find these by rocking side-to-side) and concentrate on stacking your hips, ribs, chest and head on top of each other like building blocks. Exhale powerfully while pulling your abdominal muscles inward toward your spine. Then pull your shoulders back gently. Take several deep breaths.

Finally, sit up tall, while picturing the tops of your ears stretching upward. This elongates the spine and improves respiratory function. Tighten your abdominals inward and upward toward your spine while exhaling forcefully three to five times.

THE COMPASS

Benefits: Strengthens your postural muscles (to improve coordination and balance)…and reduces fatigue and stress on the legs, hips and back.

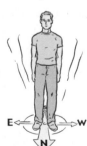

Good for: Relieving muscle soreness from extended standing as well as improving performance in all sports and physical activities.

What to do: With your feet flat on the ground about 12 inches apart, pretend you're standing in the middle of a large compass. With exaggerated movements, shift your entire body toward each of the four main points on the compass—north (forward), south (backward), east (to the right) and west (to the left)—pausing momentarily at each point. Do this three to five times. Contract your abdominal muscles and notice how your control improves.

Gradually make your movements smaller and smaller. Do this for 30 seconds. End by standing still and feeling your body weight evenly distributed.

THE PELVIS AS A FISH BOWL

Benefits: Centers the hips and places the pelvis in neutral alignment, reducing stress on the legs, back and neck.

Good for: Lifting…getting in and out of bed… and swinging a golf club or tennis racket.

What to do: Standing with your feet about 12 inches apart, contract your stomach muscles and 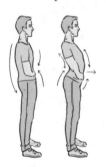 draw them inward and up toward your spine. Picture your hips as a fish bowl filled with water, with the bowl's rim at your waistline.

Now tip your hips forward slightly and visualize water spilling out of the front of the fish bowl. Next, tip your hips backward slightly and visualize water sloshing out of the back of the bowl. Finally, balance the fish bowl so that the rim is perfectly level. This is your pelvis's "neutral" position. Throughout the day, do this position as you stand up and sit.

SHOULDER BLADE, ARM, FINGERTIP

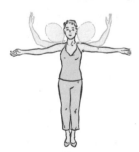

Benefits: Teaches you to initiate arm movements from your trunk muscles (including your shoulder girdle muscles) for more power and control.

Good for: Relieving muscle tension caused

by driving a car or speaking on the telephone…and playing golf and racket sports.

What to do: While standing, lift your arms to your sides at shoulder level. Then lift your arms higher, in the shape of a "U," while sliding your shoulder blades downward. Imagine that you have a balloon next to each ear. Initiate these movements from the shoulder blades. Lower your arms, then repeat three to five times.

Illustrations by Shawn Banner

Don't Let Cold Weather Sabotage Your Fitness!

Denise Austin, an influential fitness and health professional for 40 years. Known for her at-home workouts, Denise hosted the longest-running TV fitness show in history. She is the author of 12 books on fitness, including *Fit and Fabulous After 40.* DeniseAustin.com

E ven though it can be tempting to curl up under a cozy blanket on the couch and hibernate on those cold winter days, you know that will undermine your fitness—and your overall health.

Good news: It takes only a few tweaks to your daily routines (both outdoors and indoors) to stay active during the winter…and even—dare we say it?—make it fun. *What you need to know…*

WHY YOU NEED WINTER EXERCISE

Physical activity is crucial no matter what the season, but wintertime exercise offers unique benefits…

•**Increased immunity.** Research published in *British Journal of Sports Medicine* found that adults (ages 18 to 85) who got about 20 minutes of aerobic exercise (done intensely enough to break a sweat) at least five days a week for 12 weeks had only about half as many colds as those who were sedentary.

•**Reduced risk for lethargy, low mood and irritability.** These are telltale symptoms of seasonal affective disorder (SAD), but getting natural light outdoors helps guard against it.

•**More vitamin D.** Sunshine accounts for up to 90% of our annual intake of vitamin D—a key nutrient for bone health, muscle strength and other vital functions. Even though you'll get more winter sunshine in some southern and western states, exercising outdoors—no matter where you live—allows you to get more vitamin D than you would if you stayed indoors.

THE JOYS OF OUTDOOR EXERCISE

If you live in an area where the mercury plummets during the winter, there's something undeniably invigorating about crisp outdoor air. Classic winter sports, such as skiing and ice skating, are great heart-pumping, muscle-strengthening forms of exercise.

But if you're not keen on hitting the ski slope or ice rink, there's an alternative that works for most people, regardless of their fitness level. You guessed it…good old-fashioned walking. It's a convenient way to get both a cardio workout and weight-bearing exercise for stronger bones.

My advice: During winter, walk at least 20 minutes a day to promote circulation and burn fat.

Note: To warm up your muscles, light arm pumping and walking inside your house, or march in place, for three to five minutes, before going outdoors.

Helpful: Listen to your favorite music if you like, but stay alert to your surroundings. I like upbeat songs like "Walking on Sunshine."

If walking doesn't excite you, liven it up by grabbing a neighbor or friend to join you for a brisk jaunt. Or if solitude is more your thing, head for a state park, where the beauty of a recent snowfall or the glint of winter sunlight can enrich the experience.

STAY SAFE OUTDOORS

While outdoor exercise has undeniable benefits, it can be dangerous if you don't do it correctly. If you have any lung problem (such as asthma), heart disease, diabetes or any other chronic condition, check with your doctor before exercising outdoors in cold weather. *In addition…*

•**Wear moisture-wicking fabrics closest to the skin when layering your clothing.**

Also: Forgo cotton—it stays wet if you perspire.

•**Avoid tight clothing.** It can inhibit blood flow and lead to loss of body heat.

•**Cover your head, ears and fingers.** Your body focuses on keeping your core warm, so your extremities are vulnerable. Also, you never want to walk with your hands in your pockets—that can throw off your balance. And don't forget sunglasses—especially in snow, which reflects more UV rays.

•**Opt for bright colors so that you stand out in cloudy, gray or dim surroundings.** Fluorescent yellow-green is the safest choice for daytime exercise.

•**Moisturize exposed skin to prevent chapping, and don't forget sunscreen.**

Sock It to Me: Easy-to-Do Moves That Keep You Young

Barbara Bushman, PhD, is a professor in the department of kinesiology at Missouri State University in Springfield, a fellow of the American College of Sports Medicine (ACSM) and editor of *ACSM's Complete Guide to Fitness & Health.*

Need to sit down to put on socks? That's a common sign of what happens as we age—balance, coordination and agility fade. Fortunately, we can boost those skills with simple moves that fit into the fancy-sounding category of neuromotor exercise training. The point is to reduce the risk for falls and injury and enhance "functional fitness," or the ability to go about our daily business.

•**Sock Stand.** Barefoot, stand on your right foot. Bending your left knee, lift your left foot and put on a sock without sitting or using any other support…then, left foot still lifted, remove the sock. Repeat several times, trying not to touch your left foot to the ground, then switch legs.

As you improve: Try putting on, tying and then removing a shoe as you stand on one leg.

If you're a beginner: Just practice standing on one leg for 20 to 30 seconds, then rest and repeat several times…then switch legs.

•**Chair Squat.** Stand in front of a sturdy chair, facing outward, and hold your arms straight out in front of you. Slowly bend your knees and stick your rear end out, lowering yourself toward the chair as if about to sit. Allow your rear end to touch the chair seat only very lightly—without resting—then slowly rise to standing again. Repeat. This activity builds strength as well as balance.

•**Paper Towel Tube Pickup.** Place the empty cardboard tube from a roll of paper towels on the floor about 12 inches in front of you. Stand on your right foot, lifting your left foot out behind you. Carefully lean forward, bending your right knee…reach down to pick up the roll…then stand up straight. Repeat several times without touching your left foot to the ground, then switch legs.

As you improve: Use a smaller object, such as a pencil, instead of the paper towel tube.

If you're a beginner: Standing on your right foot, lift your left foot slightly. With the toes of the left foot, touch the floor in front of you…then touch the floor to your left side…then touch the floor behind you. Repeat several times, then switch legs.

•**Ball Toss.** Sit or stand and toss a tennis ball repeatedly back and forth from one hand to the other.

As you improve: Toss the ball higher…hold your hands farther apart…use a larger, heavier ball (such as a softball)…and/or stand on one leg while you toss. Try not to drop the ball!

Fast Fitness: For a Strong Core, Carry a Suitcase!

Amy Roberts, CPT, personal trainer and fitness writer in New York City. She is certified by the Road Runners Club of America (RRCA) as a running coach.

One of the best things you can do for your body is to carry luggage. Really! I'm not talking about grunting your shoulder bag through the airport. Instead you can utilize a suitcase or travel bag for a short super-simple exercise that strengthens the body's core, improves posture and helps prevent back pain. You can do it in the comfort of your own home—and, of course, any time you travel. Make lugging luggage a fun workout, rather than a chore!

I often teach this "suitcase carry" to my personal training clients. It trains your side muscles (the obliques), which support the lower back and spine, so that they are less likely to torque (twist) and bend in ways that could injure your back. (One popular exercise that makes me wince is the standing side bend with a dumbbell. Deliberately allowing the muscles that support your spine to bend under a load is a lower-back injury waiting to happen!)

What's good about the suitcase carry: We often carry lopsided loads, whether it's shopping bags from the car to the kitchen or a carry-on across an airport. This exercise makes you intently focus on your form while you do it so that your side core muscles—specifically, the ones opposite the load—have to engage to keep your whole body level. In the process, you also strengthen your shoulders and your spinal erector muscles, which keep your posture upright. Plus, you get a few more paces in on your step count for the day!

How to do the suitcase carry…

• **Fill a sturdy bag with handles, a cooler**—or, heck, a suitcase—with some books, cans of food, or even a few dumbbells. You can also use a gallon of water, which weighs about eight pounds and is a good starting point. The weight should feel heavy enough that you need to focus on keeping your posture straight but not so heavy that doing so is a struggle.

• **Stand to one side of the bag,** and bend your knees to pick it up with one hand.

• **Keeping your shoulders broad and square,** without leaning to either side, stride forward with purpose down a hallway…across a basement or garage…down a driveway or across the yard—wherever you can find a long, straight path.

• **At the end of your pass—ideally a minimum of 10 paces—bend your knees to lower the bag to the ground.**

• **Switch to stand on the other side of the bag,** pick it up with your other hand and return to your starting point.

• **Do up to three round trips,** as long as you can keep good form. Increase the weight when three round trips becomes too easy. (Remember to also practice good form whenever you're carrying other things, such as groceries.)

• **To burn more calories and give your obliques more of a workout,** try doing this exercise while walking up and down a hill.

• **Practice the suitcase carry three days a week,** and you'll see your core strength increase in just a few weeks.

• **Stop if you feel pain or discomfort** in your shoulders or back or anywhere else in your body. Try again in a few days and see how you feel.

Note: It's best to avoid the suitcase-carry exercise if you have problems with your back, hips or knees.

For additional exercises for strengthening your core, see pages 64-67, chapter 4, "Improve Your Workout."

Hoop It Up for Better Fitness

Joanne Wu, MD, physical medicine and rehabilitation physician who specializes in integrative and holistic medicine in Rochester, New York. Dr. Wu is certified to teach hoop movement through Hoopnotica and has created fitness programs integrating hoop and yoga fusion. Fit2BWell.com

You may remember kids playing with hula hoops decades ago, but the exercise known as "hooping" is now gaining popularity among adults of all ages who find that it adds variety and fun to their fitness routines.

Hooping is more than just a welcome respite from the tedium of a treadmill workout. There's scientific evidence supporting its benefits—and it's safe for many people, regardless of their fitness level.

HOOPING FOR BETTER HEALTH

You may be surprised to see the number of ways that hooping can improve your overall fitness.

Hooping has cardiovascular benefits on par with boot-camp classes, step aerobics and cardio kickboxing, according to research conducted by the Exercise and Health Program at University of Wisconsin in LaCrosse for the American Council on Exercise (ACE).

Besides its aerobic boost, hooping slims down the waist and hips. A study published in *The European Journal of Obesity* found that six weeks of daily hooping beat out a comparable amount of walking in some key health markers. For example, hooping led to more muscle in the core area and a loss of about 1.2 inches in waist circumference. Unlike walking, hooping also decreased LDL "bad" cholesterol "significantly," according to the study.

Hooping is a good calorie-burner, too—about 210 calories during a 30-minute workout. Because hooping improves core strength and mobility, it also may help prevent or treat back pain caused by stress or strain on muscles of the vertebral column. When done regularly, it can help prevent falls by improving balance and *proprioception* (one's perception or awareness of the position and movement of the body).

GETTING THE HANG OF HOOPING

Hooping can be your primary cardio activity or a lively add-on to your usual heart-health workout. When performed at an easy pace, hooping also makes a good warm-up or cool-down for any type of cardio exercise or before strength training or stretching.

Whenever you need a break from sitting, hooping is a great way to add five- or 10-minute chunks of exercise to your daily total. *To get started…*

•**Choose the right hoop.** There's a wide range of hoop sizes available. If you're a beginner, choose one between 37 and 45 inches in diameter.

To find the right one for your height: When you hold the hoop vertically on the ground, it should reach between your waist and your mid-chest. If you're buying online, use a tape measure to measure the distance from your feet to the midway point between your waist and your mid-chest and buy a hoop in that range.

Note: Don't worry if the size is not exact—a hoop that is slightly bigger or smaller will work.

You can find a good-quality hoop online for less than $30 or make your own with inexpensive PVC piping—check YouTube for videos to learn how to do this.

Some fitness hoops are also weighted, usually between one to four pounds. However, inexperienced hoopers may injure themselves if they use a weighted hoop, so start with one without any added weight.

•**Ease into the technique.** If you're a newcomer to hooping, give yourself time to master it. Some fitness centers offer classes to fast-track learning, but you can get the hang of it on your own.

What to do: Step into the hoop, and position it against your back. Then use your hips to keep it in motion and parallel to the ground as your hands let go. The key is pushing back into the hoop at the point of contact on your body to keep the momentum going. This motion can be forward to backward or side to side, depending on what works for you. The big mistake that people make is moving the body in a circular motion. If you have a favored side, switch your lead leg for a balanced workout.

•**Set some goals.** When first learning, you may be able to keep the hoop off the ground for only a few seconds or rotations at a time. Set a gradually increasing number of rotations as your goal. For example, do one rotation and catch the hoop…do two rotations and catch it. Keep adding rotations until you find your rhythm. Of course, the longer you can keep the hoop up, the more calories you'll burn and the more you'll raise your heart rate to contribute to your aerobic fitness.

Once you get the hang of it, you can gradually build up to a 30-minute session. Depending on your fitness goals, you can add hooping to your exercise regimen a few times a week.

To keep your hooping workout interesting, alternate direction every five minutes and/or use a combination of fast and slow rotations. Above all, don't give up—it takes practice, but half the fun is learning how.

HOOPING WITH MODIFICATIONS

Even though hooping is great exercise for most adults, traditional stand-up hooping isn't recommended if you have weakness or severe pain in your hips, knees and/or ankles that makes you unstable or at a high risk of falling…have a fracture or instability in the spine due, for example, to a condition such as osteoporosis…or have an open wound.

Depending on your personal situation, individuals with these conditions may be able to work with an experienced teacher or physical therapist on a modified routine. If you have any concerns, check with your doctor before starting.

Park Bench Fitness—5 Strength-Building Moves

Maurice Williams, MS, CSCS, NASM-Master Trainer and owner of Move Well Fitness, Bethesda, Maryland.

Once the weather turns nice, you would probably rather be getting your exercise outdoors in the fresh air than cooped up indoors. Running, biking and walking all are great outdoor ways to get aerobic exercise—but what about strength training when you don't have weights or machines handy?

No problem. If you have a park nearby, you can tone your muscles using a picnic table or a park bench, your own body weight—and these five strength-building moves.

FRONT PLANK ON A BENCH

The plank is a great all-round move to strengthen your body's core muscles. Why wait until you get home? Try this the next time you're taking a walk or a run in your neighborhood park.

How to do it: Start by placing the palms of your hands flat on the seat of a picnic bench or park bench, shoulder-width apart. Keeping your arms straight and shoulders directly above your hands, walk your feet back from the bench until your body is fully extended. Keep your head, neck, back and hips all in a straight line. Hold this position for six to 20 seconds. Rest and repeat nine times, working up to doing two to three sets of 10.

Alternate move: Reduce stress on your shoulders by leaning on your forearms instead of your hands.

SIDE PLANK ON A BENCH

While the side plank is harder to do than the front plank, the benefits are worth it, since the exercise is so good at strengthening not just your core and gluteal (butt) muscles but also the obliques on the sides of your torso.

How to do it: Turn so that your left side faces a picnic or park bench. Place the palm of your left hand on the seat of the bench and, keeping your left arm straight and left shoulder directly above your left hand, walk your feet to the right, away from the bench, until your body is fully extended. You will be resting on your left hand and the side of your left foot. For stability, place your right foot directly in front of your left foot. You can rest your right arm along your right side or extend it straight up. Your shoulders, hips, knees and left foot should all be in a straight line. Hold this side plank for six to 20 seconds. Then switch and do the move on your right side. Rest and repeat nine times on both sides…working up to doing two to three sets of 10.

Alternative move: An easier version that also reduces stress on your shoulder is to lean on your forearm on the bench instead of your hand.

PUSH-UPS AGAINST THE BACK OF A BENCH

The venerable push-up needs no introduction. You can also do this using a picnic table.

How to do it: Stand facing the back of a park bench. Place your palms on the top edge, a little more than shoulder-width apart, and walk your feet back as far as you can. Then, keeping your arms perpendicular to your body, your shoulders directly over your hands and your back completely straight, bend your elbows to slowly lower your chest toward the edge of the table until your elbows form 90-degree angles. Return to starting position by pushing your body away from the bench until your arms are extended again. Start with 10, and work your way up to doing 20.

SQUATS OVER THE BENCH

The squat is a great lower-body strengthening exercise. Use a park bench to gauge just how far to bend.

How to do it: Stand about four inches in front of a bench with your back to it, feet shoulder-width apart. Keeping your head in line with your spine, bend your knees while raising your arms straight out in front of you to shoulder level as you slowly lower your butt to just tap the bench. Straighten your legs and lower your arms to return to starting position. Throughout the move, keep your weight evenly over both feet and do not let your knees extend beyond your toes. Do 10 to 15 squats, working up to two to three sets of 10 or 15.

STEP-UPS ON THE BENCH

This exercise is great for leg strength—and it's aerobic, too.

How to do it: Stand facing a bench, and place your right foot on the seat. Press through your right foot as you step up onto the bench, bringing up your left foot to place it on the bench next to the right. Now, standing on your left foot, lower your right foot to the ground...and then lower your left foot to the ground, too. Keep the whole movement smooth and controlled. Repeat a total of 12 times starting with the right foot...then do 12 starting with the left foot. Work up to two to three sets of 12 with each leg.

Now that you know what to do, you'll never look at a park bench the same way again!

Get More Exercise... By Acting Like a Kid!

The late Toni Yancey, MD, MPH, former professor of health services at the University of California, Los Angeles, School of Public Health, and codirector of the UCLA Kaiser Permanente Center for Health Equity. She is the author of *Instant Recess: Building a Fit Nation 10 Minutes at a Time.* Toni-Yancey.com

No more dragging yourself to the gym—here's how to have fun while staying fit.

Do you get at least 30 minutes of moderate to vigorous exercise most days of the week? That's the amount of physical activity recommended by most major health groups. But according to statistics published in *Medicine & Science in Sports & Exercise*, fewer than 5% of people over age 20 consistently reach this goal. In fact, the average American engages in just six to 10 minutes of moderate-to-vigorous activity each day.

With all the well-known life-saving benefits conferred by exercise, why is it so difficult for us to follow this one powerful health recommendation?

The reasons are complex, but based on my more than 20 years of research on the subject, there are ways to give yourself the best possible odds of successfully incorporating physical activity into your daily life. *My secrets for creating an exercise plan that you can stick to...*

SECRET 1: **Think like a kid.** A daily exercise program will never be effective if it involves doing activities that you find tedious or uncomfortable. That's why it helps to think like a kid. Perhaps you enjoyed playing catch, jumping rope, throwing a Frisbee or using a Hula Hoop.

If you draw a blank, make a list of types of physical activity you enjoy or find relaxing.

Examples: Dancing, gardening, strolling through an art museum, or activities such as washing the car or dog or raking leaves or cutting the grass. Be sure to include the locations (at home, in a park, etc.) and times of day that work best for your schedule.

SECRET 2: **Lower your expectations.** Rather than telling yourself you're going to start exercising 30 minutes a day, set your sights a little lower in the beginning. If, like the majority of Americans, you're currently getting at most only about 10 minutes of activity per day, adding just 10 minutes of daily exercise will double your activity level.

Once you settle into this routine, start working on adding another daily activity break. If you can get in a total of two additional 10-minute daily activity sessions, you'll be getting about 30 minutes daily.

SECRET 3: **Plan activities that don't require a change of clothes.** It's risky, in my opinion, for your exercise plan to depend on a single window of opportunity, such as getting to the gym at a certain time of day. Give yourself multiple options—some of which don't require special clothing or equipment.

Good choices: Do a short aerobics session when you wake up...cycle on a stationary bike during your favorite TV show or while reading...take a walk in your neighborhood after dinner. If you work in an office, do some midmorning calisthenics instead of taking a coffee break...take a brief walk with colleagues at lunchtime...schedule a "walking meeting" in the midafternoon.

Free-form dancing is another excellent activity that can be done in street clothes. If you're in a place where the music might disturb others, use headphones. If possible, have a short group session with a leader everyone can follow—and choose energizing music with 100 to 120 beats per minute.

Fun options: Highly energetic forms of Latin dance provide excellent aerobic exercise, as do ballroom, square dancing or line dancing. All are widely available in most parts of the country. Check your local fitness or community center.

SECRET 4: **Remove the loophole.** Structure your day so that you don't have the option of not exercising. *For example...*

- **When paying bills...**stand at the kitchen counter.

- **When surfing the Internet or checking e-mail...**sit on an inflatable therapy ball.

- **If you regularly go places within walking distance...**such as a mall or drugstore, tell yourself that driving is no longer an option.

- **If you take public transportation...**buy a monthly pass that drops you off five to 10 minutes from your destination.

- **If you regularly go out to eat...**choose a diner or sandwich shop that's a five- to 10-minute walk.

- **If you use a computer at work...**connect it to a printer at the other end of the office so you'll have to take a short walk anytime you need to retrieve printed materials.

SECRET 5: **Make it social.** Studies show that social interaction is among the most important factors in determining whether adults perform regular physical activity. When people view exercise as a social activity, they're much more likely to do it.

Cultivating opportunities to meet up with regular exercise companions—from your neighborhood, place of work, etc.—should be a key part of your exercise menu.

Examples: Organize walking tours of museums or go antiquing.

Don't Feel Like Exercising?

Gabe Mirkin, MD, a sports medicine physician, former associate clinical professor at the Georgetown University School of Medicine in Washington, DC. He is the author of more than 20 books, including *The Healthy Heart Miracle: Your Roadmap to Lifelong Health.*

We all know that regular physical activity is crucial for good health—it reduces our risk for heart disease, diabetes, stroke, certain types of cancer, mental disorders, including depression and anxiety, and even premature death.

Problem: Nearly nine out of every 10 people who start an exercise program drop out within six weeks, typically due to injuries and/or lack of social reinforcement. But these aren't the only reasons that people give for skipping workouts.

In my decades of practicing sports medicine, I've heard all kinds of excuses for not exercising. *Here are the most common excuses and the rebuttals I give my patients to get them back on track…*

EXCUSE: I'm so out of shape that I wouldn't know where to begin.

My rebuttal: No matter how out of shape you might be, you'll immediately begin getting fitter once you engage in any regular physical activity. If you haven't exercised in a long time, start by simply getting a bit more physical activity each day and gradually increasing it.

The most popular recommendations are to park a block from where you're heading and walk the rest of the way and/or to take the stairs instead of the elevator.

Other possibilities: Do gardening or yard work…vacuum and wash your car…walk around the inside and/or outside of your house…tackle a cleaning project you've been putting off…ride a bike to nearby destinations instead of driving… and/or stroll around a park or mall.

When you're ready to start a more formal exercise program, don't choose an activity that requires a great deal of skill or strength you don't yet have, such as in-line skating, jumping rope or rock climbing. Instead, try a low-risk activity that you already know how to do. Walking is great for most people.

Other good choices: Swimming, cycling, jogging and/or dancing (aerobic or ballroom).

Start with just a few minutes a day. Begin very slowly and continue until your muscles start to hurt or you feel uncomfortable, then quit for the day. Do this every day until you can exercise continuously for 30 minutes daily without feeling sore. You can always add more challenging activities to your program later.

EXCUSE: I'm afraid that I'll strain my heart.

My rebuttal: It's true that heart rate and blood pressure rise during exercise, but this doesn't pose a danger for most people. A recently published Johns Hopkins study of healthy older people with mild hypertension (130–159 mmHg/85–99 mmHg) found that the short-term spike in blood pressure they experienced during moderate exercise (the equivalent of brisk walking plus weight training) didn't harm their hearts in any way. Since regular physical activity helps lower your heart rate and blood pressure when you're not exercising, being physically fit actually results in less overall strain on your heart.

Important: Always check with your doctor before starting any exercise program. If you ever develop chest pain, shortness of breath or dizziness during exercise, stop at once. If your symptoms go away as soon as you stop, check with your doctor as soon as possible. If symptoms continue, consult a doctor immediately.

EXCUSE: I can't find time in my schedule to exercise.

My rebuttal: There's no "best" time to exercise. The ideal time is any time that you will do it. It really doesn't matter whether you exercise first thing in the morning, during your lunch break or sometime in the early evening. And you don't have to exercise for long stretches at a time to get tremendous benefits. Multiple short bouts of exercise can be as effective as long sessions in strengthening your heart. Perform longer workouts (one hour or more) on the weekends, when you are more likely to have the time.

For some people, keeping an exercise diary is helpful. Use a calendar to schedule your workouts. After every workout, jot down what you did, how long you did it and how much distance you covered, if applicable. Tracking your progress will give you a sense of accomplishment and keeps you focused on your goals.

EXCUSE: I started to exercise once but got injured.

My rebuttal: It's true that almost two-thirds of people who start an exercise program end up dropping out because of an injury. Jogging is especially hard on your knees, hips and other joints because your feet hit the ground with a force greater than twice your body weight. However, the more slowly you run, the lower the shock. If you approach your exercise prudently, you probably won't get injured.

Examples…

•**Take up swimming or tai chi.** These activities put little or no stress on your joints—while delivering significant fitness benefits. Swimming improves cardiovascular health, while tai chi strengthens muscles.

•**If you enjoy cycling, consider buying—or getting your gym to buy—a recumbent stationary bike,** which provides back support while you pedal.

Typical cost: $500. You can use it year-round indoors, and it's considered one of the safest types of exercise equipment available. This type of exercise is ideal for most people with back problems.

EXCUSE: **I get bored.**

My rebuttal: Exercise can be a great social activity itself—and can lead to a more interesting social life in general. Studies have shown that the people who stick to their exercise programs are more likely to meet regularly with other exercisers in some formalized way.

You don't have to exercise with others every day—but try to meet one or more people at least once a week. Join a walking, running or cycling club that has regular weekend events…agree to meet with one or more friends at a regular time each week for a group walk, swim, bike ride or gym workout…or set up a weekly session with a personal trainer. Ballroom dancing and cycling are both great activities for couples. You won't be bored.

My "No-More-Excuses" Exercise Plan

Jamison Starbuck, ND, a naturopathic physician in family practice, Missoula, Montana, and writer and producer of "Dr. Starbuck's Health Tips for Kids," a weekly program on Montana Public Radio, MTPR.org. DrJamisonStarbuck.com

Whenever I encourage a patient to start exercising, I brace myself for the inevitable comeback: "I've tried, but I just can't stick with it."

It's no secret that regular exercise reduces the risk for heart disease, diabetes and cancer—and that it speeds weight loss, lessens menopausal symptoms and alleviates depression. But there are some secrets to creating an exercise program that can be maintained.

Here's what I recommend…

•**Set a goal.** Keep it simple. Perhaps you'll walk two miles per day three times per week with the hope of hiking a nearby mountain this summer. If you like, hire a personal trainer to give you specific strength and cardiovascular goals…learn a new sport…or join a recreational team. Devise a program that's within your physical limits, affordable and enjoyable.

•**Avoid injury.** To keep your muscles limber, alternate aerobic workouts, such as biking or using a treadmill, three times weekly, with stretching exercises, such as yoga or qi gong (a combination of postures, breathing techniques and meditation), twice weekly.

•**Get enough protein.** Low blood sugar impairs athletic performance and can make you feel fatigued, light-headed or dizzy during a workout. Blood sugar levels tend to be low in the early morning before breakfast and in the late afternoon. If you exercise at these times, consuming a small amount of protein powder 30 minutes before your workout will help stabilize your blood sugar. Whey, soy and rice protein powders are available at health-food stores. Mix a portion that contains about 20 g of protein into water, milk or soy milk.

•**Take minerals.** If you exercise regularly, consuming minerals each day is important for aiding muscle contraction and heart function. In my opinion, mineral-fortified sports drinks, such as Gatorade and POWERade, contain too much sweetener and too many synthetic ingredients to be healthful. The average adult who exercises regularly should take one or more daily mineral supplements that contain approximately 300 mg of magnesium, 600 mg of calcium, 99 mg of potassium, 25 mg of zinc, 200 micrograms (mcg) of chromium, 200 mcg of selenium and 2 mg of copper.

- **Use topical arnica.** Keep homeopathic arnica (available at health-food stores) on hand for occasional sprains, strains or tendinitis. This remedy speeds the healing of musculoskeletal injuries by supporting circulation and immune function. If you sustain a minor injury, rub arnica onto the affected area twice daily for up to one week.

- **Soak in Epsom salts.** This is one of my favorite post-exercise treats. Epsom salts help relax muscles and soothe mild muscle injuries. Add one cup to your tub and soak for 15 minutes daily, if desired. A quick cold rinse at the end of the bath will improve circulation. Taking an Epsom salt soak before bed also will help you sleep well.

Experience the Immediate Mood Lift of Exercise

Michael W. Otto, PhD, a professor of psychological and brain sciences at Boston University. He is coauthor, with Jasper A.J. Smits, PhD, of *Exercise for Mood and Anxiety: Proven Strategies for Overcoming Depression and Enhancing Well-Being.*

Exercise is hands-down one of the best things you can do for your health. So why is it so difficult to stick with it?

Recent development: Even though the many physical and mental benefits of exercise are undeniable, researchers are now making surprising discoveries about common psychological barriers that can sideline even the most health-conscious individuals…

THE EXERCISE HABIT

One of the most powerful ways to establish an exercise habit is to always do it at the same time of day—this way, your whole schedule becomes arranged in a way that lets you exercise without "juggling." This could mean getting up a little earlier each day and going for a brisk walk or going directly to the gym after work.

Other ways to make exercise a habit for you…

Avoid "inertia zones." Once you park yourself in front of the TV or pick up the newspaper, it will be much harder to get moving. So, when you get home after a long day, remember that exercise is far more likely to help you feel better than watching television.

Helpful: Put the TV remote in a drawer and tell yourself you can't get it out until you've exercised.

LOOK FOR THE RIGHT REWARD

You would think that exercise's promised health benefits would be enough to motivate anyone to get moving. Not so.

The reason: It usually takes weeks—sometimes months—before you'll see results on the scale or your waistline…and perhaps even years before the health benefits pay off in a big way.

These delayed rewards hold little appeal for humans, who are hardwired to respond more readily to immediate gratification, such as sleeping an extra half-hour or stretching out on the couch after work.

What most people fail to realize: Exercise does offer its own immediate reward—it improves mood. Within five minutes of finishing physical activity, most people feel happier and less stressed.

However, until you experience this mood shift for yourself, you may not believe it. So make a conscious effort to tune in to your emotional state—you may be surprised by the dramatic mood boost that exercise can provide.

Need proof? For two weeks, keep a written record of your mood before and after you exercise. This should give you hard evidence to show how much better you can feel after exercising.

Also helpful: Structure your workout so that the ending is pleasurable. If you're getting tired, coast for a bit, then finish with a victory sprint. Studies show that we tend to remember the end of an experience more vividly than the beginning or middle. Ending a workout on a positive note allows you to recall those good feelings later on.

6

Improve Your Game and Fun Ways to Get Fit

What Older Athletes Can Teach Us About Staying Young

Vonda Wright, MD, orthopedic surgeon and expert on active aging and mobility, founding director of the Performance and Research Initiative for Master Athletes (PRIMA) at the University of Pittsburgh Medical Center. She is author of *Fitness After 40: How to Stay Strong at Any Age*. VondaWright. com

Olympic swimmer Dara Torres won three silver medals in Beijing in 2008 and set an American record in the women's 50-meter freestyle. At 41 years old, she was nearly twice the age of many of her competitors.

Torres is not the first athlete to compete at an elite level after age 40. Baseball Hall of Famer Nolan Ryan threw a no-hitter at age 44…golfer Jack Nicklaus won the Masters Tournament at age 46…quarterback George Blanda remained in the NFL until age 48…tennis star Martina Navratilova won a US Open mixed doubles title at 49…and hockey player Gordie Howe played professional hockey until he was 52.

Here's what older athletes can teach us all about remaining physically active into middle age and beyond…

•**Fight the real enemy.** The enemy isn't age—it's inactivity. The widely held belief that physical decline is inevitable once we pass 30 is a myth. There is no scientific reason why we cannot continue to perform at or near our peaks into our 50s. Serious declines often can be staved off until our late 70s.

Most people over age 40 experience more precipitous physical declines not because their bodies fail them, but because they fail their bodies. The vast majority of Americans get less and less exercise as they age. This inactive lifestyle, not the passage of time, is the single greatest cause of their physical deterioration.

•**Push hard, but not all the time.** Older athletes must make a few concessions to their advancing age, but easing up on the throttle during workouts is not one of them. Don't just go for a walk…go for a jog. Don't just try to repeat the same performance in each exercise session…shoot for faster times and additional reps. (Always check with your doctor before starting an exercise program.)

People over age 40 or 50 should not attempt to go all out all the time, however. Older bodies take longer to recover from strenuous workouts than younger bodies. Schedule a rest day without guilt after a physically challenging day.

Example: If you plan a weeklong hiking trip with the grandkids, schedule challenging hikes only every other day, with days off for relaxing at campsites in between.

If you can't see yourself taking a day off from exercise, at least select an activity that challenges a different muscle group.

●**Try to never get out of shape.** Getting back in shape is good, but never getting out of shape is better. Athletes who remain physically competitive after age 40 usually don't have to worry about getting back in shape—most of them have never allowed themselves to get out of shape.

Example: Dara Torres was swimming competitively just three weeks after giving birth.

For those who are in great shape, staying in shape is like taking a well-tuned sports car out for a spin. But for those who are out of shape, exercising is like pushing a broken car up a hill. Their hearts and lungs are inefficient, and their muscles are weak. Exercise is unpleasant, so they avoid it.

The psychological challenge of getting back in shape can be equally daunting. Once middle-aged people let their fitness levels slide, they tend to assume that this decline is natural and inevitable, which makes it easy for them to surrender to the process. Those who never get out of shape continue to think of good health and physical fitness as their natural state and exercise as a natural part of their lives.

As difficult as rebounding from a period of inactivity can be, it will only become more difficult the longer this inactivity lasts. If you are out of shape, the best time to begin your return to fitness is today.

●**Ignore advancing age.** Successful older athletes don't think of their age as a disadvantage— most don't even think of themselves as old. They feel young, think young and react with surprise when others suggest that competing at their age is unnatural.

Example: When now-retired NHL hockey player Chris Chelios turned 47 while he was still playing professionally, he was asked how someone so old managed to stay in the league, he said, "I don't feel old."

When successful older athletes think about their age at all, they tend to focus on its advantages—decades of experience and improved technique. They believe that their younger competitors are at the disadvantage.

●**Work on injury-prevention muscles, not cosmetic muscles.** Leave the bulging biceps to the younger athletes. The muscles that matter the most to those over 40 are the ones that help us avoid aches and injuries. *Among the most important…*

●Rotator cuff muscles. Injuries of the rotator cuff (the muscles and tendons inside your shoulder) are extremely common among those over 40. These injuries make it painful to swim, swing a golf club or tennis racket, throw a baseball or do virtually anything else that involves the shoulder. To strengthen the rotator cuff, use an exercise band, placing one end under your right foot and the other end in your right hand. Raise the band slowly in front of your body, keeping your elbow straight. Do one set of eight-to-10 reps. Work up to two sets. Repeat on the left side.

●Abdominals and pelvic muscles. The secret to a healthy back is a healthy front. Keep your abs and pelvic muscles toned, and back pain is less likely. A key exercise is the plank. Lie on your stomach, hold in your abs and raise your body on your elbows and toes. Begin by holding for 30 seconds, and work up to two minutes.

●Quads. Knee pain is not always caused by a problem with the joint itself. Strengthening the four large quad muscles on the front of your thighs can make your knees feel as good as new.

Quad exercise: Place your back against a wall with your feet about 18 inches in front of the wall. Place two rolled towels between your knees, and squeeze them with your knees. Then lower your back down the wall until your knees are bent about 60 degrees. Hold for 10-to- 30 seconds, and work up to doing it 10 times. Keep your stomach pulled in.

●**Don't forget flexibility and balance.** Successful older athletes almost invariably understand that stretching and "equilibrium training" are just as important as aerobic exercise and strength training.

Our muscles become shorter and stiffer as we age. This shortens our stride when we run and makes full, fluid 360-degree shoulder motion difficult when we swim, golf or play tennis. Daily stretching can allow us to move as we did when we were young.

Stretch the major muscle groups for 30 seconds every day, not just before physical activity. After age 65, double this stretching time to 60 seconds per stretch per muscle group.

Our natural equilibrium begins to decline in our 30s, but most people do not realize that their balance is slowly failing until they start to fall down, typically in their 60s or 70s.

The best way to slow equilibrium loss is to practice balancing every day.

An easy way: Stand on one foot as long as you can while doing the dishes or brushing your teeth, then switch.

Better Your Golf Game (Without Leaving Home)

Joel Zuckerman, freelance golf and travel writer. He is the only two-time winner of the Book of the Year Award, bestowed by the International Network of Golf. Zuckerman is author of eight books, including *Pete Dye Golf Courses: Fifty Years of Visionary Design.* VagabondGolfer.com

You don't have to actually be on the golf course to improve your game. *Here are eight ways to sharpen your golf game at home…*

●**Improve your grip.** It is said that the legendary golfer Ben Hogan, who early in his career fought a pronounced hook shot, once spent an entire winter just learning how to affix his hands to the club properly, doing nothing more than holding the club. This makes sense because the only connection a player's body has to the club is through the hands. You can purchase a form-fitting grip, or training grip, at any golf shop and attach it to any golf club. Let your hands get familiar with the proper positioning on the club, and it will be comfortable to replicate when you're on the course. Hold

the club for five to 10 minutes a day, four to five times a week.

●**Strengthen your hand muscles.** Strengthen your wrists and the dozens of tiny muscles in your hands and fingers by laying a dishrag flat on a hard surface, then crumpling it into a tight ball, letting it go and repeating a dozen times with each hand. Do this three or four times weekly. You also can use one of those spring-loaded grip-strengthener devices, although it won't use all the tiny muscles as effectively as the dishrag.

●**Use an exercise ball.** Oversized exercise balls (Swiss Ball is a well-known brand) assist with balance, stability, flexibility and core strength. Beginners simply can sit on the ball with their feet on the floor for a few minutes a day. This helps with balance and core strength, both key components of the golf swing. Lying back on the ball puts the spine into extension, as opposed to the flexion we experience all day long sitting at desks, driving, etc. This helps to lengthen and stretch the spine, making it much more comfortable to get into the forward-bending posture required for a golf swing. For more exercises, go to SwissBall.com.

●**Increase clubhead speed.** The faster you swing the club, the more you also compress the golf ball and, assuming a solid (as opposed to off-center) strike, the straighter and longer that ball will fly. A great product that helps to increase clubhead speed is called the Speed Whoosh (about $80, Momentus Sports.com, click on "Golf" and then "Speed Whoosh"). It is a long, skinny, flexible antennae-like apparatus that can be swung much faster than a conventional club. Swing it a dozen times a day when you can't play golf, and then when you pick up a club on the course, you will be swinging it several miles per hour faster than before.

● **Use therapeutic bands.** These stretchy bands are good for stretching and strengthening shoulder and chest muscles in ways that expensive and cumbersome gym equipment does not. Shoulder muscles, particularly rotator cuffs, are easily injured and will keep you off the golf course for extended periods if they become injured. A strong chest is needed for an effective golf swing. Hold the band overhead with both hands so that you feel some tension in the band. You can increase or decrease tension in the band as needed by gripping it widely or narrowly. Slowly bring the band behind your back, then back up over your head and down to your belt line. You can even tie a band securely to a doorknob and practice your golf swing. Hold the position at both backswing and follow-through for a beat or two to build strength.

•**Work on flexibility.** A more flexible body allows a golfer to make a bigger, more powerful turn from the hips and torso to generate the tension in the body to hit the ball a long way. There are any number of effective ways to increase flexibility, but one of the best is the program devised by Roger Fredericks. A former PGA professional turned flexibility guru, Fredericks offers beginner, intermediate and advanced stretching programs on DVD that help golfers learn to get their bodies into positions that will allow them to play the game more effectively, with less stress on the body and a reduced chance of injury (FredericksGolf.com).

•**Sharpen your mental focus.** It's long been said that the most important six inches in golf are between the ears. To that end, there are a number of relevant books that help the golfer sharpen his/her mental focus and perform better under pressure. These books include the best-selling *Golf Is Not a Game of Perfect* by Bob Rotella, PhD, which offers some excellent visualization techniques. *Every Shot Must Have a Purpose* and *The Game Before the Game* by Pia Nilsson and coauthor Lynn Marriott also offer valuable information on effective practice techniques and how to use mental focus to play your best.

•**Daydream about golf.** Daydreaming about the game has been proved to have a positive effect on performance. Recent scientific studies have shown that while physical practice is the most beneficial technique, mentally practicing your swing and desired ball flight and outcome is more beneficial than doing nothing at all. Picture the sound and feel of solid contact from the tee, the flight of the drive, the club you choose for your approach shot, the contour of the green, the speed of the putt, etc. Play the first several holes

in your mind until you start to lose focus. Then try again the next day.

Smarter Strategies to Shape Up for Golf

Edward Jackowski, PhD, founder and CEO of Exude Fitness, a New York City–based fitness company that teaches people how to make proper fitness part of their lives. He is author of several books on fitness, including *Fit to a Tee.*

M any golfers aren't sure how to get in shape for the game or have misconceptions about how to do it. *Also, men and women tend to have different weaknesses that they need to focus on...*

MEN

Men often believe that adding muscle is the secret to adding distance to their drives. Actually, adding flexibility and range of motion is more beneficial. Men usually lack the flexibility to rotate their bodies through a golf swing, robbing them of the torque that produces long drives. Older men are especially likely to lack flexibility, but this need not be so. With proper stretching, you can have nearly as much flexibility in retirement as you did in your 30s.

Perform three simple stretches before beginning a round of golf or hitting at the driving range...

•**Hamstring stretch.** Lie on the floor with your legs extended in front of you, feet about two feet apart. Reach toward your toes by bending at the waist. Hold the stretch as far as you can reach for 15 to 30 seconds. Do not "bounce" the stretch to hold on closer to your toes—that could cause a hamstring injury.

•**Shoulder stretch.** Windmill your arms in large, slow arcs around your shoulders. The arcs should be as large and complete as you can manage. Do five to 10 circles in each direction. If you have a bad shoulder, it is safest to focus on each arm individually. Otherwise, it is okay to do both arms at once.

•**Torso stretch.** Sit on the floor with legs extended straight in front of you, then cross your left leg

Healthy Way to Improve Your Golf Swing

Lean from the hips, not from the waist. Your drives will be longer and your back healthier if your spine is straight, in its normal, slightly arched lumbar curvature, during your swing. This might feel uncomfortable at first, but stay with it and you'll get used to it.

Michael Yessis, PhD, professor emeritus of kinesiology at California State University, Fullerton, and an expert on sports technique, conditioning and training. He is author of *Explosive Golf: Using the Science of Kinesiology to Improve Your Swing*. DoctorYessis.com

over your right. Slowly turn your upper body to the left as far as you can with your right elbow against your left knee, and hold for several seconds. Then reverse positions, and stretch in the opposite direction. Repeat three times in each direction.

Men who lift weights usually lift the heaviest weights they can in order to build bulky muscles. But bulky muscles add little to a golf game and might even hurt your swing if the muscle makes you less flexible. Instead, use lighter weights but lift them more times, which builds muscle endurance rather than size. Select weights light enough so that you can do 50 reps of a particular exercise. For most men, that will be weights of no more than 10 to 20 pounds.

WOMEN

Female golfers tend to lack upper-body strength. Push-ups are the best way to correct this. Start by doing push-ups from your knees if you cannot do them from your toes. Don't become frustrated if you can complete only a single push-up the first day. Just do as many push-ups as you can, and try to do more with each passing day, working up to two sets of 15 to 25 push-ups.

Other ways women can get in shape for golf...

●**Build hand strength.** Women golfers tend to lack hand strength. Your distance and accuracy will suffer if the club moves around at all in your hand during your swing. Use a simple "hand grip" exer-

ciser or squeeze a tennis ball to build hand strength. Do this every other day for five to 10 minutes.

●**Jump rope.** Many female recreational golfers have trouble consistently centering the ball on the club face, resulting in poor accuracy. Jumping rope is one great way to overcome this hand-eye coordination problem. Using a jump rope forces the hands, eyes and body to work together, much as they should during a golf swing.

How to Prevent Golf Injuries

Frank Rabadam, DPT (doctor of physical therapy), who is certified by Back to Golf, a PGA- and LPGA-approved fitness and golf biomechanics program. He also is a certified Yoga for Golfers instructor. He is clinic director, Excel Physical Therapy and Fitness in Bala Cynwyd, Pennsylvania.

The sedate pace of golf would seem to leave little room for injuries—but that's not so. According to one study, as many as one-third of the more than 25 million golfers in the US sustain significant injuries of the back, spine, shoulders, elbows or wrists while playing the sport. *Important...*

●**Warm up properly.** A study in *British Journal of Sports Medicine* found that nearly 46% of golfers don't warm up. Those who do warm up usually perform little more than a few "air swings" before hitting the ball. Inadequate warm-up is a leading cause of injury.

Allow two to five minutes of aerobic warm-up activity—jogging in place, fast walking, etc.

Follow the aerobic workout with five to 10 minutes of gentle stretching—torso twists, chest stretches, etc. Include neck turns. Neck stiffness interferes with smooth body rotation during swings. Also, do stretches that target the hamstrings, such as lying leg lifts. Poor hamstring flexibility is a common cause of back pain.

Stretch one or two muscle groups at each hole while waiting for your turn. For more information on the best stretches and exercises for golfers, go to YogaForGolfers.com, which is run by fitness consultant Katherine Roberts. She is author of the book *Yoga for Golfers*.

•**Be careful when lifting.** Golfers often get hurt before the first tee because they jerk their clubs out of the car trunk. Use your legs as well as your back when lifting the bag. On the course, pick up balls by kneeling rather than bending.

•**Practice good balance and posture.** Most neck and shoulder stiffness occurs when players hunch over the ball excessively, with their neck and shoulders too far forward. Work with a golf pro to optimize your posture and stance when addressing the ball. You want to maintain a neutral spine position, without excessive bending or extension.

•**Limit your swing.** Amateur golfers tend to "overswing"—using greater force than necessary. Instead, shorten your swing. End the backswing at about the 1:00 position, instead of 3:00.

•**Strength train.** Lifting weights to increase strength and endurance can significantly reduce the risk of golf injuries. Focus on strengthening the shoulders, upper back, and "core" muscles in the abdomen and lower back.

•**Consider graphite clubs.** They have more "give" and generate less vibration and shock than clubs with steel shafts. This is important when you accidentally hit the ground during hard drives, a cause of wrist and elbow injuries.

Don't Hit the Ball So Hard... Secrets from a Tennis Pro

Greg Moran, director of tennis at the Four Seasons Racquet Club in Wilton, Connecticut. A teaching pro for more than 30 years, he is author of *Tennis Beyond Big Shots.*

Nearly 80% of points in amateur tennis are lost on missed shots, not won on great shots. To win more, stop trying to hit the ball as hard as you can or drop it on the lines. Instead, play patiently and wait for your opponent to make mistakes. *Also…*

SINGLES

•**Rethink your serves.** Most amateurs blast their first serves as hard as they can and frequently miss. Then they lay in soft second serves, which their opponents anticipate and return aggressively. Instead, hit both your first and second serves half to two-thirds as hard as you are capable of serving. This will allow you to get most of your first serves into play. As long as you vary the placement—and spin, if you can—of your serve to keep your opponent off balance, you will be in good shape to win most of your service points. If you do miss your first serve, hit your second serve just as hard.

The perfect toss: Bad serves often are the result of bad tosses. Pretend that the ball is a glass of water that you are balancing on the palm of your hand. Lift your hand upward, releasing the glass upward when your arm is fully extended. Begin your swing when the ball pauses at its apex so that you hit it just as it starts to descend.

•**Stop trying to hit winners when you return a first serve.** Instead, try to return first serves safely down the middle of the court, five to seven feet above the net (one to two feet above the net and at the server's feet if the server charges the net after service). The server has the advantage on the first serve. If you try to hit quick winners, you are likely to fail more often than you succeed.

•**Be more aggressive against a second serve.** Move three feet forward, then try to drive your return deep crosscourt.

•**Hit most ground strokes cross-court in singles tennis.** The ball crosses over the net at the net's lowest point, the middle, when you hit crosscourt, reducing the odds that the ball will hit the net. Because hitting crosscourt lets you aim at the long diagonal dimension of the court, it also reduces the odds that you will hit long—and increases the distance that your opponent must run.

•**When in trouble, hit up.** When your opponent has you on the run, lob your return high and deep. Lobbing forces him to retreat to the backcourt and gives you a chance to regroup.

DOUBLES

•**Avoid the one up, one back formation against skilled opposition.** This conventional doubles formation is reasonably effective against teams of limited abilities, but skilled opponents will exploit the huge gap that it creates between you and your partner. Instead, play both up if you are skilled at volleying and covering lobs…play both back if you are not. Both back is the best way to remain competitive against a doubles team of greater skill.

•Don't try to "hit 'em where they ain't." It is very difficult to hit a shot where neither opponent can reach it when two opponents are patrolling the court. *Instead, aim…*

•At your opponents' feet. These shots are very tricky to return.

•Right down the middle of the court. Your opponents will have trouble finding a winning angle on their return, and there might be a crucial moment of confusion as your opponents decide who will return the shot.

•Over your opponents' heads if both opponents are up at the net.

Exercise to Heal Tennis Elbow

Timothy Tyler, PT, ATC, sports medicine specialist, consultant, Nicholas Institute of Sports Medicine and Athletic Trauma, Lenox Hill Hospital, New York City, and coauthor of a study of elbow pain.

Buy a ribbed, pliable, eight-inch-long rubber bar, such as TheraBand FlexBar—commonly sold for general physical therapy for about $25 online (TheraBand.com).

Hold the bar upright at your side, using the hand on the same side as your sore elbow. Grasp the bar near the top with your hand on the uninjured side. Twist the top hand while bringing the bar in front of your body to hold it parallel to the ground. Then use the hand on the sore side to untwist the bar slowly by flexing your wrist. Start with three sets of five repetitions per day, adding more as the exercise gets easier, up to three sets of 15 repetitions daily.

Try Paddle Tennis!

Patrick Netter, known as The Gear Guru, is a sports, health and fitness expert. Based in Los Angeles, he founded the fitness equipment store High-Tech Fitness and created a guide to fitness equipment of the same name. GearGuru.com

If you haven't played paddle tennis, you might want to give it a try. It's great for people of all ages and skill levels. Most find it easy to learn, and it is less physically demanding than other racquet sports, such as squash and regular tennis—with fewer chances of sustaining an injury, particularly to the rotator cuff (shoulder).

HOW IT DIFFERS FROM TENNIS

Paddle tennis is similar to traditional tennis but varies in some significant ways…

•**The court is smaller**—20 feet by 50 feet versus 36 feet by 78 feet. That means less running around, making it easier for out-of-shape or less agile players.

•**Paddle.** Unlike strung tennis racquets, paddles have solid heads, with small, aerodynamically drilled holes. Paddles also are smaller than tennis racquets—9.5 inches wide by 18 inches long. Once all wood, paddles now are made of high-tech composite materials that are lighter and give more power.

•**Ball.** One standard tennis ball, which you puncture to reduce the bounce, is used for each set.

•**Serve.** Unlike with tennis, there is one underhanded serve per point, and players cannot begin the serve higher than 33 inches or lower than 31 inches from the ground. The server can strike the ball directly or let it bounce first before striking it, but he/she cannot change methods of serving during a set.

•**Scoring.** The same as tennis (four points to win a game), but matches generally tend to be shorter, with sets often played in only 15 to 20 minutes.

PLATFORM TENNIS

There is a variation of paddle tennis, called platform tennis, which is played on a court that is about one-quarter the size of a tennis court and enclosed by a tensioned fence that looks like chicken wire.

The ball remains in play even when it is hit off the fence on a bounce.

Platform tennis offers the benefit of yearlong play. The court is on a raised foundation—which makes it easier to have a heated floor to melt snow and ice in the winter. Platform tennis is particularly popular in the Northeast for tennis players who want to play outside during winter months.

MORE INFO

There are a growing number of public and private paddle and platform tennis courts in the US. For information on paddle tennis, search online for courts in your area. For information on platform tennis, go to PlatformTennis.org.

Racket Sports May Be Best for Health

Nine-year study by European and Australian researchers of 80,306 people, published in *British Journal of Sports Medicine.*

Racket sports were associated with the greatest reduction in death from any cause (47%) and death from cardiovascular causes (56%). The next best reductions came from swimming—28% from any cause and 41% from cardiovascular causes. Aerobics was associated with a 27% reduced risk for death from any cause and 36% from cardiovascular factors. The study did not prove cause and effect but did indicate that participants' risk for death dropped more when they exercised more often.

Pickleball for All

Lance Dalleck, PhD, coauthor of the study "The Acute and Chronic Physiological Responses to Pickleball in Middle-aged and Older Adults" published in *International Journal of Research in Exercise Physiology.*

In a pickle about what exercise to do that's not only good for you but fun, too? Consider pickleball. Yes, pickleball—an official, if under-the-

radar, sport complete with national championships and even a brand-new Hall of Fame.

The backstory: The game was invented in the 1960s by three dads, including six-term US representative from Seattle Joel Pritchard, to amuse their bored kids while summering on Washington's Bainbridge Island. Pritchard simply grabbed what he had on hand—Ping-Pong paddles, a Wiffle-type ball and a badminton net. Bill's wife, Joan, a rower, is credited with naming the game…after the term used to describe the slowest boat in a race, the pickle boat.

While pickleball's popularity might have been slow to start, it's anything but a slow sport. Pickleball is a great fitness activity, perfect for getting the heart and lungs pumping and for burning calories. For an American Council on Exercise study, researchers recruited 15 men and women, ages 40 to 85, to participate in six weeks of matches. Each one played in four 15-minute matches on each of three days a week.

They found that participants burned about 300 to 400 calories an hour, which is comparable to other aerobic exercises. What's more, after six weeks of games, participants saw favorable changes in both high-density lipoprotein (HDL) and low-density lipoprotein (LDL) cholesterol, their systolic and diastolic blood pressure and VO2 max, the amount of oxygen they're able to take in. All of this equates to a positive impact on cardio-metabolic health.

Another important aspect of pickleball: It's a social activity, offering the same positive emotional boost you get from exercise classes and group activities. Playing with friends who depend on you is also a great motivator to keep you exercising.

PLAYING THE GAME

A single game tends to last about 15 minutes—the first side to score 11 points with at least a two-point margin wins, but many enthusiasts play for as long as two hours at a time. The ability to enter tournaments makes pickleball appealing to people who are more competitive. The energy output isn't as strenuous as some other racquet sports, yet it's still challenging. And while you can learn new strategies to become a better player, it's fun no matter your level of skill. Those are some of the factors that draw people to it.

The paddles are now bigger than the original Ping-Pong paddles and instead of wood they're made of lightweight composite materials. The pickleballs still are made from molded plastic and have uniformly sized holes, but they come in more varieties now, some better suited for indoor or outdoor games or for tournament play. The pickleball "court" measures 20 feet by 44 feet—it's far smaller than a tennis court but has similar right/even and left/odd service courts and non-volley zones. The game can be played as singles or doubles.

One caution for beginners: The researchers found that at first falling can be common while learning to play. If you have balance or agility issues, be sure to learn the proper techniques of the game with an instructor. For more ways to improve agility, read "Agility Exercises That Prevent Falling" on page 172.

While more popular in the southeastern US, you can find a court in every state. For locations, rules and more, check out the website of the USA Pickleball Association, USAPickleball.org. Pickleballs and paddles are sold online from many vendors.

Up Your Fitness Game at Circus School

Rachel Stegman, master coach and owner of Circus School of Arizona in Scottsdale.

Carrie Heller, MSW, LCSW, RPT, founder and executive director of the Circus Arts Institute in Atlanta, professional trapeze artist, circus teacher and a licensed clinical social worker and registered play therapist.

Are you finding it hard to gear up for another session of push-ups and burpees? What about swinging on a trapeze and climbing aerial silks instead?

You don't have to actually join the circus to get as fit as an acrobat—circus schools are coming to you. Through their classes, you can achieve physical feats you never thought you would and gain

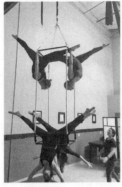

Mixed aerial class with the quad trapeze at Circus School of Arizona

strength, stamina, balance and flexibility while having the time of your life.

A real surprise: You don't have to already be in great shape to take and enjoy circus fitness classes, said Carrie Heller, founder of the Circus Arts Institute in Atlanta, one of the dozens of circus schools in cities across the country. You will need to ultimately lift your body weight during class, but at first there are many moves you can do in circus fitness classes if you're not at that point. And teachers will work with you and help you advance.

Many students who, for example, struggle to climb the soft rope called a Spanish web on their first day of class find they can do it after just a few weeks...and progress like that is very satisfying.

GETTING STARTED

Beginner classes include an introduction to foundational skills and positions low in the air and sometimes, depending on the school, may include ground based skills such as low-wire (low tightwire) walking, other balancing skills, and yes, trapeze. Know that there are also many forms of trapeze, including the static trapeze and the flying trapeze, which are completely different skillsets and are often not even taught at the same circus schools, explained Rachel Stegman, owner of Circus School of Arizona in Scottsdale, in part

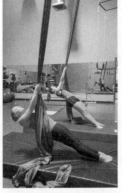

Aerial class at Circus School of Arizona

because the flying trapeze apparatus requires a much larger space.

Beginning students might also learn and practice juggling, which is fantastic for fitness and fantastic fun.

Most circus fitness students take class once or twice a week, and for best progress, it's important to also get cardiovascular exercise outside of class. Brisk walking, jogging, swimming or cycling will help you excel at circus fitness by making you stronger and building your endurance.

One of the goals as you progress is to be able to climb higher and higher heights—literally—but that doesn't rule out people who are afraid of heights. In fact, fear is actually a good thing when it comes to circus fitness because a respect for heights is important, said Rachel Stegman. You'll start on the ground and advance to low heights and then higher once you know the techniques and have the strength and confidence—all on your own schedule.

Also, going high isn't always the goal. A move done low to the ground confers as much fitness as the same move done higher, Stegman says.

In addition to basic circus fitness, some schools offer aerial fitness classes or aerial conditioning classes, in which students climb and do tricks on one or two pieces of hanging fabric, and aerial yoga classes, in which you'll execute stretching-focused yoga poses while hanging in a hammock, an especially good way to experience a wide range of motion that you can't always get on the ground.

COST AND GEAR

The cost of circus fitness classes varies widely by school and region of the country. On average, expect to pay between $20 and $30 for each one-hour class. Some schools offer punch cards with five or 10 classes for a lower per-class cost. Circus schools don't tend to require that you commit to a certain number of sessions.

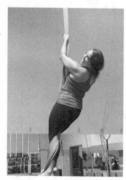

Being able to pay per class means you can take one or two classes to see if you like it without making a financial commitment. But try to give yourself at least a few weeks, the time it takes to see improvement in strength and fitness.

Suggested attire is form-fitting clothes—think leggings and a top that clings

Aerial class at Circus School of Arizona

or can be tucked in because you'll be going upside down. Avoid wearing clothes with Velcro, zippers,

buttons or sequins (save that for prime time!), any jewelry and anything with laces because they could damage or become entangled in the equipment, creating a safety hazard.

HOW TO STAY SAFE

If you're sold on finding a circus fitness class, there's one more thing to keep in mind: your safety. *As you look for a school or studio near you, ask these questions…*

●**Is the school a member of the American Circus Educators Association and have they participated in its Circus Arts Safety Network program?** Member schools must meet safety practice standards and standards of quality of instruction and training of their staff, and also follow safe rigging practices for their equipment, Carrie Heller said. You can find a member directory at AmericanCircusEducators.org/directory/

●**Are the instructors highly skilled in the circus?** For aerial acrobatic training, someone with only a yoga, dance or gymnastics background won't

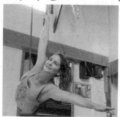

Carrie Heller of Circus Arts Institute.
Credit: Nick Arroyo

have the technical skills of someone with circus training, Stegman said. She suggests looking for instructors who have many years of circus and acrobatic training. (If a teenager is leading a class, that's an automatic red flag.)

●**Are there spotters?** This is an important safety measure, especially for beginners. A spotter's job is to direct a student in and out of moves correctly, help her learn to problem solve should she make a wrong turn and make sure her head and neck are protected at all times. Heller has one spotter for every person in the air.

There's one final caveat, often suggested before starting any new fitness program, but very appropriate here: Check with your doctor first. If you have a condition that precludes putting your body weight on a joint, for instance, or being upside down, circus fitness isn't for you. But once you have your doctor's thumbs up and you're game, swing by a circus school or studio.

Paddleboarding for Fun and Fitness

Cedric X. Bryant, PhD, chief science officer, American Council on Exercise, San Diego, California.

Paddleboarding, also called stand-up paddling, can be a terrific form of exercise. Because the sport requires you to stand and balance on a board while paddling on the open water, the muscles of your core (your abdominal muscles) and those of your sides (your external obliques), are constantly engaged in helping you to stay erect. Engaging in the sport regularly will strengthen the muscles in that region. Other benefits include better balance and relief from any lower back pain, since it's your abdominal muscles that support your back. A recent study has shown that these core-strengthening benefits go up substantially as you master the sport. Researchers theorize that more skilled stand-up paddlers exercise at a higher intensity, moving and twisting their bodies more to propel their boards faster through the water.

While there are some cardiovascular benefits associated with paddleboarding, they are more limited. In a second study, only those who had mastered the sport and paddled at a perceived rate of exertion of 15 (on a scale of 20) exercised at a level of intensity that would improve cardiorespiratory function.

Many outdoor sports shops have paddleboarding classes, but some people don't even need one to get started. If you can't find a class in your area, look online for tips on mounting the board, keeping your balance and learning to fall. Always use a leash—sold separately from the board—which tethers you to the board and keeps it within reach should you fall.

Important: Though paddleboarding is a safe, low-impact sport suitable for those of any age, people with shoulder, back or balance issues should approach the sport cautiously at first to be sure they are not aggravating any existing issues. Always wear a life vest, slather on a waterproof sunscreen and wear a brimmed hat and sunglasses to protect yourself from the sun.

America's Greatest Bike Paths—Safe, Beautiful Trails from City to Countryside That Everyone Can Enjoy

Joan Rattner Heilman, a dedicated cyclist, inveterate traveler and seasoned journalist, based in Mamaroneck, New York, is the author of more than a dozen books and hundreds of magazine and newspaper articles. She specializes in 50-plus travel.

Millions of Americans now are cycling for transportation, exercise and fun. In response, many areas in the US have special paved bike paths. Here are some of the best. (Of course, you can find paths in other areas by searching online for "bike paths" and the name of the city.)

MIDTOWN GREENWAY
MINNEAPOLIS

Minneapolis has 85 miles of off-street bike paths (plus 81 miles of on-street bike lanes) that are plowed in the winter, lit at night and open 24 hours a day. A major section is the Midtown Greenway, a 5.5-mile former railroad corridor that runs through the center of the city parallel to Lake Street, a commercial strip with hundreds of businesses. It is a quick way across town. The Greenway connects on the west with other paths, including the Minneapolis Chain of Lakes Trail, and on the east with trails that run along the Mississippi River.

Information: MidtownGreenway.org

SILVER COMET TRAIL
GEORGIA

One of the longest paved paths of its kind in the US, the Silver Comet Trail runs from Smryna, Georgia, outside Atlanta, for 61 miles to the Alabama state line. It follows the old railroad line once traveled by the Silver Comet passenger train past small towns, farms, wetlands and forests. Most of the trail is flat, although there are some serious hills at the end. Dotted here and there along the way are restrooms, picnic tables and parking areas.

Information: SilverCometGa.com

Bonus: When the Silver Comet Trail reaches the Alabama border, it connects with that state's 33-mile-long Chief Ladiga Trail.

MOUNT VERNON TRAIL
VIRGINIA

The Mount Vernon Trail, one of the most scenic bike paths in the country, begins in northern Virginia, just across the Potomac River from downtown Washington, DC, and follows the river for 18 miles to George Washington's estate, Mount Vernon. There are restrooms and water fountains along the way. Bikers get spectacular views of the DC monuments, and when they reach Gravelly Point at the north end of Washington National Airport, they can hop off and watch the planes take off and land thrillingly close by. The trail goes past Arlington National Cemetery and the Lyndon Baines Johnson Memorial Grove and through the heart of Old Town Alexandria, the city's historic district (this section includes a short stretch of on-street biking). Continuing along the river and under the Woodrow Wilson Bridge, cyclists reach a fairly steep but brief climb as they approach Mount Vernon. A tour of the first president's famous mansion and a leisurely turn around the grounds should not be missed.

Information: BikeWashington.org

CHICAGO LAKEFRONT TRAIL

As you ride along the edge of Lake Michigan on this 18.5-mile asphalt bike path, you'll get a great view of the city's famous array of historic early skyscrapers. You can make a stop at the Museum of Science and Industry, relax on one of the many sandy beaches, view exotic fish at the Shedd Aquarium or pedal on all the way to the Navy Pier, one of the city's most popular visitor destinations, to ride the Ferris wheel or play miniature golf before heading back downtown. The trail is popular with commuters who use it for speed and safety getting in and out of town.

Information: ChicagoParkDistrict.com

MANHATTAN WATERFRONT GREENWAY

You can bike around the entire island of Manhattan in one swoop—it's a marvelous journey on a 32-mile paved path. But for most people, it's best done in segments because you will want to make plenty of stops to take in the sights. You can start just above the George Washington Bridge on the West Side, then ride south with the Hudson River on your right, West Side Highway on your left, all the way to the Statue of Liberty and the Staten Island Ferry. Next time, cover the East Side, starting at The Battery and traveling up the East River past the South Street Seaport and the United Nations and under the city's famous bridges.

Information: NYCGovParks.org

JEDEDIAH SMITH MEMORIAL TRAIL
SACRAMENTO

Also known as the American River Bike Trail, it runs for 32 miles on mostly flat terrain from Sacramento to Folsom Reservoir. It hugs the American River as it passes quaint towns, parklands, woodlands and the campus of Sacramento State University. There are restrooms and water fountains along the way. Among the sights, each worth a stop, are Discovery Park in Sacramento, the pedestrian-only Guy West Bridge (a small replica of the Golden Gate Bridge) and the Nimbus Fish Hatchery, where in the fall you can watch salmon spawning.

Information: ARPF.org

Take Advantage of the Great Outdoors

Liz Neporent, MA, CSCS, exercise physiologist based in New York City and author of *Fitness for Dummies* and *Weight Training for Dummies*. Her articles have been featured in *The New York Times*, *Shape* magazine, the *Daily News* and *Fitness* magazine. She is a contributor to ABC National News and serves as emeritus on the executive board of the American Council on Exercise.

When the weather turns nice, it's always fun to take advantage of the healthful sunshine. What to do?

Everything you've been doing on exercise machines can be done moving through space—instead of standing (or sitting) in one place. Biking, walking and jogging are great ways to exercise, and you can actually see the scenery, so you don't have to rely on bad movies on TV or headphones. Even the muscular workout from an elliptical machine can be replicated in a similar way outdoors. Just find some hill courses for walking.

FITNESS COURSES MAKE IT FUN

In the absence of equipment, how can you exercise all muscles to keep them toned? Look for par courses, which are widely available in many cities. They are set up so you can do a full-body workout—plus they're fun.

A par course is basically a pre-designed fitness trail, with different exercise stations set up along the way. The starting point is clearly marked, so you usually begin there with a run (or walk or jog) to the first "station" (which usually takes two to five minutes, depending on what par course you are at or how fast you go). The stations typically have clear instructions and often pictures of the exercises to be done there.

For example, first might be a place for you to do push-ups, with instructions to do as many as you can within one minute. Then you'd get up and continue your jog to the next station. Typically these courses include a station for squats, a place for a stretch and a chin-up bar. Most par courses give you the ability to do some really difficult exercises at a beginner level. For example, if you can't do a full chin-up, you can squat down and use just part of your body weight.

THE DO-IT-YOURSELF VERSION

If you can't find a nearby par course, you can design your own, based on the concept of circuit training, which many experts consider one of the most effective ways to get a full-body workout in a reasonable amount of time. For example, you might run, walk or jog for five minutes, then stop by a park bench and do triceps dips for a set of 15. Then continue on your run for another five minutes and stop and do squats, standing in place. Five minutes more and you stop for push-ups.

This kind of workout is infinitely flexible. You can vary the intensity and duration. For example, do the first cardio exercise at a "warm-up" pace for five minutes, then the first "strength exercise" (push-ups, for example), followed by a "wind sprint" interval of 30 seconds to one minute before getting to the next "strength training" exercise. You can carry a jump rope with you and skip rope for one of your cardio exercises.

Hopping on one leg might be the best all-around calf shaper there is. Plus it allows you to work on balance and coordination. Since some body parts—like biceps and the back—are harder (but not impossible) to exercise without equipment, carry one or two exercise bands with you. They're lightweight and won't interfere with your run and they give you an infinite number of possibilities for every body part.

As for abs, planks can easily be done as one of the outdoor strength training exercises. Balance on your forearms and toes, making your body straight, just like a plank. It makes your whole middle body work because you are supporting the position with core muscles. At the end, you'll feel your whole abs work.

A TYPICAL WORKOUT CIRCUIT

1. Walk (or jog) five minutes at a very moderate pace to warm up.

2. Stop at a park bench and do one set of triceps dips (see next page).

3. Do 30 seconds of jumping jacks.

4. Sprint for 30 seconds—full out. (Beginners, just walk faster, pushing your own "personal envelope.")

5. Jog for five minutes at moderate pace.

6. Stop and do a set of lunges—10 reps per leg (see next page).

7. Jog for five minutes at moderate pace.

8. Stop and do a "plank." Beginners, hold for 10 seconds, working up to 60 seconds (advanced).

9. Jog for three minutes at a moderate pace.

10. Stop and do one set of push-ups. (Beginners, do as many as you can…advanced, go for as many as you can perform in one minute, even if you have to stop and pause every so often. It's okay to do the "assisted" version where your knees are on the ground.)

11. Sprint for 30 seconds—full out. (Beginners, just walk faster, again pushing your own "per-

sonal envelope.") Then jog at a moderate pace for three minutes as your heart rate comes back down a bit.

12. Stop and do a set of squats. (See below.)

13. Do 30 seconds of jumping jacks.

14. Jog at a moderate to slow pace as you "cool down" for five minutes.

15. Stretch.

The possible variations are endless, especially if you take the exercise bands with you. Alternate this circuit with walking, jogging, kayaking, biking, swimming and all the other great outdoor activity options.

HOW TO DO THE EXERCISES

● **Triceps dips (off a bench.)**

Sit on the edge of a bench with hands firmly holding the edge of the bench, fingers facing out. Lift your butt up and away from the bench and lower it toward the floor by bending your arms at the elbows. Don't go lower than your shoulders. Push back up. Repeat for 10 to 15 repetitions.

● **Lunges.**

Stand straight and take a large step with your left foot, placing the left foot heel first on the ground. Then lower your hips down (bending the left knee) until the right knee almost touches the ground. Left knee should stay above left ankle. Come back up and repeat for 10 reps. Repeat on opposite side.

● **Squats.**

Stand with feet shoulder width apart, toes pointing forward. Using the big muscles of your thighs, lower down until your thighs are parallel to the floor (resembling a sitting position). Keep knees above ankles. Repeat for 15 repetitions.

● **Planks.**

Get on your hands and knees, then lower the top half of your body till you're resting on your forearms. Fully extend legs back (toes and forearms touching ground). Keep your back straight like a plank and hold the position (it's hard!). Beginners—10 seconds. Advanced—try for 60 seconds.

Hike Your Way to Health

John Davis, PhD, professor of human anatomy and exercise physiology, Alma College in Alma, Michigan.

Seth Levy, media sales manager, Trailspace.com, Portland, Maine, and former manager of the Western Public Lands Initiative at the American Hiking Society.

The dictionary dryly defines a hike as "a long walk," but it's much more than that. Going for a hike involves leaving behind the hustle-bustle of life and heading into nature, whether a park, local woods or a mountain. It's refreshing and restorative because hiking is both mentally and physically engaging. According to Seth Levy, media sales manager at Trailspace.com, an outdoor gear review site, and former manager of the Western Public Lands Initiative at the American Hiking Society, the sport of hiking is becoming more popular. "Hiking engages us in the natural world by enabling us to explore an endlessly changing environment, the shifting seasons, natural quiet and variable terrain," he said. It can also be a good workout, he noted. "More people are finding that hiking helps build aerobic capacity, burn calories, increase muscle mass and increase bone density, while also enhancing mental health. While some of these benefits are true of exercise in general, what makes hiking unique is that it is accessible, self-explanatory, inexpensive and fun."

FIRST STEPS FOR NEW HIKERS

Spring and fall are probably the most popular times of year to go hiking—but any season is good for walks in the wilderness, as long as you're well-prepared. *Here are some tips to get you started…*

● **Wear appropriate shoes and clothing.** Wear shoes that support your foot and ankle, with a firm sole and a deep, durable tread for traversing uneven terrain. Always wear socks, even if the weather is hot, choosing ones that fit snugly and comfortably, preferably made of either wool or synthetic fibers— never cotton as it can cause blisters. Wear comfortable synthetic clothing, which keeps you cool by wicking moisture in warm weather, but insulates when it is cold. If you are going into the mountains, be prepared for rapid changes in weather by dressing in layers.

●**Drink up.** Hydration during exercise is always important and in the mountains even more so. The ideal beverage should have sodium in it to aid in fluid retention.

Begin slow and easy. "Start slow, enjoy the scenery, and increase your pace as your fitness and level of comfort increases," Levy advised. The first time you go hiking is not a time to set difficult goals. Keep in mind that hiking a mile on uneven terrain is different than simply walking a mile on city sidewalks. The strain will be greater and it will take longer, so plan accordingly.

●**Set realistic fitness goals.** "You can use the same formula for planning your hiking workout as with walking or running," Levy noted, assuming you have some basic level of fitness, no health risk factors and are hiking at fairly moderate altitudes (under 8,000 feet).

●**Go exploring.** You can find hiking trails near you by contacting your state and/or local parks and recreation department or you can go to the American Hiking Society's website, AmericanHiking.org. Many of these resources provide trail maps and suggestions for day hikes, including mileage and a description of terrain. Outdoor stores such as REI and Eastern Mountain Sports generally sell hiking magazines and books listing trails and hike details for different regions of the country.

INTERESTED IN SPEED HIKING?

Those interested in kicking it up a notch might want to consider speed-hiking, a sub-sport of hiking that is gaining momentum. It combines the benefits of fast-paced aerobic exercise with the muscle-strengthening benefits of altitude climbing (or hill climbing, for those who hike on flatter terrain). As with other forms of exercise, hikers can alter their experience to boost heart rate, burn fat, build muscle and enhance aerobic capacity.

Hikers average about two miles an hour, while speed hikers generally cover around four to five miles/hour. On a typical outing, a speed hiker may combine jogging, running, and, if hills or mountains are part of the terrain, uphill climbs and downhill sprints. There's no "right" pace at which to hike, Levy notes. "You might boost the challenge of a day hike by increasing your pace, where other hikers want to surpass official or unofficial records for hiking certain trails in certain amounts of time. Choose a pace, comfort level and goals that are right for you."

For more on the physiological impact of speed hiking, we spoke with John E. Davis, PhD, a professor of exercise and health science at Alma College in Alma, Michigan. He said that between four and five miles an hour is considered the "break point" where you begin to derive some cardiovascular benefit—and if you are going uphill, even better.

Of course, as with any form of exercise, it is important to take certain precautions in order to minimize your risk of injury. *Risks of speed hiking can include…*

●**Falls.** Moving quickly on uneven terrain makes it easy to fall, so the proper footwear is even more important. "Hikers who have balance issues and elderly hikers might want to seek out trails that don't have a lot of obstacles," said Dr. Davis. Look for trails that are well maintained.

●**High-altitude or mountain sickness.** "At altitudes greater than 8,000 feet, the barometric pressure is lower, the amount of oxygen that you breathe in is less, and as a result exercising becomes more difficult," said Dr. Davis. (Examples of these high altitudes would be in the Rocky Mountains range, the Sierra Nevada and the Cascades.) Symptoms of high-altitude sickness include headaches, breathlessness, fatigue, nausea or vomiting, and swelling of the face, hands and feet. If hiking while on vacation, be sure to adjust to the altitude before hiking, and make sure you are well hydrated.

HIKE YOUR OWN HIKE

While speed hiking may seem like a challenging and fun way to get a great workout, it should not be done at the expense of enjoying your hike. "The quality of your hiking experience, whether it is for enjoyment or to achieve your fitness goals, does not necessarily depend on your pace," said Levy. "Hike at whatever pace is comfortable or effective for you.

There is a saying in the hiking community that expresses this well: 'Hike your own hike!'" For more information about hiking and safety tips, contact the American Hiking Society, American Hiking.org.

National Parks You've Never Heard Of

Joan Rattner Heilman, an inveterate traveler and seasoned journalist based in Mamaroneck, New York, is author of more than a dozen books. She specializes in 50-plus travel.

If you love exploring national parks but hate contending with the hordes of people you find at places such as Yellowstone and the Grand Canyon, you can visit some of these lesser-known undiscovered treasures. You'll have them pretty much to yourself!

CAPITOL REEF NATIONAL PARK, UTAH

Located in Utah's south-central desert, Capitol Reef is noted for its nearly 100-mile-long Waterpocket Fold, a buckling of the Earth's crust that occurred about 65 million years ago, exposing 270 million years of geologic layers of rock and sediment. The prehistoric layers have been eroded by wind and water over the centuries, forming sheer multicolored cliffs, massive domes, twisting canyons, spires and arches, huge red rock monoliths and narrow winding riverbeds. You can view them on a 16-mile round-trip paved scenic drive starting at the Visitor Center in the town of Torrey. Add some bumpy rides on unpaved spur roads into Grand Wash and Capitol Gorge for closer views, and hike for miles, if you like, from the trailheads into the rocky canyons. Campers can set up in a 71-site developed campground near the entrance or in more remote areas.

Information: Open daily. $10 per person for seven days, $20 per vehicle for seven days, $20 per campsite per night. 435-425-3791, NPS.gov/care.

WIND CAVE NATIONAL PARK, SOUTH DAKOTA

This park features a spectacular underground cave in South Dakota's Black Hills. The Wind Cave, named for its whistling winds, has about 130 miles of passages that contain rare geological formations such as "boxwork" (paper-thin calcite fins that look like honeycombs), "cave popcorn" (small white, knobby formations) and "frostwork" (needlelike growths that resemble big ice crystals). Be sure to take at least one of the ranger-guided tours of the cave, and drive the paved roads through the rest of the 33,000-acre park's mixed-grass prairies and dense pine forests where you are likely to spot bison, prairie dogs and other wildlife. The park has a campground, which is open year-round.

Information: Open daily, except Thanksgiving, Christmas and New Year's Eve. There is no entrance fee, but cave tours range from $10 per adult to $30 (half price for children ages six to 16 and holders of Senior Access Passports), depending on length and difficulty. Campsites are $18 per night in warmer months...$9 the rest of the year. 605-745-4600, NPS.gov/wica.

BISCAYNE NATIONAL PARK, FLORIDA

Within sight of downtown Miami, Biscayne National Park is 95% underwater, and the rest consists of a few tiny islands and a narrow piece of mangrove shoreline on the mainland. Its clear turquoise water teems with colorful fish and sea grass and is home to the world's third-largest coral reef and the remains of many shipwrecks, so it is one of the best places in the country for snorkeling and diving. Unless you have your own boat, you must shuttle to the islands or reefs from the mainland on a boat operated by the park's concession. You also can sign up for glass-bottomed boat tours or snorkel and dive trips or rent a canoe or a kayak. In addition, park rangers offer free guided canoe or kayak trips along the coastal edges and shallow bay waters. There are no overnight accommodations, but tent camping is available on two of the park's islands.

Information: Open daily. Campsites are $25 per night for up to six people and two tents. Round-trip ferry to the campsite is $59 per person, with a two-passenger minimum. 305-230-7275, NPS.gov/bisc.

ISLE ROYALE NATIONAL PARK, MICHIGAN

Isle Royale National Park consists of one large island surrounded by more than 450 smaller islands in the northwest part of Lake Superior. It is a rugged, unspoiled wilderness preserve close to Minnesota and Canada, and it is one of the few national parks to close in winter. Accessible only by ferry, private boat or seaplane, it has no roads and no wheeled vehicles but 165 miles of hiking trails, a marina, a lodge, myriad campgrounds and miles of scenic coastline. Although it is among the least visited parks in the country, its campers stay an average of 4.1 days, the longest for any national park.

Information: Closed November 1 to April 15. User fees: $7 per adult per day, free for children age 15 and under…individual season pass, $60… There are four passenger ferries and one seaplane that offer service to and from the park. Fares and schedules vary, and reservations are recommended. 906-482-0984, NPS.gov/isro.

LETCHWORTH STATE PARK, NEW YORK

Long known as the "Grand Canyon of the East," Letchworth State Park, 35 miles south of Rochester, New York, may not be a national park, but it is as remarkable as many of them because of its waterfalls—three magnificent major waterfalls in a deep narrow gorge of the Genesee River and about 50 smaller ones along its tributaries. Hiking paths parallel the river, where you'll see an abundance of migratory birds in the spring and fall.

The park has a museum (open from May 1 to October 31) that includes artifacts from the area's original Seneca Indian inhabitants and early pioneers. There also are original log buildings, including a cabin built by Mary Jemison, an Irish immigrant kidnapped as a teenager by Shawnees and later adopted by the Seneca tribe. A historic restored inn on a cliff overlooking one of the large falls offers rooms and meals. The park also has a state-run lodge, cabins, campsites, swimming pool and snowmobile and horse trails.

Information: Open daily 6 am to 11 pm year-round. *Entrance fee:* $10 per vehicle weekends in early May to Memorial Day and daily from Memorial Day through October. Museum fees are $1 for adults and 50 cents for children age 12 and younger. Campsites are $24 to $26 per night. 585-493-3600, LetchworthPark.com.

Beyond the Beach

Donna Heiderstadt, travel expert who has visited nearly 100 countries and traveled to all seven continents. During her 24 years writing about travel, her work has appeared in TravelAndLeisure.com, Fodors.com, ShermansTravel.com and RobbReport.com.

There aren't many vacations that beat a sunny beach escape. But if you crave something more—such as hiking in a rain forest or across lava fields…rock climbing beautiful limestone cliffs…or snorkeling with stingrays—here are five tropical destinations that offer the perfect combination of sun and fun physical activity.

FOR SUN & ADVENTURE

•**Hapuna Beach on the Big Island of Hawaii.** Sometimes the most satisfying way to unwind is with an adrenaline rush—whether it's zip lining over lush treetops or mind-expanding star-gazing from atop a 13,803-foot dormant volcano covered in snow. You can do both (and so much more) on the Big Island of Hawaii, while also taking time to relax with your toes in the sand. Hapuna Beach, located in the north on the island's Kohala Coast, is your home away from home to enjoy a roster of land activities—horseback riding with paniolos (Hawaiian cowboys) in Waimea or Waipi'o Valley, mountain biking past waterfalls and hiking across lava fields in Volcanoes National Park—as well as the aforementioned zip lining at Skyline Eco-Adventures and star-gazing from atop the volcano Mauna Kea.

Where to stay: Choose a spot that is right on the beach at the 252-room Mauna Kea Beach Hotel (MaunaKeaBeachHotel.com), with its award-winning golf course. *Nightly rates:* From $529.

Insider tip: Just around the point, the 249-room Westin Hapuna Prince Resort (WestinHapunaBeach.com) has nightly rates starting at $299.

FOR SUN & WILDLIFE

•**Playa Manuel Antonio in Costa Rica.** Beaches rank among nature's most inviting creations, but add in a bunch of equally awesome creatures—from two- and three-toed sloths to prehistoric-looking iguanas—and your vacation is suddenly a whole lot more exciting. They re-side in 4,900-acre Manuel Antonio National Park, located on Costa Rica's Pacific coast and home to two beaches, including Playa Manuel Antonio. The park's trails are inhabited by such curious species as howler monkeys (who live up to their their name) and white-nosed coatis (a member of the raccoon family known for their exceptionally long ringed tails). You can enjoy a guided morning walk followed by a refreshing ocean dip in the afternoon.

Where to stay: The 38-room Arenas del Mar Beachfront & Rainforest Resort (ArenasDelMar.com) allows you to effortlessly enjoy eco-friendly amenities and indigenous wildlife on 11 beachfront acres within walking distance of the park. *Nightly rates:* From $330.

Insider tip: Book for early December or early May (dry season) for the lowest rates.

FOR SUN & CULTURE

•**Akumal Beach in Riviera Maya, Mexico.** Riviera Maya, about an hour south of Cancún on Mexico's Caribbean coast, is known for all-inclusive resorts set on beautiful beaches and three legendary Mayan cities dating back more than 1,000 years—Tulum, where city ruins overlook a photogenic beach…Cobá, where you can climb the Nohoch Mul pyramid for a panoramic jungle view…and Chichén Itzá, home to one of Mexico's largest Mayan temples, Kukulkan.

Where to stay: The 420-room Luxury Bahia Principe Sian Ka'an or the 978-room Grand Bahia Principe Tulum (Bahia-Principe.com). Located in the same 983-acre complex near Akumal, both offer great value, with adults-only Sian Ka'an tucked amid jungle foliage and family-friendly Tulum on the beach. *All-inclusive nightly rates:* From $186 and $150 per person, respectively.

Insider tip: Visit the beach from November to February to avoid the seasonal sargassum seaweed, which can spoil swimming.

FOR SUN & ROCK CLIMBING

•**Railay Beach in Krabi, Thailand.** Thailand's geologically stunning Krabi is a global hot spot for rock climbing. There are more than 700 bolted climbing routes on the limestone cliffs near Railay Beach. Local outfitters offer full- and half-day tours (both private and groups) for every level of climber—even beginners.

Where to stay: The 240-room Dusit Thani Krabi Beach Resort (Dusit.com) is located about eight miles from Railay. *Nightly rates:* From $124.

Insider tip: The best time to visit is December to March, and it's easy to combine a stay in Krabi with visits to stunning Ko Phi Phi Leh (where the Leonardo DiCaprio film *The Beach* was filmed) and other islands in the Andaman Sea.

FOR SUN & SNORKELING/DIVING

•**Seven Mile Beach in Grand Cayman.** Whether you're a beginner snorkeler or an expert diver eager to take your next plunge, the sparkling turquoise waters of the Cayman Islands' largest island and most famous beach offer all kinds of adventure, from just-offshore coral reefs to intriguing wreck dives. Grand Cayman has more than 300 dive sites—notably Babylon, Devil's Grotto and the wreck of the USS Kittiwake—while a small reef is accessible about 100 yards off Seven Mile Beach in the area known as Governor's Beach. A great family outing is a catamaran sail to Stingray City, where the unintimidated can snorkel with playful southern stingrays that congregate here for food handouts. Seven Mile Beach (and yes, it is almost that long at 6.3 miles) offers a roster of water sports—wakeboarding, Waverunner safaris, kayak rentals and parasailing.

Where to stay: Book a room at the 285-room Margaritaville Beach Resort Grand Cayman (MargaritavilleResort GrandCayman.com) for a laid-back vibe inspired by the music of Jimmy Buffett. *Nightly rates:* From $126.

Insider tip: This property has some of Grand Cayman's lowest prices in high season.

7

Best, Easy Ways to Strength Train

Weight-Training Smarts for Everyone—How to Get the Most Out of Your Strength-Training Workout

Wayne L. Westcott, PhD, a professor of exercise science, researcher and chair of the exercise program at Quincy College in Quincy, Massachusetts. He is coauthor of several books, including *Strength Training Past 50*.

It's well known that 30 minutes of aerobic exercise three to five days a week helps prevent cardiovascular disease. My favorite ways to fit this in are brisk walking or bicycling, because I love being outside in good weather. If that's not an option, I hit the elliptical machine. What's less well known—or at least less practiced—is that strength training (e.g., lifting free weights or using weight machines) is equally important to good health, especially as we grow older. The American College of Sports Medicine (ACSM) recommends that adults perform two to three strength-training sessions each week.

According to Wayne Westcott, PhD, chair of exercise science at Quincy College in Quincy, Massachusetts, strength training not only boosts metabolism and keeps blood pressure and glucose levels stable, it is also the only way to prevent the five-pound loss in muscle mass that we experience each decade as we age. Dr. Westcott explains the health benefits of strength training, and offers some useful tips on how to safely and effectively work out with weights...

STRENGTH TRAINING: THE KEY TO SUCCESSFUL AGING

Lean muscle mass naturally decreases with age, but strength training (especially training with weights) can help reverse this trend. As you grow stronger and muscle mass increases, benefits multiply—you'll find that you are more energetic, have more stamina and feel better overall.

Strength training...

•**Lowers blood pressure**, which reduces the risk for cardiovascular disease. After two months, regular weight training can cause incremental drops in both systolic (top number) and diastolic (bottom number) blood pressure.

•**Encourages muscles to utilize glucose more efficiently.** This means less glucose circulating in the bloodstream, which lowers your risk of diabetes.

•**Stimulates the skeletal system**, which helps maintain bone density. This becomes increasingly important as we age, to prevent bone-thinning osteoporosis.

•**Enables you to manage weight more effectively.** Your best bet is to combine aerobic and strength-training exercise to raise your metabolism and burn off excess calories.

GETTING STARTED

Weight training with progressively heavier resistance is far and away the best way to build strength and muscle mass. But if you're not familiar with free weights or weight machines, what's the best way to get started? Join a beginner's weight training class at the local gym, or schedule a session or two with a personal trainer who is knowledgeable in weight training. There are also helpful how-to books, such as Dr. Westcott's own *Strength Training Past 50*. If you're over 40 or have health issues, also see your health-care provider before taking on a new fitness program.

As for whether to choose free weights (barbells or dumbbells) or weight machines, such as Nautilus or Cybex, try both forms and see which you prefer. Free weights and machines work equally wellt—though, of course, free weights can easily be done at home, without investing in expensive equipment or a health club membership. Muscles can't tell the difference.

GETTING THE MOST OUT OF YOUR WORKOUT

Once you learn how to work with weights, you'll want to focus on maximizing benefits of your workouts. An average strength-training regimen consists of two to three sessions a week, with one to three sets, using sets of resistance exercises to cover all the major muscle groups. *For optimal results…*

•**Begin with eight to 10 repetitions of a series of resistance exercises.** Consult a fitness trainer at the gym to determine appropriate starting weights, which should call on approximately 65% to 75% of your maximum resistance. At the gym, it's often not necessary to book a session with a personal trainer since many have "floor trainers" available to answer questions and offer advice on proper weight levels and lifting technique. At home, most women exercise with five- to 15-pound free weights, and most men lift 10 to 25 pounds.

•**Learn to lift weights properly, in a slow and controlled fashion.** It's not the amount of weight you lift, but how you lift it that counts. As a general rule of thumb, each repetition should last five to six seconds, and a series of 10 repetitions should take 50 to 60 seconds. When in doubt about technique, seek advice from a fitness professional.

•**Be sure sessions last 20 to 40 minutes.** Weight training should be performed three days a week, on non-consecutive days, at first. As time goes on and you grow more experienced, you can cut back to only two sessions a week, three days apart. This allows the muscles ample time to recover and prepare for the next workout.

•**Remember to breathe.** Holding your breath during weight training can lead to a dangerous elevation in blood pressure. Exhale when you lift, and inhale when you lower weights.

•**Vary your exercises.** For example, do one set of repetitions to the shoulders, move down to the abs, and then on to the legs. Don't overwork any one muscle group, as this can contribute to muscle fatigue and the risk of injury.

•**Increase weight when you successfully work your way up to performing 15 reps with proper technique and without fatigue.** However, to avoid strains and sprains, don't add more than 5%—of pound weight—at a time.

•**Stretch the muscles you just worked after each strength exercise**—or, if you prefer, following your entire strength workout.

MORE STRENGTH-TRAINING OPTIONS

Other forms of strength training also work well, if you don't enjoy weights or want to incorporate some variety into your fitness regimen. *Classes or activities you might consider include…*

•**Circuit training.** This handy, all-in-one exercise program combines strength training with aerobic activities such as the treadmill and stationary bike.

•**Pilates.** This approach emphasizes slow-moving stretches and resistance exercises (including using popular exercise resistance bands) to increase flexibility and strength.

•**Body sculpting.** While body sculpting—the modern day version of calisthenics with some light weights—does not pack the same oomph as other strength-training exercises, it will help slow muscle loss and moderately increase strength.

For optimal fitness, make it a point to add strength training—with weights, Pilates or whatever other strength-training exercise you enjoy the most—to your regular fitness routine. You'll feel better, look better and enjoy your later years with greater strength, energy and independence.

Strength-Training Myths

Vikr Khanna, PA, MHS, clinical exercise specialist, health educator and chief exercise officer of Galileo Health Partners, based in Ellicott City, Maryland. He is coauthor, with Henry Brinton, of *Ten Commandments of Faith and Fitness: A Practical Guide for Health and Wellness.*

No form of exercise is more essential to muscle and bone strength than strength training. Strength training involves lifting weights and/or using exercise bands or tubing. Strength training improves just about every measure of health, including the ability to stay active and independent in your later years.

Many people think that strengthening is less important than walking or other forms of aerobic exercise. Not true. Aerobic exercise is important, but people with weak muscles don't have enough strength to adequately work the cardiovascular system.

Other strength-training myths…

MYTH: **I'll get too bulky if I lift weights.** Just about every woman with whom I've worked has said something like, "I don't want to look like Arnold Schwarzenegger."

You won't. That kind of physique is largely determined by testosterone. Few women produce enough testosterone to produce bulky muscles. For that matter, few men will ever look like Arnold in his heyday no matter how much they work out.

Genetics has more to do with bulking up than how much you lift. I'm a good example. I've been lifting weights for more than 30 years. I weigh 150 pounds, exactly the same as when I started.

When you start strength training, about 30% of the initial improvement occurs because of improved efficiency between your muscles and central nervous system. After that, your muscles start growing—but maximizing muscle size requires specific training, which most people don't need.

MYTH: **Strength training takes too much time.** Actually, it's among the most efficient forms of exercise. People are told, for example, to walk or get other forms of aerobic exercise for at least 30 minutes most days of the week. With strength training, you need to spend only about 20 minutes twice a week.

Many of my clients are busy executives. I typically advise them to go to the gym, warm up with five to 10 minutes of light cardio work (such as walking or running on a treadmill) and then strength train for 15 to 20 minutes. That's long enough to work all of the main muscle groups.

MYTH: **I can get just as strong with yoga or Pilates.** No, you can't. These activities are beneficial, but they provide only light-to-moderate workouts. They're useful if you're just starting to exercise after being sedentary. After that, people tend to "top out" within a few months because the exertion levels don't change.

With strength training, you can constantly change the intensity of workouts by changing the weight and/or repetitions as your strength increases. People who lift weights can double their strength within a year.

MYTH: **"Free weights," such as barbells, give a better workout than machines.** They give a different workout. When you lift a barbell or dumbbell, you have to balance the weight in multiple planes. For example, you not only have to lift the weight but also have to prevent it from swaying from front to back or from side to side. This brings additional muscle groups into play.

Weight machines allow you to lift in a more controlled manner. There's no side-to-side or front-to-back movement. There is less stress on the joints, which generally is preferable for older or less fit adults. The machines isolate particular muscle groups, which can give notable gains with less stress.

A Simple Strength Training Program for Those Over 50

Brad Schoenfeld, PhD, certified strength and conditioning specialist and an associate professor of exercise science at Lehman College in New York City where he directs the Human Performance Lab. He is the author of *Science and Development of Muscle Hyperthophy.* BradSchoenfeld.com

Have you been shying away from weights? You're not alone. Less than 15% of older adults regularly do strength training, according to a study published in *Clinical Interventions in Aging.*

Yes, cardio is a must for heart health, and those tai chi classes are terrific for mind-body wellness and balance. But when it comes to building up the muscles that will help you be independent and flexible, strength training is the ticket.

Unexpected bonuses: In addition to improving key biomarkers, such as blood sugar and blood fats, research shows that strength training even improves executive functioning and memory.

With all those benefits, what's stopping you? While it's easy to lace up your walking shoes, many people just don't know how to get started with a strength-training regimen.

The good news is, it's never too late to start—and strength training can be easy to do. However, if you're new to strength training, it's wise to book an appointment with a personal trainer, who can assess your abilities, show you proper form and customize a routine for you with body-weight, free-weight and/or machine exercises.

It takes only about 10 to 15 minutes two or three times a week to obtain benefits in health and functional capacity with a strength-training workout. To gain muscle strength, you need to do as many repetitions (reps) as it takes to reach exhaustion. One set (eight to 12 reps) of each exercise usually does the trick if the weight is heavy enough. To continually challenge your muscles, add weight and/or reps as you progress.

To get started, here's a simple strength-training program…*

*As with any new exercise program, consult your doctor before starting.

GET STRONG WITH THESE 6 SIMPLE EXERCISES

•**Squat.**

Target: Quads (front of thighs), glutes (buttocks) and hamstrings (back of thighs).

What to do: While standing with your feet shoulder-width apart and slightly turned out, contract your core (abdominal and back) muscles and slowly lower your body as though sitting down in a chair until your thighs are parallel to the floor. Once you reach the "seated" position (or as low as you can safely go with proper form), straighten your legs to return to start.

Goal: When you're just beginning, do the exercise without hand weights and work up to using weights that challenge your muscles.

Good rule of thumb: If you aren't struggling on the last repetition, then the weight is too light.

•**Front plank.**

Target: Core.

What to do: Lie on your stomach with your forearms on the floor and feet together. While keeping your spine straight, lift your body off the floor, balancing on your forearms and toes and contracting your core muscles. Hold for up to 60 seconds.

Goal: To make the exercise more challenging, work up to balancing on your hands instead of your forearms.

•**Chest press.**

Target: Pectorals (upper chest).

What to do: Lie face up on a bench with your legs on either side, feet flat on the floor and holding a hand weight in each hand. Bring the weights to your shoulders, palms facing away and upper arms pressed to your sides. Then extend your arms straight up, bringing both weights together until they touch when your arms are fully extended.

Alternative: If you don't have a bench, you can lie on the floor when performing this exercise—but it will limit your range of motion and somewhat lessen the results.

•**Lateral raise.**

Target: Deltoids (shoulder).

What to do: While standing with your feet shoulder-width apart, grasp a hand weight in each hand, palms facing your body and arms at your sides. Keeping your elbows slightly bent, raise your arms out to the sides and lift the weights to shoulder level. Be sure not to raise your shoulders as you lift the weights.

●**Single-arm row.**

Target: Back.

What to do: Place your left hand and left knee on a flat bench with your right foot firmly on floor. Grasp a hand weight in your right hand, palm facing your body and arm at your side. Raise the weight straight up until it's just below your armpit. Contract the muscles in your upper back as you lower the arm back down. Complete reps on one side, then repeat on the other side.

Alternative: If you don't have a bench, you can grasp any secure object. If it's a chair, be sure that it's very sturdy to avoid injury.

●**Calf raise.**

Target: Calves.

What to do: While steadying yourself with a handrail, stand on a stair tread with your weight on the balls of your feet, heels hanging off and below the stair. Rise up as high as you can onto your toes until your ankles are fully extended. Contract your calves, and then slowly return to starting position.

You Don't Have to Heave Heavy Weights to Strengthen Your Muscles

Brad Schoenfeld, PhD, a certified strength and conditioning specialist and an associate professor of exercise science at Lehman College in New York City, where he directs the Human Performance Lab. Dr. Schoenfeld is also the assistant editor in chief of the National Strength and Conditioning Association's *Strength and Conditioning Journal,* and the author of *Science and Development of Muscle Hypertrophy.*

To get the biggest bang from your exercise regimen, strength training is a must. It not only builds muscle and bone but also helps manage your weight and control chronic health problems such as diabetes and heart disease.

But not everyone relishes the idea of heaving heavy weights. And the practice can be risky for people with arthritis, osteoporosis and other conditions.

Good news: Researchers have now discovered that people who repeatedly lift light weights get nearly the same benefits as those who do heavy-weight workouts.

Why this matters: Whether you're using hand weights or exercise machines, the lighter-weight approach can make strength training safer and more enjoyable.

Men and women who lift light weights instead of heavy ones are also less likely to experience joint, tendon or ligament injury. Plus, the workouts are easier for older adults…those with arthritis or other health problems…and those who are new to weight lifting.

THE NEW THINKING

According to traditional thinking, you need to lift heavy weights to build your muscles. In practice, this meant identifying your one-repetition maximum—the heaviest weight that you could lift just one time. Then you'd design a workout that required lifting 65% or more of that weight eight to 12 times.

This approach is still favored by many elite athletes because lifting at the edge of your ability targets fast-twitch muscle fibers, the ones that grow quickly and create an admirable physique. But studies now show that slow-twitch fibers, the ones that are stimulated to a greater extent by light lifting, can also develop and grow.

Important finding: In a recent meta-analysis published in the journal *Sports Medicine,* people who lifted lighter weights for six weeks achieved the same muscle growth—although not quite as much strength—as those who lifted heavy weights.

Heavy lifting is still the preferred approach for people who need to develop their strength to the utmost—top athletes, construction workers, movers, etc. But those who simply want to look better and improve their functional capacity—the ability to carry groceries, work in the yard, play recreational sports, etc.—will do just as well with lighter loads.

Bonus: Building muscle mass also helps control blood sugar.

LESS WEIGHT, MORE REPS

Muscle growth occurs only when muscles are exhausted—when you simply can't move the weight one more time. So to get comparable benefits to a traditional heavy-weight workout requiring eight to 12 repetitions, you'll need to do 20 to 25 reps with lighter weights. Your weight workouts will take a little longer, but your muscles will be just as tired when you're done.

A LIGHT-WEIGHT PLAN

Lighter-weight workouts are easier on the joints than those done with heavy weights, and the results are still relatively fast—you'll likely notice an increase in strength/muscle size within a few weeks. *To start…*

•**Choose your weights wisely.** Instead of calculating percentages—a heavy-weight lifter, as described earlier, may aim to lift at least 65% of his/her one-repetition maximum—keep it simple. Forget the percentages, and let repetitions guide your starting weights. For example, do each exercise 20 to 25 times. If you can't complete that many, you're starting too heavy. Conversely, if you can easily do 20 to 25 reps, the weight's too light.*

Important: You're not doing yourself any good if you can easily lift a weight 25 times. You need to strain. On a one-to-10 scale of effort, the last few reps should rate nine-and-a-half or 10.

•**Do multiple sets.** You'll progress more quickly when you do three sets of each exercise—for example, bicep curls. Complete 20 to 25 repetitions… rest for two minutes…do them again…rest…and repeat one more time. If you don't have the time—or the desire—to do three sets, opt for a single-set approach. You'll still notice increases in strength and muscle size, but your gains won't be as great as with a multi-set approach.

•**Work out at least twice a week.** You want to work each muscle group—arms, legs, chest, mid-section, etc.—at least twice a week. Three or four times weekly will give even faster results.

Important: Don't work the same muscles two days in a row. Growth occurs during the recovery phase…and injuries are more likely when you stress already-tired muscles.

If you work out every day: Alternate muscle groups—for example, do leg and back exercises on Monday…arm and chest exercises on Tuesday… then more leg and back work on Wednesday, etc.

EXERCISES FOR REAL LIFE

The strength-training exercises below will give you more confidence and power when doing your daily activities—follow the advice above for choosing your weights, repetitions, exercise frequency, etc.…

•**Bicep curls.** Exercising this upper-arm muscle will make carrying groceries a bit easier.

What to do: Hold a hand weight in each hand. While keeping your elbows near your sides and your shoulders back, curl the weight toward your shoulder, then lower it back down.

•**One-arm triceps extensions.** This exercise will strengthen your triceps (muscles on the backs of the upper arms), which help balance the biceps—and give your arms a toned appearance. It will help when moving furniture or shoveling snow.

What to do: While sitting, hold a hand weight over your head, with your arm straight up and your elbow close to your head. Bend your elbow and lower the weight just behind your neck, then raise it back up. Repeat with the other arm.

•**Lunges.** This versatile exercise targets the buttocks and thighs, along with the arms, making climbing stairs easier.

What to do: With a weight in each hand, stand with your feet about shoulder-width apart. Take a long step forward with your right foot. As your foot lands, bend the knee until the thigh is nearly parallel to the floor. Pull your right leg back to the starting position, then lunge with the left foot.

*Hand weights are available in neoprene, iron and vinyl at many retail stores and online. I recommend holding various weights in a store to choose the one that feels best.

Which Strength Training Program Is Best for You?

Wayne L. Westcott, PhD, a professor of exercise science, researcher and chair of the exercise program at Quincy College in Quincy, Massachusetts. He is coauthor of several books, including *Strength Training Past 50*.

Thirty minutes of aerobic exercise, such as walking or cycling, three to five days per week has long been known to help prevent cardiovascular disease.

Strength training is equally important for maintaining healthy cholesterol levels and blood pressure—and even more critical for preventing diabetes and boosting the body's metabolism, which helps burn calories and prevent weight gain.

Why is this type of exercise so important? Researchers have found that regular strength training is the only way to prevent the five- to seven-pound loss in muscle mass that all adults—except trained athletes—experience each decade beginning in their mid-20s.

That's why the American College of Sports Medicine (ACSM) now recommends that, in addition to regular aerobic workouts, all adults perform two or three strength-training sessions per week. Each workout should last 20 to 40 minutes and consist of eight or more exercises that work all the major muscle groups of the body.

There's just one problem: If you walk into a health club or local YMCA, you're likely to encounter a bewildering array of strength-training classes that claim to "firm and tone your body," "build lean muscle mass" or some combination of the above. Which type of class is right for you?

Any class you're considering should be supervised by a trainer who has been certified by a national fitness organization, such as the ACSM or the American Council on Exercise. When properly supervised, strength training is one of the safest forms of exercise there is—even among elderly and frail adults.

Caution: Your muscles require 48 to 72 hours to recover from each strength-training workout. Adults age 50 or older should strength train every three days.

What you need to know about strength-training classes…

BODY SCULPTING

What it does: Tones muscles, while moderately increasing strength and muscle tissue.

These classes include a variety of strength-building exercises, using elastic resistance bands, dumbbells, medicine balls (handheld, weighted exercise balls) and calisthenics. A typical body-sculpting class consists of eight to 15 different exercises that work all the body's major muscle groups. Each exercise should involve 20 repetitions or less, and take no more than two minutes.

While body-sculpting classes don't produce as much gain in strength and muscle mass as other types of strength-training exercises, they will increase lean muscle tissue somewhat, and are highly effective at increasing functional muscle strength (used for lifting and carrying).

PILATES

What it does: Strengthens the "core" muscles of the low back, front abdominal muscles and oblique muscles that run from the back of the abdomen to the front.

Pilates classes use slow-moving stretches and resistance exercises to increase flexibility and strength. These moves are performed using Pilates equipment (pulleys and weights set on a frame) or without equipment on a floor mat.

Caution: If you have back pain, check with a doctor before taking Pilates classes to be sure you have no structural abnormalities that might be exacerbated.

Note: Core-training classes offer benefits that are similar to those of Pilates and typically consist of a variety of resistance exercises using calisthenics, medicine balls, lightweight dumbbells, resistance bands and inflated stability balls (which you sit on while exercising)—all designed to activate and strengthen the low-back and abdominal muscles.

WEIGHT TRAINING

What it does: Builds strength and muscle mass.

When it comes to increasing strength and muscle mass, no other form of strength training comes close to matching standard weight training. Weight training typically involves about 10 different resistance exercises covering all the major muscle groups. They can be performed with weight machines (such as those made by Nautilus or Cybex) or free weights (barbells and dumbbells). In each exercise, a weight is lifted eight to 12 times in a slow, controlled fashion.

Research has found that weight training increases the glucose uptake of the body's muscles by nearly 25% (reducing the risk for diabetes), and lowers blood pressure by an average of 4 mmHg systolic (top number) and 2 mmHg diastolic (bottom number) over periods of two to four months. By stimulating the skeletal system, it also can help maintain bone density.

CIRCUIT TRAINING

What it does: Combines the maximum strength- and muscle-building benefits of weight training with an aerobic workout that benefits the cardiovascular system.

In a circuit-training class, exercisers perform about 10 weight-training exercises for one minute each. Between these strength exercises, a minute or two of aerobic activity (such as riding a stationary bicycle or walking/jogging on a treadmill) is performed.

These classes are excellent time-savers, since they offer the benefits of weight training and an aerobic workout in a single session of 30 to 45 minutes. Due to the aerobic component, circuit training also burns about 50% more calories per workout session than standard strength-training classes.

Build Muscle With This "Rubber Band" Workout

Stephanie Mansour, certified personal trainer, Certified yoga and pilates instructor, and host of *Step It Up with Steph* on PBS. StepItUpWithSteph.com

I f your image of a powerful muscle workout includes a lot of shiny and expensive equipment at an expensive health club, think again. You can get a full-body workout with a set of rubber resistance bands that costs less than $20 and can be stashed in a drawer when not in use or even packed in a suitcase when you go on vacation.

Rather than using weight, these stretchy tools use resistance that you must move against to strengthen your muscles.

Bands actually can be more effective than hand weights in terms of toning and injury prevention because their constant tension engages multiple muscles simultaneously through the range of motion, particularly the smaller, stabilizing muscles in the back, hips, quads and glutes. And resistance bands can be used to work your leg muscles as well. Try doing that with a dumbbell!

Resistance bands are available in various forms, such as flat strips and tubes with handles on the ends. But your safest bet are minibands—circular rubber bands that loop around the arms and legs. You don't need to worry about losing your grip…or about strips flying out of closed doorjambs and snapping you in the face…and you can purchase them in multipacks for varied resistance, changing them out as your fitness level advances.

Bands come in bright colors. The resistance tends to increase as the color gets darker.

Example: A yellow band offers less resistance than a blue band. *Two brands that I like…*

Gaiam Restore Mini Band Kit: $9.98 for a set of three bands.

4KOR Fitness Resistance Loop Band Set: $18.95 for a set of six bands.

RESISTANCE BAND WORKOUT

The following six moves will work all the major muscle groups in your body. Turn them into a circuit workout by performing them in the order listed, repeating the entire sequence three times. It takes 20 minutes or less, depending on the number of reps.

Do the exercises at least three times per week for maximum benefit. Start with 10 reps per exercise. As you gain strength, increase to 15 reps. Once this becomes simple—probably in two weeks—move on to a higher-resistance band level.

●**Half Squat.**

Muscles worked: Quads, hamstrings, gluteus (buttock) medius, stabilizing muscles around the ankles.

Get ready: Step into the miniband, positioning it a few inches above both knees. Stand with toes forward, feet hip-width apart, creating a bit of tension around the band. Place your hands on your hips to help with balance.

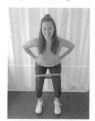

Go: Begin squatting down as if you were about to sit in a chair, but stop midway. As you lower down, contract your abdominal muscles by pulling your navel toward your spine, and gaze downward to ensure your knees are aligned with your second toes, which will keep your hips, thighs, knees and ankles in proper alignment and ensure that the correct muscles are being activated.

Once you are halfway through the squat, press down through your heels to stand up, squeezing your glutes at the top. Be sure to stand fully upright at the top of each rep looking straight ahead with shoulders relaxed and glutes engaged. Strive to maintain outward tension on the band throughout the exercise.

Step it up: Squat all the way down, with knees bent at a 90-degree angle, as if tapping your butt in the imaginary chair.

●**Side Step.**

Muscles worked: Quads, gluteus medius, gluteus maximus, stabilizing muscles around the ankles.

Get ready: Begin in the half-squat position as above with the band a little above the knee. Place your hands on your hips to help with balance.

Go: Step your right foot about six inches to the right (band tension will increase), then step your left foot to the right the same amount (band tension will decrease a bit but should never go slack). Complete 10 steps to the right, then repeat the sequence to the left. Your navel should stay pulled in, abdominals contracted, as if you're steeling yourself for a punch to the stomach. Doing this will help protect your low back throughout the move. If you do experience low-back discomfort, stand up and try the Side Step with just a very slight bend in the knees.

Step it up: You can grab some dumbbells and do bicep curls as you step to the side to work your arms…or reach your arms up to the ceiling without weights to challenge your balance.

●**Lying Down Bridge.**

Muscles worked: Transverse abdominis (the deepest layer of front abdominal muscles—beneath your "six-pack" muscles), rectus abdominis core (the more superficial abdominal muscles—the ones that form the six pack), glutes. If you perform the advanced version, you also will work the gluteus medius, which is notoriously weak in many people and critical for stability when you move, such as walking and climbing stairs, and keeping the body in proper alignment to prevent hip and knee problems.

Get ready: Sitting on the ground, position the miniband a few inches above both knees as in the exercises above. Lie down, bending your knees so feet are flat on the ground, hip-width apart, and heels are positioned so that when you lay your arms by your sides and reach along the ground toward your heels, your fingertips touch or almost touch your heels. Strive to maintain tension in the band throughout the exercise.

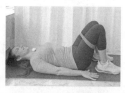
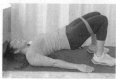

Go: Inhale deeply, filling your stomach with air. As you exhale, tilt your pelvis up, pressing your low back into the ground. Now, press down through your heels and lift your tailbone off the ground, followed by your low back and middle back, squeezing your butt tightly at the top. Your butt will be a few inches off of the ground.

Hold for two or three counts before slowly returning down, starting with the middle back, then the low back and finally the tailbone. Rest for a count, then press back up until you complete all reps.

Step it up: At the top of each bridge, open your thighs out and in three times, pushing against the band's resistance.

●**Banded crunch.**

Muscles worked: Transverse abdominus, rectus abdominis.

Get ready: Assume the same starting position as in the Lying Down Bridge, miniband above your knees, knees bent, heels close enough to your 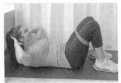 butt that you can touch (or almost touch) them with your fingertips. Tilt your pelvis so your low back presses into ground.

Go: Place your hands behind your head, and lift your head and neck a few inches off the ground. Pulse up and down through your repetitions without resting on the ground in between. Keep your elbows out, and avoid pulling on your head. Maintain tension on the band throughout.

●**Shoulder Blade Squeeze.**

Muscles worked: Shoulders, upper back.

Get ready: Standing with feet hip-width apart, 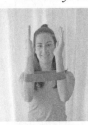 place the miniband around your forearms and extend your arms in front of you at shoulder height, palms facing in but pulling apart from one another to create tension in the band.

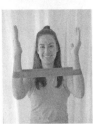 *Go:* Concentrate on keeping your shoulder blades back and down, as if you are squeezing a ball between them. Then spread your arms apart as far as you can. (Depending on your band's resistance, you'll be able to move them six inches to one foot apart.) Return to the starting position, not allowing the band to collapse as you continue through all repetitions.

●**Modified Banded Lat Pull Down.**

Muscles worked: Lats, core, biceps.

Get ready: Choose a looser band for this exercise. Standing with feet hip-width apart, knees 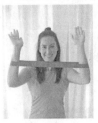 softly bent, place the miniband around your forearms and extend your arms overhead, palms facing in but pulling apart from one another to create tension in the band. Avoid hunching your shoulders as you do this move, and keep your ribcage still throughout rather than bobbing up and down.

Go: Pull your navel in toward your spine, and contract your abdominals as you pull your elbows down to the sides and slightly behind you—almost like cactus arms—as if you were performing lat pulls down at the gym. Return to the starting position. Repeat for all reps.

3 Resistance Band Exercises Everyone Should Learn

Jacque Crockford, MS, CSCS, certified personal trainer and exercise physiology content manager at American Council on Exercise (ACE), San Diego.

If you've been resisting resistance bands, it's time to give in. These lengths of stretchy tubing with handles, which challenge and train muscles through a full range of motion, are an amazingly convenient and effective way to build strength.

They're safe, inexpensive, portable and easy to use. You can work out with them anytime and anywhere. Learn just a few resistance band exercises, and you can incorporate them into your workouts at home—and you'll always have a routine when you travel.

Here are three exercises everyone—whether you're a fitness novice or an elite athlete—should be doing to strengthen the upper and lower body and improve balance and flexibility.

SQUAT

Why it's essential: The squat increases flexibility and strength in both the upper and lower body.

How to do it: Place your resistance band under both feet. Standing with your feet hip-width apart, hold the handles at shoulder level.

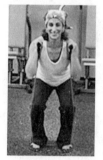

Keeping your chest straight, squat down as if you were sitting, moving your hips back and down until your thighs are parallel to the floor.

Stand back up, pushing through your heels. If you want more resistance, you can extend your arms straight up above your head as you stand back up.

Repeat. Your goal is to work up to 20 reps.

SEATED ROW

Why it's essential: Rowing engages the back muscles that help pull the trunk and shoulders into better alignment—while strengthening your upper-body muscles.

How to do it: Loop your resistance band around a sturdy anchor (such as a couch leg or a stair

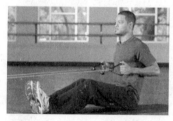

bannister), and sit on the floor with your knees slightly bent and your feet together. Keep your back straight and your abs tight throughout the movement. Hold the handles of your band with your palms facing each other.

Without leaning back, pull the handles toward you until they reach your sides, keeping your elbows close to your body. Slowly straighten your elbows as you return to your starting position.

Repeat. Your goal is to work up to 20 reps.

Note: You can also perform this exercise standing.

STANDING ROTATION

Why it's essential: Rotating helps us maintain our balance and create more efficient movement patterns. This exercise strengthens your abdominals.

How to do it: Tie your resistance band to a sturdy anchor (again, such as a couch leg or stair banister) so only one handle is available. Stand sideways to your band with your feet hip-width apart, and hold

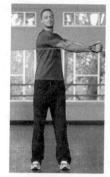

the handle with both hands, arms fully extended before you at chest level.

Keeping arms straight and abdominals tight, rotate your torso away from the anchored band as far as you can. Your head and torso should move together. Hold briefly, and then rotate back to starting position.

After performing several repetitions, turn to face the opposite direction and repeat the movement, rotating to the other side. Work up to 20 reps.

As with any new exercise routine, it's always a good idea to check with your doctor before getting started…and that's especially true if you have any joint problems or other physical challenges. And as with any physical activity, if it starts to hurt, stop.

Note: The images in this story that demonstrate each exercise are used with permission, courtesy of the American Council on Exercise. You can see more in their Exercise Library at AceFitness.org. Search "Exercise Library."

A Complete Strength Training Workout for Seniors (Beginners, Too)

Cedric X. Bryant, PhD, chief science officer, American Council on Exercise, San Diego. Hemns in fitness magazines and exercise science journals and is author or numerous books, including *Strength Training for Women.*

Being strong is essential for good health and vitality. Here's an easy muscle-building routine suitable for seniors and newbies.

Best part: You can do it at home with just one inexpensive piece of equipment.

You have a lot to gain from this simple routine. Strength training not only builds muscles, it also improves bone density, speeds up metabolism, promotes balance and even boosts brain power. You'll also gain mobility.

Translation: This routine will help make everyday movements—such as getting in and out of a car, reaching overhead, bending and climbing stairs—much easier for you.

And not to worry...you won't be straining under heavy barbells. All the exercises below use just your own body weight or a simple elastic tube for resistance.

Recommended: Opt for a light-resistance tube with handles, available at sporting goods stores and online for about $10 (I like the durable SPRI brand, SPRI.com).

What to do: Get your doctor's OK first, as you should before beginning any new exercise routine. Perform eight to 15 reps of each of the following moves two to three times per week on nonconsecutive days—muscles need a day between workouts to repair and strengthen. Always move in a slow, controlled fashion, without jerking or using momentum. When you can easily do 15 reps of a particular exercise, advance to the "To progress" variation.

NO-EQUIPMENT-NEEDED EXERCISES...

•**Wall Squat**—for legs and buttocks.

Start: Stand with head and back against a wall, arms at sides, legs straight, feet hip-width apart and about 18 inches from wall.

Move: Keeping head and torso upright and your back firmly pressed against the wall, bend knees and slide down the wall about four to eight inches. Knees should be aligned above ankles—do not allow knees to extend past toes. Hold for several seconds. Then, using thigh and buttock muscles, straighten legs and slide back up wall to the start position. Repeat.

To progress: Bend knees more, ideally to a 90° angle so thighs are parallel to floor, as if sitting in a chair.

•**Wall Pushup**—for chest, shoulders and triceps.

Start: Stand facing a wall, feet hip-width apart and about 18 inches from wall. Place hands on wall at shoulder height, slightly wider than shoulder-width apart.

Move: Tighten abdominal muscles to brace your midsection, keeping spine and legs straight throughout. Slowly bend elbows, bringing face as close to wall as you can. Hold for one second, then straighten arms and return to the start position. Repeat.

To progress: Start with feet farther from wall... and bring face closer to wall during pushup.

•**Supine Reverse March**—for abdominals, lower back and hips.

Start: Lie face up, knees bent, feet flat on floor, arms out to sides in a T position, palms up, abs contracted.

Move: Slowly lift left foot off floor, keeping leg bent...bring knee up and somewhat closer to torso...when left thigh is vertical to floor, stop moving and hold for five to 10 seconds. Then slowly lower leg and return foot to floor. Repeat. Switch legs.

To progress: As knee moves upward, raise both arms toward ceiling...lower arms as leg lowers.

MOVES WITH TUBES...

•**Seated Row**—for back, abs and biceps.

Start: Sit on floor, torso upright, legs out in front of you, knees slightly bent, feet together. Place center of elastic resistance tube across soles of feet and hold tube handles in hands, arms extended in front of you, elbows straight.

Move: Bending elbows, slowly pull handles of tube toward chest (do not lean backward, arch back, shrug shoulders or bend wrists). Hold for several seconds, then slowly straighten arms and return to the start position. Repeat.

To progress: To increase resistance, rather than placing center of tube across soles of feet, anchor it firmly around an immovable object one to three feet in front of you.

•**Lateral Raise**—for shoulders.

Start: Stand with feet hip-width apart, anchoring center of elastic resistance tube under both feet. Hold tube handles in hands, arms down at sides.

Move: Keeping elbows very slightly bent and wrists straight, slowly lift arms out to sides so palms face floor and hands reach shoulder height (or as high as you can get them). Lower arms to the start position. Repeat.

To progress: To increase resistance, widen your stance on the tubing.

Fine-Tune Strength Training for Specific Goals

Jacque Crockford, MS, CSCS, certified personal trainer and exercise physiology content manager at American Council on Exercise (ACE), San Diego.

You know that strength training does great things for you. But you probably don't know that you can tailor your strength workouts to meet very specific health and fitness goals—goals that are much more precise than just how strong you are. And the beauty is that it doesn't take more days at the gym. All it takes are tweaks to the amount of weight you lift and how many times you lift it, a simple formula called total training volume.

In strength training terms, each exercise is done for a certain number of sets with a short rest break in between. A set, in turn, consists of a certain number of times you repeat an exercise—repetitions or reps. The number of sets and reps, along with the length of the rest periods between sets—the total training volume—are different for different goals.

*A note on the amount of weight to lift…*No matter what your goal, choose a weight that you can lift in good form for the minimum number of reps given —it should feel challenging toward the final reps of each set.

Jacque Crockford, an American Council of Exercise certified personal trainer, describes how weight training programs differ for four popular fitness goals including some exercises to add to your current plan…

GOAL: AVOID MUSCLE LOSS WHEN DIETING

Exercise goal	Sets	Reps	Rest
Avoid muscle loss when dieting	2 to 3	8 to 12	At least 60 seconds between sets.

When you're dieting, you want to drop fat, but lean muscle is often a casualty. Strength training with medium, moderately hard to lift weights using the above routine can keep your body from metabolizing muscle when you cut calories.

Sample training program: Romanian deadlift, Squat to overhead press, Lateral lunge to high row, Kneeling hay baler, Renegade row and Push-up.

GOAL: BURN MORE CALORIES AT REST

Exercise goal	Sets	Reps	Rest
Burn more calories at rest	5 to 6 done as circuits	10 to 15	60 to 90 seconds after each circuit

Muscle naturally uses more energy to maintain its natural function when compared to fat, which means the more muscle you have, the more calories you burn. To maintain these calorie-burning muscles and burn more calories, even after the workout is over, try a high intensity workout with short rest periods. "Circuits" are an ideal approach. With a circuit, instead than doing all the sets of one exercise before moving to the next exercise—the normal way to train approach, you do one set of each exercise without any break between exercises. Then you rest for a minute and repeat the entire circuit. Circuits are time efficient. If, for instance, you do five different exercises with 10 reps each, it should take you about five minutes per circuit…so you'll complete five circuits, with a minute or so of rest in between each circuit, in about 30 minutes.

Sample training program: Kettlebell swing, Forward lunge, Chin-up, Push-up, Rainbow medicine ball slams

GOAL: DEVELOP OVERALL STRENGTH TO STAY INDEPENDENT

Exercise goal	Sets	Reps	Rest
Develop overall strength to stay independent	2 to 4	4 to 6	30 to 60 seconds

Having strong muscles from head to toe is key to supporting your joints and keeping you mobile throughout your life, not to mention all the daily activities we take for granted when we're younger. Strength training in a balanced way, not missing any important muscles, helps preserve your independence, especially when you do exercises that mimic real life movements such as twisting, moving side to side and going backwards. A comprehensive program has 2 to 4 sets with 4 to 6 reps each using a weight that allows you to maintain correct form for 6 reps—when you can complete 6 with correct form, it's time to slightly increase the weight.

Sample training program: Deadlift, Reverse walking lunges, Cable single-arm press, Sliding transverse lunge, Cable wood chop and TRX single-arm row

GOAL: DEVELOP A SPECIFIC BODY PART

Exercise goal	Sets	Reps	Rest
Develop a specific body part	3 to 6	6 to 12	30 to 90 seconds

When we lift weights, we stimulate production of certain hormones, including testosterone and growth hormone, that help trigger muscle growth and help muscles recover from exercise. The more we lift, the more of these hormones are produced, yes in women, not just in men, but definitely not to the same degree, so women shouldn't fear becoming over-developed. High total volume is what's needed to develop a specific body part. That means a higher number of sets—between 3 and 6—with a weight that's challenging but manageable.

Sample training program for triceps: Chest press, Cable triceps extension, Dumbbell pullover press and Reverse grip pressdown.

TRAINING TIPS

Stretch before and after your workouts to keep your muscles flexible and prevent injury…

Dynamic stretches are done while moving and should be performed as part of your warm-up. An example would be walking lunges while reaching your arms overhead. This promotes lower body flexibility while also lengthening the muscles of your trunk.

Static stretches are done without movement (no bouncing!) and are typically held for about 30 to 60 seconds. Do these after your workout as part of a cool-down. An example would be a rear calf stretch for the back of your lower leg.

Self-myofascial release is a form of self-massage that promotes length and relaxation in the muscles and connective tissues in your body. It can improve muscle pain and soreness. Do this on days you're not exercising or as part of a warm-up or cool-down.

Finally, give your muscles a break. Strength training causes small tears in muscle tissue, and that's a good thing because as they repair themselves, your muscles get stronger. But give your muscles at least two days to recover between each strength-training session—meaning no more than three strength-training sessions per week.

7 Ways to Plank for Strength, Flexibility and Balance

Lee Jordan, certified American Council on Exercise (ACE) health coach and personal trainer based in Jacksonville, Florida.

Jim White, registered dietitian, certified fitness instructor, and owner, Jim White Fitness & Nutrition Studios, Norfolk, Virginia.

The Plank. We're not talking about carpentry or what pirates make prisoners walk off, but an amazing exercise that *simultaneously strengthens many of your body's most critical muscles*—your core.

It tightens your belly…provides better support for your lower back…increases flexibility in your shoulders and the arches of your feet and your toes…improves your posture…and helps you keep your balance when you're out and about during your busy day.

How can one single exercise that you do for only 30 seconds to a minute do all this? We'll tell you. *And we'll show you seven ways to do it, from easy to challenging, with variations to strengthen different muscle groups...*

PLANK 101

The main focus for any plank pose is on the area between your hips and your shoulders—your core. All of the plank positions below work your core, and all but the last one work your gluteals—your butt muscles. The variations target specific muscle groups—to strengthen the muscles in your chest, shoulders, arms, legs and back.

The first one, the *High Plank*, is the basic form. It's the best one to get started with—and also the easiest one to customize. If you want a little more challenging core workout, try the *Front Plank*.

With each position, start by holding it for 10 to 15 seconds. As you get stronger, increase the time—aiming for a goal of one minute. Start with the stationary poses first. Once you can hold a stationary pose for one minute, challenge yourself with one or more of the mobile poses. It's fine to increase your planking time if you want even more challenge!

STATIONARY PLANKS

High Plank.

Tones your core and gluteals (butt muscles).

Lying on your stomach, lift your body so that you're supported on your hands (flat on the floor)

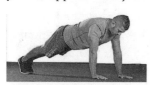

and your toes, arms straight. It looks like a push-up. Pay attention to keeping your abdominals taut and maintaining your body in a straight line from your head to your ankles.

Front Plank.

Tones your core and gluteals and also your chest, shoulders, arms and legs.

Lying on your stomach, lift your body so that you are supported by your forearms and your toes. Your

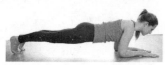

elbows should align under your shoulders. Maintain your body in a straight

line from your head to your ankles, making sure not to lift your head or arch or curve your lower back. Squeeze your gluteal and abdominal muscles while pressing your elbows into the floor.

Side Plank.

Tones your core and gluteals and also your obliques (muscles on the side of the torso that help you turn from side to side) and hips.

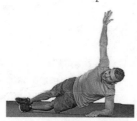

Lying on your right side, prop yourself up on your right elbow and forearm, with your elbow aligned directly under your shoulder and your feet stacked. Now tighten your abdominals and lift your hips off the floor. Your head, shoulder, hips and feet should line up straight. As you lift your hips, push your elbow into the floor for stability.

Switch sides and repeat.

MOVING PLANKS

High Plank with Alternating Shoulder Touch.

Tones your core and gluteals and also your upper chest, back and legs.

Start with the High Plank. In a smooth, alternating movement, balance on your left hand only and touch your right hand to your left shoulder...then bring your right hand down, and touch your left hand to your right shoulder. Repeat for one minute (or however long you can).

Plank Jacks.

Tones your core and gluteals and also your legs.

While holding a Front Plank position, continuously move your legs together and then apart—as if you were doing jumping jacks. Keep your upper body stable, maintaining a straight line...avoid raising your hips out of alignment.

Mountain Climber Plank.

Tones your core and gluteals and also your upper

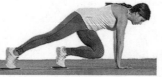

arms and legs.

While holding a High Plank position, bring your left knee in toward your chest, pointing your toe, and then extend it back to its starting position. Bring your right knee in toward your chest and extend back to start. Continue alternating legs in a smooth movement while maintaining your upper body in a stable position.

Twisting Plank.

Tones your core and also your obliques, shoulders and arms.

Begin in a Front Plank position. Then turn your body so that you're supported on just your right forearm and lift your left arm straight up toward the sky. Bring your arm back down into the Front Plank…then turn and do the same on your left side, lifting your right arm toward the sky. Alternate side to side, aiming for a goal of holding for 30 seconds on each side.

Here's to happy planking—and a stronger, more supple, flexible and injury-resistant body!

Note: The images in this story that demonstrate High Plank, Front Plank, Side Plank, and Mountain Climber Plank are used with permission, courtesy of the American Council on Exercise. You can see more in their Exercise Library at AceFitness.org. Search "Exercise Library."

The Ultimate Strength Workout

Doris St-Arnaud, a Trois-Rivières, Quebec–based 25-year veteran of the fitness industry and the author of four books about using stability balls, including *Stability Ball Exercises with Weights.*

As you age, one of the simplest—yet most effective—actions you can take to maintain your ability to perform everyday activities, such as carrying shopping bags and climbing stairs, is to build muscle strength.

What you may not know: The expensive, free-standing weight machines that are found in gyms around the country are not always the best way to build strength.

Important new finding: When 30 people exercised twice weekly for 16 weeks, researchers found that those who used "free-form" equipment, such as hand weights, improved their strength by 115% versus 57% when freestanding exercise equipment, such as a leg-press machine, was used.

Why the big difference? According to exercise physiologists, weight machines primarily strengthen the muscles that are needed to move the weights in the designated range of motion, while free-form equipment works the primary muscles that lift the weight and, to a greater degree, the nearby muscles that support and stabilize the primary muscles.

For even greater benefits: While performing free-form strength-building exercises, sit or lie on an inflatable "stability ball." This helps strengthen another set of muscles, called stabilizers. These include the postural muscles in the lower back, abdomen and thighs.

The following exercises, which work all the major muscles in the body, can be performed in about 20 minutes in your home.*

To get started: Everything you need to perform these exercises is available at sporting-goods or discount stores—three pairs of hand weights (starting at about $8 a pair)…three pairs of strap-on ankle weights (starting at about $10 a pair)…and an inflatable stability ball (starting at about $20).

The hand and ankle weights you choose should be light enough so that you can do at least eight repetitions of each exercise but heavy enough so that you can't do more than 15 repetitions.

Example: A woman who is just beginning to strength-train may start with two-pound hand or ankle weights, while a male beginner may start with five-pound weights. Once you can easily perform 15 repetitions, switch to a heavier weight. Increase the weight by one to three pounds at a time depending on the strength of the muscles worked.

To choose the proper size stability ball: Follow the instructions on the package, using your height as a general guideline. Inflate the ball so that your knees and hips are at the same level when you sit on it.

*Rest at least 48 hours between workouts to allow for adequate muscle recovery, and always check with your doctor before beginning any exercise program.

For each of the following exercises, perform one set of eight to 15 repetitions unless otherwise noted...**

●**Arm curl.**

Primary muscles used: Biceps (fronts of the upper arms).

Among the secondary muscles used: Fronts of the shoulders, the upper back and sides of neck.

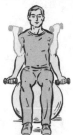

What to do: While holding a weight in each hand, sit on the stability ball with your feet on the floor, your elbows next to your waist. Keeping your elbows in this position, lift the weights toward your shoulders. Return slowly to starting position.

●**Triceps press.**

Primary muscles used: Triceps (backs of the upper arms).

Among the secondary muscles used: Fronts of the shoulders and pectorals (front of the chest).

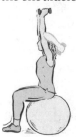

What to do: While holding a weight in each hand, sit on the ball with your abdominal muscles tightened and your back straight. Extend both arms overhead, palms facing each other and elbows slightly flexed. Keeping your elbows stationary, bend them to lower the weights to the backs of your shoulders. Return slowly to starting position with arms overhead.

●**Leg lift.**

Primary muscles used: Quadriceps (fronts of the thighs).

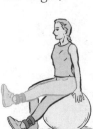

Among the secondary muscles used: Iliopsoas (muscles connecting the pelvis to the front of the hip).

What to do: Place a weight on your right ankle and sit on the ball with your palms holding the sides of the ball for added

**If you prefer not to use a stability ball, you can perform the arm curl, triceps press and leg lift while sitting in a chair...the fly while lying on your back...and the reverse leg lift and back rise while lying on your stomach (on a mat or bed).

stability. Straighten your weighted leg with your heel resting on the floor, then flex your ankle so your toes point upward. Lift your weighted leg as high as you comfortably can. Return slowly to the starting position. Perform a second set of eight to 15 repetitions with your left leg.

●**Fly.**

Primary muscles used: Pectorals.

Among the secondary muscles used: Fronts of the shoulders, triceps and biceps.

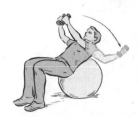

What to do: While holding a weight in each hand, sit on the stability ball and carefully "walk" forward until your lower back rests on the ball. Keep your feet and knees shoulder-width apart with your knees directly above your heels. Extend your arms above your chest, elbows slightly bent and palms facing each other. Lower your left arm to the side until it's in line with your shoulders. Return slowly to the starting position. Perform a second set of eight to 15 repetitions with your right arm.

●**Reverse leg lift.**

Primary muscles used: Buttocks.

Among the secondary muscles used: Hamstrings (backs of the thighs).

What to do: Place a weight on your left ankle, then face the ball with your knees slightly bent and lean forward to rest your trunk on the ball. Keep your feet shoulder-width apart with both hands flat on the floor for extra stability. While holding your weighted leg straight, lift it off the ground as high as you comfortably can, then slowly lower it again without touching it to the floor. Perform a second set of eight to 15 repetitions with the right leg.

●**Back rise.**

Primary muscles used: Lower back.

Among the secondary muscles used: Backs of the shoulders, and middle and upper back.

What to do: Rest your trunk on the stability ball and lower your head so your chin also rests on the ball. Hold a weight in each hand and place your hands in front of your forehead with your palms facing down. Keeping your head in line with your trunk, lift your head, shoulders and chest off the ball and pull your elbows back toward your hips.

Illustrations by Shawn Banner.

The Wall Workout: 5 Exercises to Improve Strength, Flexibility and Posture

Joel Harper, a personal trainer in New York City who designs workouts for Olympic athletes, celebrities, musicians and business executives. He created the workout chapters for the best-selling YOU series of books by Michael Roizen, MD, and Mehmet Oz, MD. He is the creator of the PBS best-selling DVDs *Firming After 50* and *Slim & Fit.* Harper is also the author of *Mind Your Body: 10 Core Concepts for an Optimally Balanced You.* JoelHarperFitness.com

Forget crowded gyms, clunky dumbbells and fancy exercise machines. If you have access to a wall, you can get a great strength workout using nothing more than the weight of your own body. Bodyweight exercises are a simple, no-frills way to improve strength, flexibility and posture. Because you use a wall for balance, you can hold the positions longer—important for improving endurance as well as strength.

Wall workouts are particularly helpful for those who aren't accustomed to exercise…for people with physical limitations (such as back pain or knee arthritis)…or when you're recovering from surgery or other physical problems.*

The workout below is designed to use every major muscle. To further improve your balance and foot strength, you can also do the routine barefoot. *Aim to do these exercises every other day for two weeks…and if you feel the benefits, continue at the same frequency thereafter…*

*Check first with your doctor before starting this—or any new—exercise program.

•**Imaginary chair.** It's a great exercise for increasing thigh and gluteal (buttock) strength, which is needed to support your spine. Unlike traditional squats, which involve lowering your body and rising back up, in this exercise you hold one position—helpful for those with knee pain or limited knee strength.

What to do: Stand with your back against a wall. While keeping your back in contact with the wall,

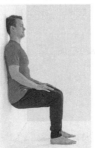

slowly slide your back down the wall while simultaneously walking your feet forward until your legs are in right angles. Go only as far as it feels comfortable for your knees. If your knees start to ache, stop moving forward… a "higher" position is easier for beginners. Once you're "sitting," count for as long as you can comfortably hold the position. Each day, try for 10 more seconds. To help improve your posture, keep your stomach taut, your chin up and your shoulders pressed against the wall.

•**Push-ups.** They strengthen the chest, biceps, triceps and shoulders—all of which promote good posture. Traditional, on-the-floor push-ups are often too difficult for beginners…or for those with limited upper-body strength. Wall push-ups involve the same basic movements but with less re-

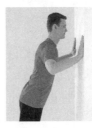

sistance—and they're good for people with back problems because they don't stress the spine.

What to do: Place your palms on a wall at about shoulder height, spaced slightly wider than the width of your shoulders. Back your feet a foot or two away from the wall—stepping farther back increases the difficulty…standing closer to the wall reduces it. Start with your elbows bent. Your face will be close to the wall.

Slowly extend your arms—while exhaling—to push away from the wall. Then inhale while returning to the starting position. Repeat as many times as you comfortably can—ideally, for 30 to 60 seconds.

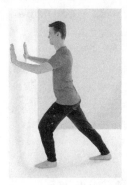

•**Calf stretches.** Strong calves will improve your ability to walk and climb stairs.

What to do: Stand facing the wall, with both hands on the wall and your arms extended but slightly bent—keep this position throughout the exercise. Step back with your right foot. While holding this position, bend your left leg until you feel a stretch in your right calf. You can also slightly bend your right knee and drive

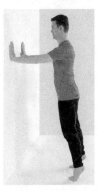

it toward the same toe to increase the stretch. Relax into the stretch, and hold it for 10 seconds or more. Then switch legs and stretch the left calf.

•**Ankle strengthener.** Ankles are a commonly injured body part. People with weak ankles are more likely to have sprains. They are also more likely to have balance problems—the ankles are involved in proprioception, the body's ability to orient itself in space.

What to do: Stand facing a wall, with your feet about hip-width apart. Put both hands on the wall for support. Rise up on your toes, going as high as you can. Hold the position for a few seconds, then slowly lower your heels back down. Do this 25 times.

•**Bridge.** It strengthens the entire midsection, along with the hamstrings, glutes and lower back—all needed for good posture.

What to do: Lie on your back, with your buttocks 12 to 18 inches from the wall. Start by planting the soles of your feet flat against the wall so that your legs make a right angle. Then, while squeezing your abdominal muscles, lift your hips

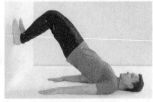

while keeping your shoulder blades flat on the floor. Lift all the way up so that there is a straight line from your knees to

your shoulders, then drop down one inch. This is the height to rise up to each time. Hold the pose for about 10 seconds, then lower back down—but don't let your bottom rest on the floor. Keeping it slightly elevated between movements will increase the intensity of the workout. Do this 25 times.

Is Your Workout Causing the Wrong Kind of Weight Loss?

Kristen M. Beavers, PhD, department of health and exercise science at Wake Forest University, Winston-Salem, North Carolina, and lead author of the study titled, "Effect of Exercise Type During Intentional Weight Loss on Body Composition in Older Adults with Obesity," published in *Obesity.*

Jacqueline Crockford MS, CSCS, an ACE (American Council on Exercise) certified personal trainer and exercise physiology content manager at ACE in San Diego.

You're on a diet, you've ramped up your aerobic exercise, and the numbers on the scale are going down. There's just one problem—this popular weight-loss formula could be causing you to lose so much muscle, as opposed to just losing fat, that you are endangering your strength, stability and, if you're older, continued independence. In fact, a new study shows that combining dieting with aerobic exercise can make people lose more muscle mass than if they didn't exercise at all!

The study: Researchers at Wake Forest University in North Carolina recruited 249 people in their 60s and 70s who were overweight and followed them for 18 months. Each participant was assigned to one of three programs—dieting with no exercise…dieting plus aerobic exercise (which, for this study, was walking)…or dieting plus weight training using weight machines. The two exercise groups worked out four days a week for 45 minutes.

The results: Diet plus aerobic exercise actually led to greater muscle loss than dieting alone. Among those who dieted only (no exercise), 16% of the weight they lost was muscle. Among those who dieted and did aerobic exercise, 20% of the weight they lost was muscle. On the other hand, among those who dieted and lifted weights, just 10% of the weight they lost was muscle.

Weight training won out in another way, too. Participants who dieted and weight trained lost 17 pounds of fat, on average, while those who dieted without any exercise lost just 10 pounds of fat. (The group that dieted and got aerobic exercise lost 16 pounds of fat.)

Now, no one, including the researchers, is saying that dieters should refrain from aerobic exercise—it's essential for heart health and for overall fitness. But this study shows just how important weight training is and why you should add it to your diet plan. For a specific routine to preserve muscle while dieting, see "Finetune Strength Training for Specific Goals" on page 123.

The benefits go beyond the scale: We all naturally lose muscle mass as we age, starting in our 30s. The additional muscle loss from dieting is greater in older people. So while losing excess weight is good for overall health, preserving as much muscle mass as you can with strength training will keep you strong and independent, prevent functional declines and help you avoid falls. Learn more ways to fight muscle loss in your senior years.

Important: If you're new to strength training, ask your doctor if it's OK for you to start, says Jacqueline Crockford, a certified trainer with the American Council on Exercise. Once you get the green light, begin working out two days a week, and as you get stronger, you can work out every other day (muscles need about 48 hours between sessions to recover).

8

Anyone Can Exercise

You Can Exercise Even If You're in a Wheelchair or Stuck in Bed

Marcie Davis, has used a wheelchair for more than 40 years, written articles on the importance of exercise for those in wheelchairs and has worked extensively with physical therapists and certified personal trainer Cat Miller of the Genoveva Chavez Community Center in Santa Fe, New Mexico. Ms. Davis is the chief executive officer of Davis Innovations, a public-health and human service organizational development firm also in Santa Fe. DavisInnovations.com

I f you use a wheelchair—or can't get out of bed because you are recuperating from an injury or long illness—it's important to exercise to maintain fitness, control your weight and prevent stiffness and muscle atrophy.

Good news: It's easy to get the exercise you need. All you need are an inexpensive set of light dumbbells (two to five pounds)…and a little determination. It doesn't take long to strengthen key muscle groups and increase your range of motion.

Important: Talk to your doctor before starting an exercise program. Then, schedule a session with a certified personal trainer or physical therapist who has experience working with people with limited mobility.

Be sure to talk with him/her about shoulder and neck protection.

Exercise-related injuries caused by improper form —or by overdoing it—can be particularly troublesome for those who depend on fewer muscle groups to get around and those who are stuck in bed.

Most people do best when they exercise for about 30 minutes, five or six days a week. If you need assistance to exercise and can schedule only two or three weekly sessions, extend your workouts to 45 to 60 minutes after you become fit enough to handle a session that long.

WARM-UPS AND STRETCHES

Always start your workout with light cardiovascular movements—such as arm circles or shoulder shrugs (if you don't have serious arm or shoulder issues)—for at least three to five minutes as a warm-up.

Stretching is important, too: Do it throughout your workout. I stretch at the beginning and end of exercise sessions, as well as in the middle. People in wheelchairs, or those who are limited to a bed, need to stretch a lot.

For example, focus on the major muscle groups in the…

•**Neck**—lower your left ear toward your left shoulder and hold for 10 seconds…repeat on the other side. Do 10 times total.

•**Chest**—lift both arms (to shoulder height if you can) and extend them out to your sides with

131

palms facing forward. Then move your arms back, pressing your shoulder blades together as much as you comfortably can. Do five times.

●**Hands and fingers**—flex your hand so that your fingers are spread out. Hold a few seconds, then make a fist for a few seconds. Extend your fingers again and use the other hand to gently pull each finger. Do this about six times, then repeat with your other hand.

EXERCISE SESSIONS

Whether you're in a wheelchair or in bed, do each exercise slowly. Unless otherwise indicated, count from one to six from the beginning to the end of each movement. Never hold your breath while exercising. Exhale when you're tightening muscles, and inhale when the muscles are relaxing. *To work the neck, back and abdominals, do…*

1. Side reaches. While sitting in a chair, with your arms relaxed at your sides, twist your torso to the right, letting your arms follow the motion of

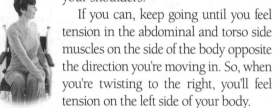

your shoulders.

If you can, keep going until you feel tension in the abdominal and torso side muscles on the side of the body opposite the direction you're moving in. So, when you're twisting to the right, you'll feel tension on the left side of your body.

Slowly repeat a right-center-left movement—stopping in the center before twisting to the other side—10 to 15 times.

If you're in bed, you can work some of the same muscles with an exercise known as a minimal crunch. While lying on your back with your arms at your sides, tighten your stomach muscles and very slightly raise your head and shoulders—don't raise them more than about an inch. Hold the stretch for a few seconds, then relax. Repeat 10 to 15 times or as many times as you can.

2. Neck extension. You can do this exercise while sitting in a chair or lying down. Keeping your

back and shoulders relaxed, gently thrust your neck forward, like a turtle. Go as far as you comfortably can, then ease your neck back. Repeat 10 times.

3. Cardiovascular exercises. Perform simple cardiovascular exercises, such as moving your arms in circles or shrugging your shoulders, for three to five minutes. You can do these move-

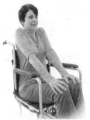

ments while sitting up or lying down. Try to do the movements quickly enough to increase your breathing/heart rate.

Even better: If you go to a gym and it has an upper-body bike (powered by your arms instead of your legs), you can use it to perform similar movements, but at a higher intensity.

To work your shoulders, biceps, wrists and abdominals, start with…

●**Dumbbell raise.**

What to do: Hold the dumbbell vertically. Lay your right hand over your left, and wrap your fingers around the top of the dumbbell. Rest it on your right thigh. Keeping your elbow close to your side, raise the dumbbell until it's almost touching the front of your right shoulder. Repeat 10 to 15 times. Switch sides.

●**Biceps curl.**

What to do: Hold a dumbbell horizontally in your right hand, with your palm up, just above your right thigh. Keeping your elbow close to your side, curl your arm upward until the weight is close to shoulder height. Then relax and lower the weight to the starting position. Repeat 10 to 15 times. Switch sides. *For variety, try…*

●**Dumbbell chop.** Hold the dumbbell vertically. Lay your right hand over your left and wrap your fingers around the top of the dumbbell. Lift the weight at your midline to chest height. Slowly lower the weight at an angle toward your left hip, as though you were chopping wood. Then raise it to the starting position. Repeat 10 to 15 times. Then do the exercise at an angle toward your right hip. Repeat 10 to 15 times.

●**Ab finder.** The goal of this exercise is to work only the abdominal muscles. First, place the fingers of one hand in the area around your belly button. Keeping your shoulders and neck relaxed, tighten the muscles in the abdomen by pulling your belly button back toward your spine. Keep contracting when you feel the muscles tighten—hold the tension for about 10 seconds, then relax. Repeat 10 to 15 times.

4 Best Exercises to Do When You Sit All Day

Tom Holland, MS, CPT, exercise physiologist and certified strength and conditioning specialistbased in Darien, Connecticut. He is the author of *Beat the Gym: Personal Trainer Secrets—Without the Personal Trainer Price Tag.* Team Holland.com

If so many of us are always busy, why are our bodies getting weaker and weaker? It's mainly because we spend so much time sitting! The less we move, the more muscle mass we lose, leaving us vulnerable to injury—not to mention increased risk for obesity, diabetes and stroke. But all is not lost.

Exercise physiologist Tom Holland, MS, CPT, who shares his four favorite exercises for people who are stuck in their chairs…*

EXERCISE #1: No-Hand Get-Ups. When we sit for prolonged periods, our powerful butt muscles or "glutes" (gluteus maximus and gluteus medius) begin to atrophy. Weak glutes can affect posture and movement, which can translate into knee injuries and hip problems as other muscles try to compensate for our deconditioned glutes.

What to do: Start from a seated position. *Then…*

•**Stand up from the chair**—without using your hands to push off or grab hold of anything. That's it.

•**Stand up relatively slowly, to a count of about two seconds.** Extend your arms straight out in front of you to help your balance.

•**Then lower yourself back down even more slowly, to a count of four seconds.** This controlled movement—working against gravity—tones your muscles.

•**Repeat five to 10 times daily.**

EXERCISE #2: Butt-Pain Stretch. When people complain of a mysterious pain in their backside,

*If you are wearing shoes with a heel greater than one inch, take them off before doing these exercises.

the cause is often due to overuse of the *piriformis*, a muscle deep inside the glute that extends from the pelvis to the outer hip. Because the piriformis is a major part of our lower-body infrastructure, that "pain in the butt" is a warning that additional pains (including hip pain and low-back pain) are yet to come if this one is ignored.

What to do: To get a good piriformis stretch and eliminate the pain…

•**Cross your right leg over your left leg so that your right ankle rests on your left knee.** You may feel some tension in the upper-back portion of your right thigh.

•**Gently press your right knee toward the ground, breathing into the stretch.** You should feel a stretch in the muscle deep in your buttocks. You should not feel any stress on the knee itself—if you do, try pressing on the inside of the lower thigh just above the knee. Stretch only as far as is comfortable.

•**Lean slightly forward, and hold the stretch for 10 to 30 seconds.**

•**Switch legs and repeat.** Do two to three repetitions per side a few times a day.

EXERCISE #3: Chair Crunches. This simple exercise works your abdominal core muscles to help prevent low-back pain and other sore muscles and joints.

What to do: To build your core, lean slightly back in your chair. *Then…*

•**Lift both knees up so that you are balanced and your feet are six to 10 inches off the ground.** (If you are sitting on a couch, scoot toward the front of the cushion, lean back slightly and start from there.)

•**Hold that position for 30 seconds…or as long as you can.** This exercise is about time, not repetition. Be sure to keep your shoulders down and relaxed, and remember to breathe normally. Do this exercise once to several times a day.

EXERCISE #4: Twist Stretch. This back stretch sounds more complicated than it is…and once you try it, you'll wonder how you ever got through a day without it.

What to do: To get started, sit up straight with both feet flat on the floor. *Then…*

• **Place your left hand on the outside of your right knee.**

• **Place your right hand on the outside of the right armrest of the chair.**

• **Rotate your upper body to the right.** You should feel a stretch in your lower back. Your head should follow along naturally with your upper body. Stretch only as far as is comfortable. Hold the stretch for a count of five, remembering to breathe throughout the stretch.

Note: If you feel pain, stop—this exercise should not cause any pain.

• **Then switch.** Place your right hand on the outside of your left knee…with your left hand, hold the outside of the left armrest of the chair…and rotate your upper body to the left.

Repeat the cycle (turning once on each side) a total of three times. If you sit for long periods (especially in a confined space, such as an airline seat), try to do this stretch at least once every 15 to 30 minutes.

5 Pilates Moves You Can Do from a Chair

Stefanie Gordon, Pilates Method Alliance–certified Pilates teacher (PMA-CPT), National Academy of Sports Medicine–certified personal trainer, corrective exercise specialist and STOTT Pilates certified instructor, based in Short Hills, New Jersey. Ms. Gordon is also a pre/postnatal Pilates specialist with The Center for Women's Fitness in Chicago.

It seems like everyone, including fitness gurus, celebrities, professional athletes—and probably some of your friends—can't say enough about the core-strengthening, flexibility-building benefits of Pilates. If you haven't tried it yet, maybe it's time! No need to sign up for a class or buy equipment—just get a steady chair (one that doesn't roll) without arms.

While Pilates might seem like a "new" trend, it actually was developed in the 1920s and gained popularity in this country during the 1960s and '70s. Designed as a complete mind-body regimen, Pilates incorporates breath and alignment principles into a full-body workout that strengthens the abdominal, back and pelvic muscles needed for nearly all body movements. Pilates also increases flexibility and helps make your movements more efficient, protecting you from injury as you go about your daily activities.

Pilates—especially more advanced moves—can seem intimidating. But many moves are perfect for beginners.

Below is an easy routine that is suitable for older people who may have less flexibility or anyone who has been sedentary and is just starting Pilates.* Except for the last move, each exercise starts in a seated position with feet flat on the floor, spine neutral (maintain the natural curve of your lower spine) and knees hip-width apart. For the most benefit, do the whole routine two to three times a week.

• **Seated Rotation.** Works the transverse abdominis (the deepest layer of front abdominal muscles—beneath your "six-pack" muscles) and obliques (side abdominals), helps pelvic stability and mid-back (thoracic) flexibility.

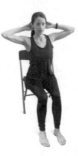

What to do: Clasp your hands behind your head and slowly exhale as you rotate your upper body to the right…and slowly inhale, pulling in your abdominals, as you rotate back to center. Then exhale as you rotate to the left…and inhale as you rotate back to center. Keep your buttocks stable on the seat of the chair. Repeat (center-right-center-left-center) eight times.

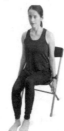

• **Seated Leg Lifts.** Also works the *transverse abdominis*, as well as strengthens hip flexors.

What to do: Keeping your hips stable, inhale as you slowly lift one foot two inches straight up from the floor (your knee should stay bent)… and exhale as you slowly lower your foot back to the floor. Then do the same with the other foot.

*Consult your doctor before starting this (or any new) exercise program.

Important: Tighten your abdominal muscles and feel the lift coming from your abs, not your leg muscles. Repeat the move (alternately lifting each foot) 10 times.

•**Seated Saw.** Encourages mid-back rotation, core engagement and stretches the upper body.

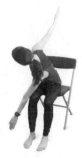

What to do: Start with arms raised straight out to your sides, making a "T" with your torso. In a smooth move, rotate your torso to the right, bending forward to reach down with your left arm to touch your left pinky finger to the outside of your right foot…then straighten back to the starting position…and rotate to the left, bending forward to touch your right pinky finger to the outside of your left foot… and return to the starting position. Repeat the whole move five times.

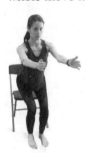

•**Sit-to-Stand.** Targets the transverse abdominis muscles and the major muscles of the legs—quads (front thigh), glutes (buttocks) and hamstrings (rear thigh).

What to do: Sit with arms held straight out in front. Take a breath and exhale slowly as you stand up. Then take another breath and exhale slowly as you slowly sit back down.

Note: Don't crash down onto the chair. If you do, you're not using your muscles enough! Repeat 10 times.

•**Hamstring Stretch.** Stretches the lower back, hamstrings and calf muscles.

What to do: Stand facing a chair, about a foot or so in front of it. Bend forward at your hips and place your hands flat on the chair seat with your

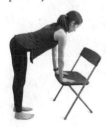

arms straight but elbows not locked. Keep your upper back flat (not rounded) with your pelvis neutral (that is, maintain the natural curvature of your lower spine) and your legs straight but knees not locked.

Take a deep, slow breath in…and then exhale slowly. Repeat the breath pattern for a total of five times.

Alternative: If you can't straighten your legs while leaning on your hands on the chair seat, raise the height of the seat with a couple of large books.

Exercise illustrations: Courtesy of Stefanie Gordon

Feel-Good Exercises You Can Do in Bed

Genie Tartell, DC, RN, sports chiropractor based in Kingston, New York, who was team chiropractor for the New York Reebok aerobic team. She is coauthor of *Get Fit in Bed.*

Think about the last time you really stretched your body. Didn't you feel great afterward?

Unfortunately, most individuals—including many who are physically active—just don't do enough to improve their muscle tone, flexibility and strength. To help people incorporate a simple workout regimen into their daily routines, I have devised a program that can be performed in a comfortable setting you are bound to visit each day—your bed.

These bed exercises not only increase your strength, flexibility and endurance, but also stimulate production of the mood-enhancing brain chemical serotonin, leaving you feeling calm and relaxed. As a result, most people find that they sleep better when they do these exercises at night, and feel invigorated if they do the routine in the morning.

The following exercises are designed for anyone but are particularly helpful for people who are confined to bed (while recovering from an illness or injury) and for those unable to find time during the day to exercise. They can be completed in just 10 minutes a day.

Important: When performing each movement, breathe in slowly for a count of four…hold for a count of one…then exhale through pursed lips for a count of four.

ALTERNATE LEG LENGTHENER

Purpose: Tones and stretches the spine and pelvis, which bears much of the upper body's weight.

What to do: While lying on your back with your body centered on the bed and your hips and legs flat on the bed, stretch your right leg forward by pushing with the heel of your right foot. Return your leg to the starting position. Do the same stretch with your left leg. Repeat five times with each leg.

HIP SIDE TO SIDE

Purpose: Tones and stretches the hips and low back.

What to do: While lying on your back with your hips flat on the bed, rock your hips gently—as far as comfortable—to the right and then to the left. Keep your upper body stable. Repeat five times in each direction.

ARMS-SHOULDER SEESAW

Purpose: Tones and stretches the shoulders and upper back.

What to do: While lying on your back, place your arms at your sides. Slide your right arm and shoulder toward your right foot. Next, raise your right shoulder toward your head, while at the same time sliding your left arm and shoulder toward your left foot. Then raise your left shoulder toward your head, while lowering your right arm and shoulder toward your right foot. Repeat five times on each side, moving your shoulders up and down like a seesaw.

ARMS TOWARD THE HEADBOARD

Purpose: Stretches the shoulders and rib cage, allowing for deeper, much more relaxed breathing.

What to do: While lying on your back, extend your arms behind your head. Stretch your right arm toward the headboard of your bed or the wall behind you. Return your right arm to your side and then extend your left arm behind you. Repeat five times on each side.

ELBOW-KNEE PISTON

Purpose: Strengthens your abdominal muscles while increasing your heart rate (improves heart muscle strength and endurance).

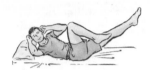

What to do: While lying on your back, raise your knees and, using your stomach muscles, lift your upper body toward them. Bend your arms so that your elbows are pointing at your knees. Bring your left elbow toward your right knee, then return to the starting position. Then bring your right elbow toward your left knee, maintaining a continuous pumping motion. Repeat six times.

COBRA

Purpose: Builds upper body strength (important for daily activities such as bathing and cooking).

What to do: Lie on your stomach with your elbows bent and palms flat on the bed next to your shoulders. Fully straighten your arms to lift your upper body so that it curves into a cobra-like position. Hold for a few seconds, then return to the starting position. Repeat three times.

MODIFIED BOW

Purpose: Tones and strengthens the back and improves muscular coordination.

What to do: Lie on your stomach with your arms at your sides. Raise your legs and upper body simultaneously (only to a level that is comfortable), then reach back with your arms as if you are trying to touch your raised feet. Hold for a few seconds, then return to the starting position. Repeat three times.

SWIMMING IN BED

Purpose: Strengthens the arms and legs, while increasing heart rate and stimulating blood flow throughout the body.

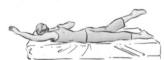

What to do: While lying on your stomach, move one arm forward, then move it back while moving your other arm forward, simultaneously kicking your legs. Repeat 20 times, counting each arm movement as one repetition.

BRIDGE

Purpose: Cools down the body and directs blood flow away from the legs to the heart, reducing risk for blood clots in the legs.

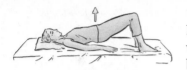

What to do: Lie on your back with your knees bent, feet flat on the bed and your arms at your sides. Tighten up your buttock muscles as you lift your pelvis toward the ceiling—until your pelvis is in line with your thighs. Then gently lower your body back to the bed. Repeat five times.

Important: If you think any of these exercises may be too strenuous for you, check with your doctor before trying them.

Exercise illustrations by Shawn Banner.

The Easy Way to Do HIIT

Robert Zembroski, DC, DACNB, a functional medicine physician, board-certified chiropractic neurologist, clinical nutritionist and director of the Darien Center for Functional Medicine in Connecticut. He is author of *Rebuild: Five Proven Steps to Move from Diagnosis to Recovery and Be Healthier Than Before.*

High-intensity interval training (HIIT) is one of the most exciting trends in fitness, but the word "intensity" can scare away all but the most committed. Exercise is already hard, you may be thinking, and now experts want to make it harder?

Actually, it's the opposite. Most people find HIIT easier than traditional cardio workouts, such as jogging, swimming or even shoveling snow. Compared with cardio training, HIIT more effectively improves your metabolic rate (for burning calories)…and improves your VO2 max—a parameter associated with cardiovascular health—according to research. In addition, it strengthens the immune system.

What most people don't realize: Even though HIIT alternates periods of all-out exertion with periods of lower-intensity exercise, the intense segments of the workout don't have to be too grueling. *Facts you need to know to get started with HIIT…*

THE MAGIC OF HIIT

With HIIT, you exercise as hard as you can for 30 seconds to a minute. (The actual exertion level and duration of the "burst" will vary from person to person.) Then you slow down to a lower intensity for a minute or two…then repeat the hard-easy sequence a few more times. The total length of the workout depends on your fitness level and physical abilities.

It's the "explosive" part of the workout that creates what can only be called "magic." People who engage in HIIT have better cardiovascular health—including improved cholesterol profiles and less insulin resistance—than those who do conventional endurance workouts, according to research published in *Experimental Gerontology.*

EASE INTO HIIT

HIIT is a safe form of exercise, which poses no more risk for sprain/strain injuries than any other exercise regimen. As with any new workout, however, it's a good idea to get the go-ahead from your doctor before starting HIIT.

I tell people who are elderly or have physical limitations—or are merely new to exercise—to start with a low-intensity version of HIIT.

Example: If you're a 65-year-old who has mainly been sedentary, you might start out with a slow walk (the easy part of the exercise at up to 3 mph), then pick up your speed—walking at around 4 mph to 5 mph while swinging your arms for the hard part. After 30 seconds or a minute of fast-walking/arm-swinging, you'd drop back to a stroll for a minute or two, then maintain the cycle for four to five rounds. *To get started…*

Choose your sport. With HIIT, it doesn't matter which activity you choose. You can do the exercise/rest cycles in a swimming pool or on a treadmill or an exercise bike—or using your own two feet. All that matters is that the activity allows you to go all-out for a brief period of time…drop down to a slower level…then go all-out once again. For most people, four of these intervals are enough to get an excellent workout.

•**Don't exercise on an empty stomach.** If you don't have enough blood sugar when you exercise, your body will pull sugar from the muscles first. That's the opposite of what you want to happen. To improve body composition, you want to preserve muscle and burn fat. The best way to do this is to exercise within one to three hours after having a small meal.

Good pre-workout meal choices: A couple of scrambled eggs with a few slivers of avocado and a side of veggies. Or a healthful protein bar such as RXBAR, Oatmega or SimplyProtein Whey Bar.

•**Work with your limitations.** Many of my patients have some physical limitations. They might be overweight...out of shape...or deal with arthritis, leg pain or other minor (or not so minor) disabilities. You can still engage in HIIT—you just have to find what works for you. A personal trainer can offer advice.

•**Go low and slow.** To start, I recommend doing an HIIT workout three days a week, for about 10 minutes each time. You'll slowly increase the total time—by increasing the number of intervals and/or the duration of the exertion/rest components— as you get stronger. Aim to work up to 20 to 30 minutes for each session.

•**Don't forget the warm-up and cooldown.** When you start your workout, whether it's biking, jogging or using a StairMaster, slowly go through these movements for the first few minutes...and shift into low intensity of the same exercise for a few minutes of cooldown at the end of the workout.

Each week, you'll find that you can gradually increase the duration and intensity of the workouts.

Aerobic Exercise for People with Limited Mobility

Karl Knopf, EdD, director of fitness therapy and senior fitness for the International Sports Sciences Association and retired director of adaptive fitness at Foothill College in Los Altos Hills, California. He is author of many fitness books, including *Stretching for 50+* and a board member of Sit and Be Fit, a nonprofit organization dedicated to healthy aging.

Everyone knows about the multitude of benefits of aerobic exercise. But anyone with limited mobility, such as stroke victims and paraplegics, cannot participate in the usual range of aerobic activity.. Fortunately, there are many practical options. *Here are some exercise choices for those with limited mobility......*

IN THE SWIM

Water can be a lifesaver—literally—for the person whose mobility is limited. Water has wonderful capabilities, not least that it presents a range of resistance to the muscles, he said. There are a variety of therapeutic pools designed exactly for this purpose—some where you can use a walker or wheelchair in the water, and also commercially available "swim spas" (also called "counter current" pools, which can often be found in physical therapy centers and are available for installation in private residences as well), where you can adjust the water flow so you can swim in place or walk with more of a challenge, he said.

Water walking can be another option. There are some people who use wheelchairs instead of walking because it's just simpler for them to get around and easier on their joints, but they actually have some ability to use their legs. By using a pool "noodle" (children use these brightly colored, foam-covered tubes as pool toys) under their arms while in the water, a "mobile wheelchair user" can actually float in one place while moving his/her legs as though walking and get a lot of aerobic benefits.

Note: To avoid drowning, exercise caution and never go in the water unsupervised. You might even consider wearing a life jacket or an AquaJogger to make you feel safe in the water.

BICYCLES BUILT FOR YOU

Pedal exercisers (like bicycle pedals but without the bicycle) are easy to find, and easy to use for the mobility-challenged person who retains some (even if not much) ability to move the legs. This unobtrusive, relatively inexpensive (prices typically range from $15 to $40, depending on the materials with which they are made) device is widely available through medical supply stores. It consists of a small frame with pedals on which a "rider" can place his feet while sitting in a regular chair and pedal away, just like a regular bicycle.

ARM-ONLY AEROBICS

For people with absolutely no use of their legs, there are several ways to get aerobic exercise. Many gyms are equipped with a device called an arm ergometer. Almost like an inverted bicycle, there is a seat on which the user sits while grasping a set of "handlebars" which rotate exactly like a bicycle pedaling device but powered by the arms. This provides an excellent aerobic workout with no leg motion necessary whatsoever.

Caution: Arm exercises generally elevate heart rate more than leg exercises, so if you're using one of these devices, don't rely on exercise heart rate to determine your intensity level. Instead, use the rate of perceived exertion. Ask yourself, "How hard is this on a level of one to 10, with one being the least possible effort (like sleeping) and 10 being the most effort you could possibly manage for a few seconds." Aim for a workout that feels moderately challenging. (It's best to get specific advice from your physical therapist or health-care provider on how hard to push yourself.) Another option would be the talk test. If you can't carry on a conversation, you are training too intensely.

YOU CAN DO THIS AT HOME

There are video options, as well. *Sit and Be Fit* (SitAndBeFit.com) is a non-profit organization that produces a television show for seniors and the mobility-challenged (it appears on PBS stations) and also sells a variety of video workouts for people facing physical challenges. With workout videos specifically for people with Parkinson's disease, arthritis, osteoporosis and MS, as well as for those who are mobility impaired, the organization and its products come highly recommended. The "Season 8 Workout" DVD, for example, has a warm-up, a seated circulation workout, seated towel exercises, seated weight workouts and optional leg strengthening and stretching exercises that require standing but not walking. While obviously not like running, these raise the heart rate enough to get substantial benefit.

Of course, for people still able to walk even just a few steps, it's possible to get a workout the old-fashioned way, by just doing it. People using walkers or even wheelchairs might still be able to exercise by walking, albeit very slowly and carefully. And for short exercise intervals, you can stand behind a walker and walk five minutes then rest—and repeat for a few times, building up endurance.

In all cases, it is important that people of limited mobility discuss their exercise strategies with their health-care professional, who can provide a recommendation to a physical therapist in your area. Even one session with a physical therapist can be helpful in planning a home-based exercise program. They are specially trained to provide exactly this sort of advice, and are quite often excellent motivators as well.

An Easy Way to Get Fit at Home

Mark A. Stengler, NMD, naturopathic doctor and founder of the Stengler Center for Integrative Medicine in Encinitas, California. He is author or coauthor of numerous books, including *The Natural Physician's Healing Therapies* and *Bottom Line's Prescription for Natural Cures*, and author of the newsletter Health Revelations. MarkStengler.com

There are all kinds of fitness products marketed to people who are recovering from a stroke or an injury or who have a chronic condition. Many of these products are not worth buying—but I have found and recommend an exercise chair that is helping many of my patients who are frail or sedentary or are recovering from an injury.

The VQ ActionCare Resistance Chair allows you to do a full-body workout from a seated position. It looks like a kitchen or folding chair except that it has several cable pulley systems attached. When you pull or push them, the cables offer smooth, low-impact resistance for building muscle strength in a more user-friendly way than lifting weights. The cables come in eight resistance levels.

Because many of the exercises can be done from a seated position, it is especially helpful for those who may have balance problems or are weak or frail. A balance bar on the back of the chair facilitates standing exercises, such as calf raises or step-ups. One of my patients, a 70-year-old woman with osteoporosis and trouble with balance, was afraid of falling. She now uses the chair and has increased strength and stability.

Other benefits: The chair, which comes with exercise guidelines for specific medical conditions, can help mobility and improve range of motion. It can be used by people who are obese (the chair holds up to 400 pounds) and those who are rehabilitating from cancer treatment or an injury. Those with chronic diseases, such as cardiovascular disease, also can benefit from using the chair. This chair is not for you if you already reap the benefits of an exercise program that includes strength or resistance training.

Optional attachments, such as a stationary bicycle apparatus, can be purchased to expand your workout options.

Important: Consult a doctor before beginning any new exercise routine. For more information about the VQ ActionCare Resistance Chair, call 800-585-4920 or go to VQActionCare.com.

Cost: $279.95.

9

Equipment and Gear Help

The Best Home Gym Equipment for Any Budget

Carol Ewing Garber, PhD, professor of movement sciences and director of the graduate program in applied physiology at Teachers College, Columbia University, New York City. She is a registered clinical exercise physiologist and past president of the American College of Sports Medicine.

There are so many makes and models of home exercise equipment that you could work up a sweat trying to choose which are right for you.

Among the questions you need to consider: Do I really need to spend big bucks to have an effective workout? Which items are built to last? And which will make me want to work out?

Here are some of the best pieces of exercise equipment for different needs and budgets*...

TREADMILLS

Construction quality and warranty length are especially important with motorized treadmills, which take a pounding.

Best overall treadmill: Precor TRM 445 is an extremely durable, gym-quality product backed by an excellent warranty. It features an effective

*Some products listed here were temporarily out of stock at press time because of increased demand and production delays. Prices are the lowest recently available.

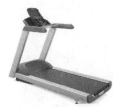

shock-absorption system that reduces stress on knees, hips and feet, and it's capable of creating inclines as steep as 15% and declines up to 2%. It's very quiet, has a 22-x-56-inch running surface and can reach speeds up to 12 miles per hour (mph)—a five-minute mile. $5,199. PrecorHomeFitness.com

Best folding/budget treadmill: Sole F80 doesn't sacrifice durability or running surface area for the sake of compact size the way some folding treadmills do. Its running surface is a big 22-x-60 inches and provides effective shock absorption—it's capable of speeds up to 12 mph and inclines up to 15%, though it does not decline. $1,600. Sole-Treadmills.com

STATIONARY BIKES

It's important that you choose a stationary bike that makes you feel comfortable. The best ones have seats and handlebars that can be adjusted in multiple ways. A "recumbent" stationary bike allows you to sit at a relaxed angle on a truly supportive seat rather than perch leaning forward on a small bike seat. Some high-end bikes offer live spin-class workouts or sessions with trainers on video screens, though that generally requires paying a membership fee. You could skip that and just mount a tablet computer in front of a lower-priced no-membership-fee bike, then use free fitness apps or stream spin-class videos and first-person-perspective rides available for free on YouTube.com.

Best overall upright stationary bike: Diamondback 510ic Indoor Cycle Magnetic Trainer, which has an extremely adjustable seat and handlebars, can fit riders from 5'2″ to 6'5″. This sturdy bike's 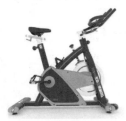 chain drive and 32-pound flywheel provide an admirably smooth ride, while its 16 resistance levels and many preset workout programs help keep those rides challenging and interesting. Its video screen displays data such as speed, distance and heart rate, but if you want a video distraction, you'll have to place it near a TV or attach a tablet. $799. DiamondbackFitness.com

Warning: Fit and comfort are crucial, as noted above, and not even the impressively adjustable 510ic feels right to everyone. Other well-made stationary bikes worth a test ride include the Assault AirBike Classic ($699, AssaultFitness.com)...Concept 2 BikeErg ($990, Concept2.com)...and Peloton Indoor Exercise Bike, which has grown tremendously popular because of its subscription-based live-video spin classes ($2,245. OnePeloton.com).

Best budget/folding stationary bike: Xterra Fitness FB150 Folding Exercise Bike is solidly built for its price range, yet also capable of folding down to an impressive small amount of floorspace when not in use—18.1″ x 18.1″. It features eight resistance settings and, unlike many low-cost models, a useful display screen that provides feedback such as speed, time, distance, pulse rate and calories burned. It's not designed for people heavier than 225 pounds or taller than 5'10″, however, though it does fit riders as short as 4'10″. $149. XterraFitness.com

Best recumbent stationary bike: Schwinn 270 Recumbent Bike is quiet and extremely versatile—with 25 levels of resistance and 29 workout programs, nine of them controlled by the rider's heart rate. There are heart-rate monitors in the handlebar grips, or an optional heart-rate–monitoring chest strap can be added. Its comfortable seat has ventilation and lumbar support, while its "step-through" frame design makes it easy to get on and off, even for riders who have limited mobility. It can support riders up to 300 pounds, though people significantly taller than six feet or shorter than 5'3″ might find it a poor fit. $649. SchwinnFitness.com

Best budget recumbent stationary bike: Marcy Recumbent Exercise Bike ME-709 has impressively solid construction quality considering its low price. Like the Schwinn, it has a step-through design and can handle riders up to 300 pounds, but the ME-709 also can handle riders with inseams of 27 to 36 inches. It has eight resistance settings and—unlike some in this price range—it includes a screen that reports time, distance, speed and calories burned. $209.99. MarcyPro.com

ELLIPTICAL TRAINERS

High-end ellipticals are more likely than cheaper ones to have adjustable stride length, making them appropriate for a greater range of heights and gaits. Better units also offer a greater range of resistance levels and exercise routines.

Best overall elliptical trainer: Sole E95S lets users set stride length from 18 inches up to 24 inches with the push of a button, a range wide enough to accommodate almost everyone. Users also can choose among 20 resistance levels and 10 workout programs, including two controlled by the user's heart rate—pulse sensors are built into the grips, or you can wear the wireless chest strap. The E95S is impressively sturdy—it's capable of handling users up to 400 pounds—and is backed by an excellent warranty. It has moving arms for a full-body workout, and its big 30-pound flywheel provides smooth, quiet operation.

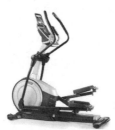

The main downside: It's so solidly built that it can be a challenge to reposition—it weighs 265 pounds. $2,199.99. SoleTreadmills.com

Best budget elliptical trainer: ProForm Endurance 720 E is sturdy and backed by a solid warranty. Its stride length is fixed at 19 inches, but it has moving arms, 20 different resistance levels and a 0%-to-20% adjustable "ramp" angle that mimics an incline. Like many ellipticals, it's heavy—335 pounds. $1,299. ProForm.com

ROWING MACHINES

Different rowing machines produce resistance in different ways. Some use hydraulic pistons, but those provide poor durability and unpleasant, inconsistent resistance. Others use magnetic resistance, which is reliable and very quiet. For a more authentic rowing feel, a few use water resistance where paddles pull through a water tank, or air resistance, where rowing spins a flywheel.

Best overall rowing machine: Concept2 Model D is an air-resistance rower that's durable enough 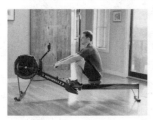 to be used in professional gyms. It separates easily into two sections, making it simple to store away if, for example, you need to convert your workout room to a guest room for the holidays. The Model D is sturdy enough to handle rowers up to 500 pounds even though the unit itself weighs a modest 57 pounds. Users with inseams greater than 38 inches might require an optional extra-long monorail. $900. Concept2.com

Alternative: The Concept2 Model E, costing $1,100, is similar to the model D but with a higher seat that's easier to get on and off.

Best for simulating the feel of rowing on water: WaterRower Classic Rowing Machine does this as well as any rowing machine on the market—resistance results from rotating a flywheel that's inside a small, sealed water tank. With its black walnut frame the WaterRower is more attractive than most exercise equipment, but it doesn't put style ahead of substance. It's so sturdy that its maximum user weight is listed at 1,000 pounds, though users with inseams greater than 37 inches might benefit from the XL Rail Option, which adds $100 to the price. $1,495. WaterRower.com

Best budget rowing machine: Sunny Health & Fitness SF-RW5515 uses magnetic resistance rather than the less desirable hydraulic resistance. Build quality is good for home use, and users with inseams up to 44 inches should find it a good fit, though maximum user weight is 250 pounds. $279.99. SunnyHealthFitness.com

Hand weights, resistance bands and stability balls can all be found for under $20 a set online.

Supercharge Your Workout with a Weighted Vest

Wayne L. Westcott, PhD, a professor of exercise science and chair of the Exercise Science Program at Quincy College in Quincy, Massachusetts. He is coauthor of several books, including *Strength Training Past 50.*

Move over dumbbells and resistance bands… and make room for the weighted vest! This underused piece of exercise paraphernalia is designed to add some heft to a variety of workouts.

Bonus: Even if you're just a casual exerciser, a weighted vest can make your muscles stronger, help you burn more calories and crank up the benefits of your cardio workout.

Important: To make sure that a weighted vest and the workouts described here are right for you, check with your doctor. Use of a weighted vest may not be appropriate for those with osteoporosis, pregnant women, obese individuals and people with orthopedic injuries, especially those affecting the spinal column.

Once you get your physician's go-ahead, a weighted vest can help you…

• **Build lean mass.** A weighted vest is a great tool to combat the age-related loss of muscle mass and strength known as *sarcopenia* and to preserve your ability to complete activities of daily living, such as climbing stairs and carrying groceries.

• **Burn more calories.** Strap on a weighted vest that equals 15% of your body weight and walk at an easy 2.5-mph pace, and you'll burn 12% more calories than a person not wearing a vest, according to research. Wearing a weighted vest has also been shown to feel less taxing than adding intensity by other means, such as increasing speed or walking on an incline.

●**Retain bone mineral density.** In a Canadian study, researchers found that a weighted vest helped reduce bone turnover (a physiological process that fuels bone loss) while reducing body fat and increasing muscle mass in postmenopausal women.

●**Improve walking ability.** Wearing a weighted vest can improve walking ability in people with gait problems caused by conditions such as Parkinson's disease and certain types of palsy.

THE RIGHT VEST FOR YOU

To choose a weighted vest that's right for you, first look for a formfitting vest that covers your chest. If it extends down toward the waist, even better. This will better distribute the weight of the vest without affecting your hip movements when walking. Wide shoulder straps are a plus—they don't interfere with your range-of-motion and put less stress on the shoulders than narrow straps. Also look for a vest that offers a relatively even weight distribution for the front and back.

When determining the weight of your vest, start with 5% to 10% of your body weight. For example, if you weigh 120 pounds, look for a vest with a starting weight of six to 12 pounds. Most vests also have pockets that allow you to add weight packets as you get stronger, but don't exceed 15% to 20% of your body weight.

Helpful: Always add weight gradually—for example, by two-pound increments, adding a one-pound weight to both the front and rear vest pockets to prevent injuries.

3 EASY WAYS TO USE YOUR VEST

If a weighted vest is new to you, it's smart to incorporate it into your existing exercise plan. Consider starting with 15-minute endurance training sessions and progressing gradually by five-minute increments to 45-minute sessions. *You can use a vest for…*

●**Warm-ups.** This will help you quickly engage muscle fibers and raise your core body temperature. Walking at a slow pace with the vest on is the perfect warm-up for weighted-vest walking at a brisk pace. While you shouldn't run with a weighted vest (it creates too much landing force), a pre-run weighted-vest walk can serve as an effective running warm-up.

●**Walking.** You can create a cross training–like program by wearing your weighted vest every other day—go at a slower pace for 20 minutes on the days with it and at a faster pace for 30 minutes on the days without it.

Bonus: On the "off" days, you'll feel lighter and find it easier to increase your pace, which is great for motivation.

Note: Weighted vests may be used in other weight-bearing exercise, such as elliptical training, but should not be used in exercises such as running, as mentioned above, and rope jumping that produce large landing forces.

●**Strength training.** Wear your weighted vest to increase resistance for standing exercises done with a straight torso, such as squats and stationary lunges.

However: To avoid overstressing your back, don't wear a weighted vest for exercises that involve bending your trunk forward or backward or that require horizontal body positions, such as planks and push-ups.

A standard strength-training protocol while wearing a weighted vest is to complete a total of three sets of eight to 12 reps with two minutes of rest between each set. Start with just the vest. You should be able to do at least eight reps in good form. Once you're able to complete 12 reps for each of the three sets, you can add weight to the vest.

Important: The additional muscle stress associated with wearing a weighted vest requires at least 48 hours recovery time between successive strength-training workouts. Although endurance training usually requires less recovery time, an every-other-day protocol is recommended to avoid overtraining syndromes.

Best Way to Track Your Steps

Tom Holland, CPT, exercise physiologist, Darien, Connecticut. TeamHolland.com

If your aim is simply to track your steps and you get frustrated with technology, buy a pedometer (under $20) and just clip it on your belt loop or waistband. Higher-end pedometers will track other metrics (such as calories burned) and will sync to your smartphone or tablet.

An electronic fitness band, worn like a watch, will count your steps, too. Most also measure your heart rate and track the hours you sleep and the calories you burn. Sync the device to your phone or computer to chart your workouts and goals on a graph. These range in price from under $100 to $200, and the battery must be recharged every few days.

Many fitness apps track the same things as an electronic fitness band but require a smartphone, smart-watch or tablet. Some apps are free, others require a fee.

Gear That Makes Exercise Safer and Much More Comfortable

Colin Milner, CEO of the International Council on Active Aging, a Vancouver, British Columbia–based organization dedicated to improving fitness and quality-of-life issues in older adults.

Let's face it. Exercise sometimes hurts. So when we fear that our bodies might rebel, we're tempted to put off exercise or even skip it.

That's a shame because it doesn't make sense to deprive ourselves of exercise—it's hands-down the most powerful health protector there is. So what's the solution?

By choosing the right workout aids, you can dramatically ease the discomfort of key exercise routines. *Here's what works best for…*

STRETCHING

Who among us isn't just a little—or a lot—stiff and achy at times? Stretching is perhaps the best exercise you can do to loosen up those tight, inflexible muscles. It will help limber you up and improve your range of motion—both of which make it easier to do day-to-day activities such as grabbing groceries off a high shelf.

But if you're not very flexible to begin with, stretching is likely to cause some discomfort.

What helps: Gaiam Multi-Grip Stretch Strap ($12.98, Gaiam.com). With multiple handholds along the strap, this product allows you to ease into your stretches with greater control than you could on your own or if you relied on a regular strap without handholds.

WALKING

Walking is the easiest, most approachable workout there is. But if you've got pain due to arthritis, back problems or a hip or other joint replacement… or balance problems, even walking can be difficult.

Adding walking poles helps reduce impact on your joints, normalize your gait and improve your balance. The addition of poles also helps to boost your cardio endurance and increase your caloric burn—with poles, your heart rate will be 10% to 15% higher compared with traditional walking, and you'll burn about 400 calories per hour versus 280 calories.

What helps: ACTIVATOR Poles ($109.99 per pair, UrbanPoling.com). These aren't just any old walking poles. They feature bell-shaped, rubber tips for added grip and reduced vibration. With a doctor's prescription, this product may be covered by insurance.

SWIMMING

Swimming is a great low-impact, whole-body exercise for people who are watching their weight, building cardio strength or looking for relief from arthritis pain.

For the average recreational swimmer, however, efficient breathing can be challenging. Many swimmers feel like they're struggling for air…or their necks tire or become painful from constantly twisting and lifting.

What helps: Finis Swimmer's Snorkel ($29.99, FinisInc.com). Unlike many snorkels, which are designed for scuba divers, this product was created specifically for swimmers. Its adjustable head bracket lets you wear it with a swim cap and/or goggles while allowing you to keep your head in a fixed position so that you don't have to remove your mouth from the water to breathe.

CYCLING

Riding a bicycle is another great low-impact exercise. It has been shown to improve muscle strength and promote lung and heart health. The problem is, traditional bike saddles (on both stationary and road bikes) place a lot of pressure on the perineum (the area between the genitals and the anus). This contributes to pain and erectile dysfunction in men and numbness in women.

What helps: ISM Cruise Saddle ($109.88, ISM seat.com). This is a noseless saddle, which directly supports your "sits" bones (at the base of the buttocks) while easing pressure on the perineum. Research has found that no-nose saddles reduce most perineal pressure in male riders and improve penile blood flow when compared with traditional bike seats. No-nose saddles also reduce numbness in women.

Could a Fitness Tracker Save Your Life?

James E. Ip, MD, associate professor of clinical medicine and director of cardiac pacing and implantable devices at Weill Cornell Medicine's division of cardiology in New York City. He is author of the articles "Evaluation of Cardiac Rhythm Abnormalities from Wearable Devices" and "Wearable Devices for Cardiac Rhythm Diagnosis and Management," both recently published in *JAMA*.

I f you are among the millions of Americans who wear a wrist device that counts your steps, you probably already know that many of these fitness trackers also can monitor your sleep patterns,

nudge you to get up and move when you sit too much and estimate how many calories you burn in a day.

But did you know that some of the newer devices are being credited with saving lives?

Consider these recent press reports...

●**A 73-year-old Connecticut woman with unexplained shortness of breath noticed that her device showed a higher-than-usual heart rate—and it kept getting higher over a period of a few days.** She went to a hospital, and it turned out she had life-threatening blood clots in her lungs.

●**A 34-year-old Utah man noticed his device was showing a much lower-than-normal heart rate.** At his wife's insistence, he went to a hospital, where he learned he had dangerous blockages in two coronary arteries.

●**A 42-year-old man who had a seizure was taken to a New Jersey emergency room, where he was found to have a rapid, irregular heartbeat known as atrial fibrillation (A-fib).** The condition can lead to stroke or heart failure. Because he was wearing a fitness device, doctors asked to see his heart rate recordings, which allowed them to time the onset of his abnormal heartbeats and choose the best treatment.

The people in all of these examples happened to be using Fitbit devices, but the data that alerted them and their doctors to their health risks are available on many devices.

The key feature in most of the devices: A sensor, called a *photoplethysmogram* (PPG), that sits against the wrist and uses light-emitting diodes (LEDs) to continuously detect blood volume changes that can be translated into a heart rate—the number of times your heart beats in a minute.

For a healthy adult who is sitting quietly and not under any unusual stress, the normal "resting" rate is 60 to 100 beats per minute. In general, younger, fitter people have lower resting heart rates.

While consumer fitness devices are not perfect heart rate monitors, they can give you a good estimate of your resting rate and your rate during exercise. When you work out, you want your heart rate to rise. How much your heart rate should increase depends on your age, fitness level and goals. A rule of thumb is that moderate-to-intense exercise should get you to 50% to 85% of your maximum heart rate, which you can calculate by subtracting your age from 220.

Here's what you don't want: A spiking heart rate when you are sitting still or a heart rate that stays sluggish even when you get moving.

What a fast or slow heart rate could mean: A fast heart rate can be caused by a number of conditions ranging from anxiety or dehydration to infection or an actual heart rhythm problem. A slow beat can signal anything from heart damage to sleep apnea to an underactive thyroid.

With most popular devices, you can see your current heart rate on your wrist and check your heart rate history—going back hours, days or weeks—on an app or a website.

At least one device, the Apple Watch, has an additional optional feature—you can set it to send you an alert if a rapid heartbeat develops at a time when the device senses you are not moving much. The watch also can send you alerts for slow heartbeats. The latest version has two more features approved by the FDA—a notification for irregular heartbeats that could signal A-fib and an app that lets you take a brief electrocardiogram (ECG)—a test of your heart's electrical activity. If results look abnormal, the device will urge you to seek medical care.

Some wearable devices, including the Apple Watch, also can detect hard falls. If the wearer seems unresponsive, it can even be set to make automatic calls to 911 or other emergency contacts.

People who may want to consider using a fitness tracker include those who have a personal or family history of cardiac problems…and those who have a medical condition such as high blood pressure or diabetes.

Important: If you have one of these devices, take the time to read through online user guides before deciding whether to turn on the various alerts.

And don't forget the cost. The latest Apple Watch will set you back $400 or more, while other smartwatches and trackers with heart rate detection start at under $100 and go up to around $350. In addition to Fitbit, popular brands include Garmin, Polar and Samsung. *Other considerations…*

●**None of these devices or features is a substitute for medical advice.** If you see something worrisome or confusing, you should always check with your health-care provider.

●**The risk for false alarms is real.** A preliminary report from a study conducted for Apple said that 16% of watch wearers who got a notice about irregular heartbeats were not actually experiencing A-fib. Doctors expect accuracy rates to vary among consumers, with young and healthy users most likely to get false alarms.

●**Risks and benefits remain unclear.** There's no study showing that wearing one of these devices leads to better medical care or outcomes. Even what seems like an obvious benefit—early detection of A-fib—comes with risks. For example, many people diagnosed with the condition are prescribed a blood thinner, which increases bleeding risks. The risks of taking the drug must be balanced against the potential benefit of preventing stroke.

●**Your doctor may not be sure how to interpret data from these devices.** Because medical systems have not yet developed best practices for incorporating the information produced by wearable devices into the patient's medical record, doctors typically handle this issue on a case-by-case basis.

However, there's reason to think wearable devices that monitor our health will only become more common and useful. Paired with data from other connected devices—such as weight scales, blood pressure monitors and blood glucose monitors—they will produce a torrent of data. Consumers and medical providers will have to work through how best to use it all.

In the meantime, if you decide to wear a fitness tracker, speak to your doctor about the data you should be collecting and how to best use it to help protect your health.

How Precise Are Fitness Trackers?

Jung-Min Lee, PhD, assistant professor, Physical Activity and Health Promotion Laboratory, University of Nebraska, Omaha. His study was published in *Medicine and Science in Sports and Exercise.*

Fitness trackers are relatively inexpensive devices that promise to tell you how much exercise you're getting and how fit you are. The idea is that you wear one of these lightweight, computerized sensors (also called activity trackers) on your body or clothing, and it records when you're moving and how you're moving, so that you can learn whether you're getting enough exercise and burning enough calories…or if you should raise the bar on your activity level.

Some fitness trackers are designed to be worn on the wrist, some around the upper arm or as a pendant or a waist clip. Such devices were once used only in research settings, but consumer models are growing in popularity, generally costing between $50 and $150.

But do they really work?

Not precisely, according to several different studies that evaluated different models. But that doesn't mean they're useless. My research team conducted a study that evaluated eight different fitness trackers that claim to use a technology called *indirect calorimetry*, a measurement of energy—or *calorie*—expenditure that uses oxygen consumption as a gauge. The eight trackers included Body-Media FIT, which is a band worn on the upper arm, DirectLife, which can be worn around the neck (or carried in a pocket or attached to a belt), the Fitbit One, Fitbit Zip and ActiGraph, which are all belt clips, and the Nike+Fuel Band, Jawbone UP and Basis B1 Band, which are wristbands.

These eight commercially manufactured trackers were compared with a professional indirect calorimetry device (a unit used in university, government and commercial research) in 60 healthy men and women who wore all of the trackers and the indirect calorimetry device simultaneously. The study participants, decked out in their array of trackers, performed a series of activities that lasted for a total of 69 minutes. They walked on a treadmill at different speeds, reclined, used a computer, ran at different speeds, went up and down stairs, played basketball, and rode a stationary bike. All this time, each device was (supposedly) measuring how many calories the participants burned.

The results: According to the professional-grade indirect calorimetry device, the average energy expenditure was 356.9 calories, but the average of readouts from the various consumer fitness trackers ranged from 271.1 calories for the Basis B1 Band to 370.1 calories for the Fitbit Zip. Although no consumer tracker hit the nail on the head, all except the Basis B1 Band came within a relatively acceptable margin, with error ratings ranging from 9% to 13%. The BodyMedia Fit, Nike+Fuel Band and Fitbit Zip were closest in accuracy to the indirect calorimetry device.

LESS ABOUT PRECISION, MORE ABOUT MOTIVATION

Although our study proved that these consumer-grade fitness trackers are only "OK" when it comes to accurately counting calories burned, they can be worth the money, but with certain caveats.

Reason: Trackers are great motivational tools. Almost all trackers have goal-setting features that allow you to program your desired activity level into them. The tracker will then give you feedback, via communication with your smartphone or whatever other electronic device you've synced it with, to keep you motivated. For example, if you've set a goal to walk 6,000 steps in a day but the monitor determines that you're sitting down, you might get a gentle reminder via e-mail or smartphone to get moving.

Even if your tracker is off by 5% or 10% or so on your calories burned, it's OK because you are also going to use your eyes and your common sense when it comes to assessing your fitness. If your tracker tells you that you are burning the same number of calories that you believe you are eating, but you are still gaining weight, you know what to do. You need to eat less and/or exercise more.

Many trackers also include bells and whistles that allow you to, for example, calculate how many calories you're eating per meal, tally up total activity time or distance traveled (yes, like a good old-fashioned pedometer) or even add up how many calories you've burned while sleeping, though I wouldn't depend on snoozercise for fitness.

There's also a style factor. Most wristbands look more like high-tech watches or jewelry than fitness gadgets. And some trackers, such as Misfit, are waterproof so that they can literally be worn all the time.

Still, about one-third of people who get fitness trackers no longer wear them after three months. Some of this loss of interest can be attributed to purchase of a model that's uncomfortable to wear or otherwise fails to meet a user's expectations.

Recommended: If you are interested in using a fitness tracker, get as much information as possible about different models. Carefully peruse online reviews of actual users to get the pros and cons, and comparison shop at sites such as Top Ten Reviews, which list and rate features, side by side, of the most popular models. Then go to a store that carries several brands to try them on and see how they feel.

Beware: Fitness Trackers Can Hurt Your Sleep

Kelly Glazer Baron, PhD, MPH, a clinical psychologist in the department of behavioral sciences, Rush University Medical Center, Chicago, and lead author of a study published in *Journal of Clinical Sleep Medicine.*

Don't rely on a sleep tracker to improve your sleep on its own. Wearable fitness and sleep-tracking devices, such as Fitbit and the Apple Watch, can help people set goals and track their sleep behaviors but also promise more than they can deliver. They cannot really measure stages of sleep or determine the difference between light sleep and periods of wakefulness. But because they seem to quantify sleep—and sleep seems to be quantifiable, with the common recommendation to get eight hours per night—some people use the devices for goal-setting. That means they go to bed with the goal of finding the next morning that the tracker displays a certain amount of a certain type of sleep.

But for some that behavior produces stress and anxiety that make it harder to get restful, restorative sleep. It can lead to a preoccupation with perfecting sleep, which has been called *orthosomnia*, which means *correct sleep* and is similar to the preoccupation with healthful eating called *orthorexia.* In fact, this fixation on potentially inaccurate or incomplete data can make it harder for therapists to help people with insomnia. Even if much more accurate laboratory sleep studies show deep, restorative sleep, a sleep tracker may indicate that total sleep "restless." A patient who believes that may not respond to treatment—or medical reassurance.

Sleep trackers can even reinforce poor sleep habits by encouraging people to spend more time in bed. That is typically the opposite of what sleep therapists recommend for people who have difficulty falling asleep or staying asleep.

The trackers are already used by 15% of US adults, and another 50% have said they might consider buying one. So the problem of orthosomnia is likely to grow.

Self-defense: Realize that even for the best of sleepers, there are ups and downs, good nights and bad nights, restful and less-restful sleep periods. That is entirely normal. And don't depend on a fitness/sleep tracker to tell you what's really happening with your sleep.

WBV Caution

Dan Hamner, MD, sports medicine physician in private practice, New York City.

Whole-body vibration (WBV) machines do not have FDA approval. Before trying a WBV machine, talk to your doctor, especially if you have a herniated disk, low-back pain, a bone fracture or you are pregnant. Prices for the machines vary widely—from about $400 (Soloflex) to $12,995 (Power Plate models).

What Whole-Body Vibration Therapy Can Do for You

Harold Merriman, MPT, PhD, physical therapist, associate professor, department of physical therapy, University of Dayton, Ohio.

There's been some "buzz" about whole-body vibration (WBV) machines. They're new, improved takes on the "jiggle belt," a weight-loss and fitness gimmick from the 1950s, 1960s and even 1970s. Compared with jiggle belts, WBV machines have sleeker designs and don't include belts. Some designs consist of a platform (sometimes called a "power plate"), and some consist of a platform with an attached stand or a handrail. The user stands on the platform while vibrations continuously pulse from the platform up through the feet to bones and muscles.

Word is that WBV machines effortlessly tone muscles, whisk away weight and get rid of cellulite in minutes per day. In short, like old jiggle belts, these gadgets promise to replace regular exercise.

It sounds too good to be true, but research shows that some of the health claims made by manufacturers of WBV machines are indeed true. But before you invest in a machine, which can range in price from $100 to $18,000, you ought to know what it actually can and can't do.

WHAT WBV MACHINES CAN DO

Research shows WBV improves balance and coordination and increases the strength and mass of muscle and bone in a way similar to traditional muscle-strengthening exercises, such as weight lifting. Weight lifting, as well as walking, stair climbing, jogging and dancing, put stress on muscles and bones, which stimulates them to grow stronger. The vibrations of WBV machines seem to have a similar effect—so much so that they are now being used in physical therapy and in sports training.

WHAT NOT TO EXPECT FROM WBV MACHINES

A major claim of both old jiggle belts and purveyors of many state-of-the-art WBV machines is that they can help you lose weight and cellulite.

Unfortunately, WBV has no direct effect on cellulite or weight loss. However, because muscles burn body fat for fuel when they are being worked, you may shed a pound to two while a WBV workout is strengthening and toning your muscles.

As for whether WBV can replace regular exercise, clearly, no. WBV will never replace aerobic exercise, such as walking, stair climbing, jogging and dancing, because it does not give your heart a workout. It can't completely replace weight training because WBV focuses mostly on your lower body and only somewhat on your core. You need to do regular weight-training exercise to fully work your core and upper body. Some physical therapy programs use WBV machines combined with other traditional forms of exercise to enhance strength and balance with less effort.

Although manufacturers of WBV machines say that 15 minutes a day at a frequency of three times a week is all that's needed to benefit, more research is needed to determine how much time should be spent on a WBV machine and that it probably differs from person to person depending on age, fitness and health status.

SAFETY CONCERNS

Home WBV machines generally are safe as long as they are used according to the manufacturer's directions, which include limiting daily use. It is known that headaches, nausea and neurologic symptoms, such as tingling and numbness, can occur in people who have jobs that expose them to repeated and prolonged vibration (forklift-truck operators, for example). Therefore, people need to limit initial WBV use to five or 10 minutes a day and then to continue at a moderate pace. To minimize the chance of side effects, physical therapists instruct users to stand on the WBV machine platform with knees slightly bent. Doing so works as a shock absorber.

So, although WBV may not get you out of "real exercising," it can be a useful muscle-toning and strengthening add-on to traditional aerobic and muscle-strengthening exercise routines.

Resistance Bands Offer an Irresistibly Fun Workout

Wayne L. Westcott, PhD, a professor of exercise science and chair of the Exercise Science Program at Quincy College in Quincy, Massachusetts. He is coauthor of several books, including *Strength Training Past 50.*

Here's a flexible way to do strength training, especially while traveling—working out with large, colorful rubber bands called "resistance bands." They're easy to use and can add variety to a strength-training regimen. As long as you use proper form and sufficient tension or resistance, they offer an excellent workout.

WHY STRENGTH TRAINING IS A MUST

Strength training—so often overshadowed by more popular aerobic exercise—is vital to our health. With each decade after age 30 we lose an average of five to seven pounds in lean body mass. Not only does strength training prevent this loss, it can reverse it and help you build new muscle... and more muscle means more stamina, more energy and better health overall. Strength training also preserves bone density, lowers blood pressure and helps you maintain a proper weight.

The American College of Sports Medicine recommends a minimum of two strength-training sessions a week and workouts should generally include eight to 10 exercises (eight to 12 repetitions each) using major muscle groups. Set aside at least one day of rest between workouts.

RESISTANCE BANDS: THE PROS AND CONS

As with all types of strength training, working out with resistance bands (also called "cords" or "tubes") can deliver significant improvements in body composition, strength and endurance. But as with any exercise, it's also a matter of personal taste. There are both pros and cons.

What's great about resistance bands...

●**They're inexpensive.** Most bands cost between $5 to $20. A kit—which typically includes several bands with different levels of resistance, along with a door attachment and an exercise chart—typically runs anywhere from $20 to $50. The more expen-sive kits include accessories like sport towels and storage bags.

●**They're portable.** This is why I love to travel with a set of resistance bands. I toss them into my carry-on bag so I can work out when I get to my hotel. Resistance bands are terrific for people who live in small spaces and for those who want to squeeze in a mid-day workout at the office.

●**They're versatile.** Resistance bands work for all fitness levels—beginner, intermediate or advanced. When it begins to get easy, just move on to a thicker band with greater resistance.

●**They're simple to use.** Working out with resistance bands is a cinch. *For example...*

To work the biceps (upper arm muscles): Stand on the band and grip handles with both hands. With knees slightly bent, slowly bend arms and bring hands toward shoulders in a biceps curl.

To perform a chest press: Wrap the band around a stable object (or use the door band attachment), and face away from it. Hold handles in both hands, and sit or stand far enough away from the object to create tension in the band. Begin with arms at your sides. Squeeze your chest as you press arms out in front of you.

On the other hand...

●**Resistance bands are more subjective than weights.** When you're working with free weights (barbells or dumbbells) or weight machines (such as Nautilus or Cybex), you know exactly what weight you're lifting, and can increase or decrease as you wish. Things aren't so clear-cut with resistance bands, which are more a matter of guesswork and how you feel.

●**Resistance bands offer a different type of resistance than free weights.** Actually, this can be seen as either a pro or a con. On the plus side, enthusiasts say that bands offer more continuous resistance (since gravity is not a factor, as it is with free weights), so you get a better, more consistent workout. But serious athletes counter that barbells and dumbbells deliver a far more intense workout.

THE RIGHT WAY TO USE RESISTANCE BANDS

It's easy as anything to get started on resistance band workouts. Pick up a kit on-line or at any sporting goods store.

Dr. Westcott's favorite: Resistance bands from SPRI Products. Bands come in a variety of resistance levels—very light, light, medium, heavy and ultra heavy. The thickness of the bands determines their level of resistance and they're often color-coded to help you remember which is which. Most beginners are fine with light bands... only relatively frail individuals would need to start with extra-light resistance bands. The bands come in different lengths, sometimes even packaged for men and women.

There are lots of types of bands, but you'll do best to start off with a few of the simple, standard long ones with handles in a variety of resistance levels. A door attachment is a must-have, since it enables you to work your leg, arm and back muscles by pulling a band attached to the door.

Note: Make sure the door is locked so nobody walks in when you're doing your exercises.

Other helpful tips include...

• **Choose the right bands.** Beginners should start with thinner, lighter-colored, lower resistance bands. If you're an experienced weight lifter, go with thicker, dark-colored bands that offer more resistance. The key is to use a band that is thick enough to fatigue the target muscle within 30 to 90 seconds of repetition of an exercise.

• **Extend bands in a slow and controlled fashion.** Begin with a series of eight to 12 reps of each exercise (depending on your fitness level), and take your time. The more you control the pace of your exercises, the more your muscles will benefit.

• **Mix it up.** As with free weights and weight machines, avoid putting undue stress on any one muscle group, which can lead to next-day soreness or even injury. Instead, start with one set of repetitions to the upper body, work your way down to the abs and on to the quads.

• **Exhale while stretching band...** inhale when band is shortening.

• **Take a drink.** Avoid dehydration. Always keep water handy during any workout.

• **Cool down.** Always follow up with gentle stretches after challenging your muscles with strength exercises.

Whatever form of strength training you choose—whether you want to give resistance bands a try, or you're loyal to your free weights—make sure you make it a regular part of your fitness plan. And for those of you who haven't yet started strength training, resistance bands may be just the right place to start.

Get Powered Up with Medicine Ball Workouts

Daniel Taylor, MS, a performance enhancement specialist (PES) and certified strength and conditioning specialist (CSCS). Taylor is a conditioning coach at Siena College in Loudonville, New York, and coauthor of *Conditioning to the Core.*

You probably don't think of yourself as an "athlete," but adopting a secret from the pros will help you stay as strong and fit as possible. More and more professional athletes, including football and soccer players, are now adding medicine ball workouts to their exercise regimens—and you can, too.

You've probably heard of medicine balls. Originally made out of animal hide, they date back to ancient times and were used for the same reason we use them today—to increase strength and cardiovascular fitness. Modern medicine balls, typically made out of rubber, leather or nylon, come in a variety of sizes and weights, ranging from one pound to 50 pounds and costing as little as $12 to about $100.

What can a medicine ball do for you? Plenty! Throwing and catching a medicine ball is a plyometric exercise—that is, it combines stretching and contracting movements to build strength, speed and endurance. Medicine ball workouts are particularly effective for people with chronic conditions that improve with consistent strength training (such as osteoporosis, back pain, diabetes or high blood pressure)...and/or those who don't have much gym experience. Barbells, machines, kettlebells (heavy weights with handles) and other gym equipment can be intimidating if you are new to them—balls are not. Medicine balls are comfortable and fun to use!

YOUR CORE CURRICULUM

Medicine ball training primarily addresses the core—all those muscles in your abdomen and lower back. Strengthening these muscles is particularly important to help prevent back pain, improve posture and make everyday movement easier.

There's no one-size-fits-all weight for the ball. You want one that you can throw...but if it doesn't require much effort to do so, then you should go a bit heavier. Most beginners start with six- to eight-pound medicine balls. People with an intermediate level of fitness can use a 10- to 12-pound ball...and those who consider themselves very physically fit may use a ball that is 15 pounds or heavier.

The following workout is a great complement to a regular exercise regimen that might include aerobic activity, such as regular walking or running, and stretching exercises. Adults at various fitness levels can perform the exercises below. Do them two to four times per week on nonconsecutive days.*

●**Push-up.**

Purpose: Strengthens the chest, shoulders and abdomen, which improves strength for carrying heavy items.

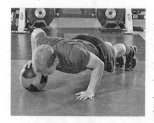

What to do: While lying facedown on the floor, position your body next to a relatively solid medicine ball. Place your right hand on the ball and your left hand on the floor. Lift your body so that your left hand and toes are the only parts of your body touching the floor while your right hand is on the ball. The

*Check with your doctor before beginning medicine ball workouts—or any new exercise program. This is especially important if you have osteoarthritis, heart disease and/or diminished hand-eye coordination.

ball may feel a bit unstable—if you can't control it, prop the ball against a wall. Then simply do a push-up with one hand on the ball and the other hand on the floor. Repeat eight to 12 times. If this is too difficult, do the push-up with your knees on the floor.

●**Overhead slam.**

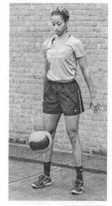

Purpose: Strengthens the shoulders, back and abdominals for core fitness.

What to do: Stand with your feet parallel and hip-width apart. Slightly bend your knees. While holding the ball, extend your arms in front of you, then raise the ball overhead. Next, throw the ball as hard as you can at the floor, then catch the rebound. Repeat eight times.

●**Side throw.**

Purpose: Strengthens the shoulders, back, side abdominals and hips for better turning movements (such as golf swings) and to help prevent falls.

What to do: Kneel on a gym mat parallel to a wall (about your body length away). Your right

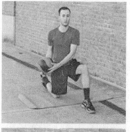

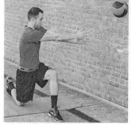

knee should be on the mat while your left leg is bent at a 90-degree angle with your foot flat on the floor. Tighten your glutes (buttocks) and abdomen to create stability. Throughout the exercise, maintain a completely straight body alignment for maximum effectiveness. Using both hands, hold the medicine ball to the side of your waist about a hand span away. Rotating through your shoulders (not your lower back), throw the ball as hard as possible in a baseball-swing fashion against the wall. Perform eight repetitions. Repeat on the opposite side.

Medicine ball photos provided by Human Kinetics

Kettlebells—A Unique Way to Get Fitter Faster

Michele Olson, PhD, professor of exercise physiology at Auburn University at Montgomery in Montgomery, Alabama. A certified strength and conditioning specialist, she is the creator of the DVD *10 Minute Solution: Kettlebell Ultimate Fat Burner.*

For a full-body workout, it's hard to beat a kettlebell, a round weight suspended below a handle. Because the weight is distributed unevenly, maneuvering a kettlebell recruits core muscles. The workout also builds other muscles, boosts bone strength and promotes cardiovascular fitness.*

To begin: Using an eight- to 12-pound kettlebell (about $30 at sporting-goods stores), start with just a few repetitions ("reps") of each move, increasing reps as you improve. Keep abdominal muscles tight...don't arch your back...don't drop the weight...do wear low-profile (not platform-soled) athletic shoes.

Resource: The DVD *10 Minute Solution: Kettlebell Ultimate Fat Burner.*

TWO-ARM SWING

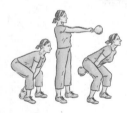

Start: Stand with feet slightly wider than shoulder-width apart, toes angled out, kettlebell on the floor between your legs, several inches behind your heels.

Swing: Bend knees, keeping spine straight and chest up...grasp handle with both hands...straighten legs, push hips forward and swing arms out in front to raise kettlebell to shoulder-height...bend knees, dropping arms so kettlebell moves between thighs... continue swinging for desired number of reps.

SHOULDER PRESS

Start in "rack" position: Stand with feet slightly wider than shoulder-width apart, knees slightly bent, kettlebell in your right hand, elbow bent, fist positioned in front of shoulder joint, kettlebell resting on the back of your forearm.

*Check with your doctor before beginning any exercise program.

Press: Straighten right arm so kettlebell is directly above right shoulder (keep wrist straight)... bend arm to return to start position...repeat. Switch to the left hand.

WEIGHTED SQUAT

Start in the rack position (described above).

Squat: Slowly bend knees, sticking out your rear end (as if taking a seat in a chair) and keeping your knees above your ankles, chest up and back straight. Continue lowering hips until thighs are parallel to the floor...slowly rise to start position...repeat. Switch kettlebell to the other hand.

STIFF-LEG LIFT

Start: Stand with feet shoulder-width apart, toes angled out slightly, arms straight down in front of you, holding kettlebell at hip-height with both hands.

Bend and lift: Keeping arms and back straight, bend knees slightly and hinge forward at hips... lightly touch kettlebell to floor in front of you... contracting buttocks muscles, straighten knees and return to start position...repeat.

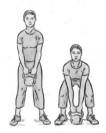

Caution: Skip this exercise if you have low-back problems or osteoporosis—it can strain a weak back or spine.

TACTICAL LUNGE

Start: Stand with feet together, arms straight at your sides, kettlebell in your left hand.

Lunge: With left leg, step back about 24 inches, landing on ball of left foot...bend both legs, lowering left knee until right thigh is parallel to floor...

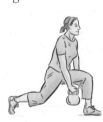

pass kettlebell beneath right thigh, switching kettlebell to right hand...step left leg forward to starting position. Repeat, stepping back with right leg and switching kettlebell to left hand.

Illustrations by Shawn Banner

Desk Chairs That Make You Healthier

Steven Weiniger, DC, a member of the postgraduate faculty at Logan University in Chesterfield, Missouri and managing partner of BodyZone.com, a national online information resource and referral directory for posture-exercise professionals. A past delegate to the White House Conference on Aging. he is author of *Stand Taller, Live Longer*.

What's not to love about a desk chair that can make you stronger and healthier?

As it turns out, there are quite a few intriguing seating options. Some chairs are designed to improve your posture…some put exercise equipment at your fingertips…and some are designed to encourage subtle, ongoing movement. Steven Weiniger, DC, a faculty member at the Logan College of Chiropractic in St. Louis and author of *Stand Taller, Live Longer* shares his expert input on some of these interesting seating choices.

FOLDING CHAIR PLUS EXERCISE CABLES

The VQ ActionCare Chair has a molded vinyl seat and back and is built on a simple metal frame. It looks something like a classic folding chair—and it actually does fold up for storage. It incorporates exercise cables attached at both the bottom of the frame and shoulder height. It is marketed as a fitness tool, since you can use the resistance cables periodically throughout the day…and as something that is useful for senior citizens who want to add more movement to their day. Though he acknowledges it to be convenient, Dr. Weiniger does not feel it works as a "desk chair," especially given its price—he suggested that as long as you aren't chair-bound because of illness or injury, you could get better results by buying a set of resistance bands and an exercise ball for less money and more functionality. Dr. Weiniger points out that sitting all day and just adding some upper-body exercise is not the solution. The lack of motion in sitting is the problem…training some muscles to be stronger is not stretching the muscles and joints, which get tight during long durations of sitting.

LIKE SITTING ON AN EXERCISE BALL

The Gaiam Balance Ball Chair combines an exercise ball and the same type of resistance cables mentioned above, and it can be really fun to sit on. Picture a black plastic frame that looks like a modern sculptor's vision of a chair…but with an exercise ball firmly planted in the seat area…exercise cables with handles attached to the bottom (to be used for bicep curls, shoulder presses and other strength-training moves)… and locking casters on its feet. Even though the casters do lock, Dr. Weiniger warns that these chairs can be unstable. The balance ball itself is removable for separate exercise, and the unit comes with a resistance cord, toning band and 105-minute workout DVD. The ball is also available in a variety of interesting colors, including sage and plum. Dr. Weiniger had some concerns about whether a person could sit comfortably for long periods in this chair. "Though the model in the advertisement is sitting straight, there's no way that she won't slump after a while," he said, adding that as core muscles tire, the pelvis will tend to rock back.

He also noted that since the ball is fixed in place in the chair, it's not able to roll. "That's the goal of sitting on an exercise ball in the first place," he noted, explaining that a rolling ball forces a reflex stabilization of deep muscles—while a stationary ball does not. You would do better simply sitting on an exercise ball, since it requires small muscle adjustments.

KNEELING CHAIRS

Kneeling chairs first became popular in the 1970s. They have no backs, and the seats are angled somewhat down, putting the sitter in a modified kneeling position. The idea is that this chair encourages better posture by distributing the weight evenly between the knees and pelvis, sliding the hips slightly forward and aligning the neck, shoulders and back. Proponents observe that a forward-angled seat promotes a more natural curve to the spine. It is also believed that the kneeling position reduces spinal compression and increases blood flow throughout the body. Dr. Weiniger's opinion? "The biomechanical idea behind this is very intelligent, but some people—those who are overweight, for example—have knee problems. This posture can create extra pressure, straining the knees." And the chair doesn't allow you to shift positions, so Dr. Weiniger says it may not be a good choice for people who sit at their desks for long hours. Available from various manufacturers and online for $89 to $379, depending on materials used.

SADDLE CHAIRS

Picture a small horse saddle on a post—like a bar stool—and you've got an idea of what a saddle chair looks like. Many manufacturers make these chairs. Their selling point is that you'll sit in a position that's halfway between standing and sitting, something akin to horseback riding. This position allows the legs to drop and spread in a very natural way. I can tell you, though, that you wouldn't want to try to sit in one if you're wearing a pencil skirt! Dr. Weiniger said that putting the sitter in a position that lets the pelvis roll forward reduces stress and facilitates motion in the low back—and added, "This is a very comfortable position that allows for easy control of your body." Made by many companies and available in office-supply stores, and online, including Amazon.com and Staples, $149 to $199.

SHOPPING SMARTS

Dr. Weiniger had a few shopping tips for anyone and everyone in the desk chair marketplace—even those looking for more traditional chairs...

•**Any desk chair you buy should allow you to easily change your sitting position,** because locking into one position is often a problem. After our review, however, it is clear that few do. That is why after sitting for a while you need to stand up and stretch. Your work habits should include changing your position in the chair during the day. This helps to distribute stress over more muscle fibers and joints and leaves you much less tense.

•**Choose a chair that allows you to sit with your back straight and shoulders wide**—meaning not pressed together across the front of the body, but open. Dr. Weiniger explained that most

people tend to sit in a "folded-in position" which, done for long periods, actually causes your chest muscles to shorten.

•**Look for a chair that has an adjustment allowing you to tilt the seat forward slightly.** "This lets you roll your pelvis forward, and forces you to lean back and engage the spinal extensor muscles as well as strengthening the lumbar curvature," Dr. Weiniger said. "Your head will be more on top of your shoulders and your torso will be on top of your pelvis, all of which makes for better body alignment."

Dr. Weiniger pointed out that "most of us know it's smart to invest in a good mattress, but the reality is many of us spend more time sitting at our desks than sleeping." It makes sense to put some thought—and even invest some money—in the chair where you spend so many of your waking hours.

Get More Fit While You Sit

Craig Horswill, PhD, clinical associate professor of kinesiology and nutrition, University of Illinois at Chicago.

Sitting for long stretches—particularly more than 60 to 90 minutes at a time—is bad news for your health. In fact, one study linked 7% of all deaths in adults age 45 and older (even for those who exercise regularly) to excessive sitting.

Many people—and companies—have spent a lot of money to equip offices with standing desks and desks connected to treadmills so that workers can stay more physically active while they work.

Recent development: A new product, tested by scientists at the University of Illinois at Chicago, helps sedentary workers burn calories by increasing movement—while sitting. The HOVR is a movable footrest that is installed on the underside of a desk to help counter the negative effects of sitting by allowing users to swing or twist their legs while working. (Another version has a floor stand that eliminates the need for installation.)

How it works: The aim is to increase non-exercise activity thermogenesis—that is, the calories you burn in non-sportslike activity, such as typing, fidgeting or climbing a flight of stairs.

In a study, the HOVR raised users' metabolic rates (the rate at which your body burns calories while at rest) by 17%, compared with 7% for those standing at a desk. The increase in metabolic rate is probably less than that for an under-desk Exercycle or treadmill desk, although the HOVR may be less distracting.

Where to buy: SitFlow.com

Cost: About $69 for the desk-mount swing and $119 for the floor stand version.

Note: There are similar types of products available online.

The Right Clothes for Every Sport

Pete McCall, MS, CSCS, independent exercise physiologist and consultant and ACE-certified personal trainer based in San Diego. He is author of *Smarter Workouts: The Science of Exercise Made Simple* and host of the *All About Fitness* podcast. McCall has taught for both the American Council on Exercise and the National Academy of Sports Medicine. PeteMcCallFitness.com

If showing up to exercise is half the battle…wearing the right gear is the other half. A simple cotton shirt can ruin a day of skiing, while an added sweat-wicking base layer could keep you hiking or snowshoeing comfortably for hours. And shoes with cleats or clips let you tackle your indoor cycling with far more gusto—and fewer injuries—than sneakers.

Fabrics and designs for sportswear have become very high-tech. Investing in a few key pieces can help you get the most out of all of your workouts…

FOR: OUTDOOR WINTER SPORTS, SUCH AS SNOWSHOEING AND SKIING.

When outdoor temperatures drop, you need to dress in clothes that draw perspiration away from your skin as you exercise, yet trap heat to keep you comfortably warm and protected from the elements.

Here's why: Not only does sweat that sits on your skin feel uncomfortable as you exercise in cold weather, it also leaves you chilled and prone to hypothermia. In the old days, even "thermal underwear" was cotton—but cotton traps moisture and remains cold and damp next to your skin, increasing the risk of chafing and making a cold day even colder.

What to wear: Aim for two to three strategically chosen layers depending on the temperature and activity level. For your base (next-to-skin) layer, choose a lighter moisture-wicking material, typically a synthetic fabric such as polyester and nylon, often labeled Coolmax or Supplex. These come in different weights to be used in different temperatures. Many brands and styles are available for between $20 and $50, but they're all very similar in quality.

Your second layer is your insulating layer, which will help preserve body heat while allowing perspiration to dissipate. Try wool or synthetic fleece, which is warm. There's a wide price range, from fleece T-shirts at Uniqlo for $15 to fleece crew neck long-sleeve shirts at LL Bean for $40 to REI wool shirts for $120.

For a third layer—especially if it's snowing or windy—add a water- or wind-repellent top layer made with a breathable fabric, such as Gore-Tex, which will keep the heat in and the wind and moisture out.

FOR: WALKING AND RUNNING

Besides staying warm, when on the move, you need to protect your muscles from overexertion and fatigue so that you don't get sidelined by injuries. For this, many athletes and trainers have taken a page from the medical world, by using compression technology to help recirculate blood and oxygen more effectively.

What to wear: Once the domain of professional competitors, compression leggings, socks and arm sleeves now are being worn by everyday athletes looking to get more out of their workouts. Not everyone agrees that they make a difference but there is mounting evidence that recovery is faster with them. These leggings and socks feel snug—far tighter than traditional leggings but not as tight as the medical compression stockings commonly worn for varicose veins. Compression leggings promote better venous return, the flow of deoxygenated blood from the muscles back to the heart. Blood and oxygen circulation is improved throughout the lower body and/or arms, which can make workouts such as walking and running feel easier.

Recent finding: In a 2019 study, subjects walked for 30 minutes on a treadmill without compression leggings and a week later while wearing ones with 20 mmHg to 30 mmHg. (The degree of compression is measured in mm, millimeters of mercury, or Hg. The higher the number, the tighter the fit.) Wearing the compression garments led to a reduction in perceived exertion, meaning that you can work out longer.

Look for a very snug but not uncomfortable fit—the goal is to squeeze blood from your legs back up toward your heart. It should be difficult to pinch the fabric and pull it away from your body, but the pants shouldn't dig into your skin or cut off your circulation.

Note: People with varicose veins or other pre-existing conditions should consult their healthcare provider before wearing compression gear.

FOR: STRENGTH TRAINING

Look around the weight room the next time you're there. Most people are in running or cross-training shoes. But these actually may put you at risk for injury. Cushiony running shoes absorb impact when running. But when worn while executing, say, a squat or a standing shoulder press, the squishy sole can throw you off balance.

Here's why: In strength training, you receive feedback from the ground through your feet. Your feet basically act like data receptors, feeling the ground beneath you and sending messages up through your nerves and muscles, telling your brain how to stabilize your body as you lift the weight.

If you have a half inch of rubber between your feet and the ground, you lose out on that important feedback. Watch someone squatting in running shoes with a barbell across his/her back, and you'll notice his feet wobbling side to side and back and forth. That also forces you to expend more energy than necessary, so you'll tire out faster. Running shoes in particular tend to have an elevated heel, pitching your body slightly forward—helpful when running but not when strength training. The tilt places excess pressure on the muscles in the front of your lower body while neglecting your hamstrings and glutes. This forward pitch also increases knee injury risk when strength training.

What to wear: Buy minimalist shoes specifically made for weight lifting, or look for a flat, lightweight, flexible shoe with a minimal heel drop (the difference between the height of the heel and the ball of the foot) and comparatively thin sole. You want a wide toe box that allows your toes to spread out, so your feet can mold to and grip the ground.

FOR: SPINNING

If you're one of the more than 35 million Americans trying indoor cycling, you know what an intense, exciting workout it can be. But if you're wearing regular gym shoes, you may be cheating yourself out of the safest, most effective workout possible.

Here's why: Cycle-specific shoes have a stiff shank, the supportive structure that sits between the insole and outsole, and cleats, a metal or plastic mechanism that secures your foot to the pedal. Both features help transfer more power from your body into the bike on the downstroke. You derive the majority of your power on the upstroke from being clipped in with your cleats. Without this, you end up working harder for the same momentum and speed.

Also: Without the security of cleats, feet can cramp as your toes and forefeet struggle to stay on the pedals.

What to wear: Special cycling shoes with cleats. In some cycling classes—such as those offered at SoulCycle—these shoes are a requirement. (If you don't have your own, they will rent them to you). Flywheel provides free shoes, or people can bring their own. Both companies' bikes are compatible with Look Delta cleats. If you're taking at least two classes a week, it's worth it to invest in your own cycling shoes.

Look for a shoe that's cycle-specific, with cleats built in.

Try: Shimano IC5 Indoor Cycling Shoes for women ($125, Zappos.com) or Flywheel Sports Indoor Cycling Shoe ($128, Amazon.com)…Gavin MTB Mountain Bike Mesh Indoor Fitness Cycling Shoes for men or women ($64.95, Amazon.com).

MORE FROM PETE MCCALL, MS, CSCS

The Way to Stay Dry Down There

Up to 20% of women have reported quitting their physical activities because of bladder leakage caused by bouncing, jumping or other high-impact moves. But a new generation of undergarments, called leak-proof underwear or absorbent underwear, uses innovative materials in the gusset (crotch) to absorb leaks while feeling dry to the touch. These materials often are antimicrobial, moisture-eliminating and odor-resistant.

Try: The Speax brand, which comes in multiple styles, from hiphugger to thong, sizes XS to 3XL (and in some styles, bigger) and can hold up to eight teaspoons of urine without feeling wet ($28 to $39, SheThinx.com).

Suit Up to Beat the Heat

Tom Holland, MS, CPT, an exercise physiologist, certified sports nutritionist and certified strength and conditioning coach. He is author of *The Micro-Workout Plan: Get the Body You Want Without the Gym in 15 Minutes or Less a Day* and hosts the podcast "Fitness Disrupted" on iHeartRadio. Team Holland.com

---

Do hot days leave you feeling listless? There's a reason—in the sweltering heat, your body must devote much of its energy reserves to maintaining a safe internal temperature, leaving you with little left in the tank for other activities.

Beyond placing yourself in front of the air conditioner, there are several surprising ways to maintain your energy levels when the mercury climbs…

●**Cool your neck and the insides of your wrists.**

For a deeper, more lasting chill, freeze a wet bandana and wristbands before donning them. Or use items specifically designed to hold the cold, such as the Mission Enduracool Reflective Cooling Headband ($14.99) and the Chill Pal 12 in 1 Multi Style Cooling Neck Gaiter Face Cover ($8.97). Instant-cold packs also are helpful to keep in your bag.

If you're stuck out in the heat without these items, buy a cold beverage in a can or bottle and hold it against your neck and/or the insides of your wrists before drinking. This helps maintain your energy in two ways—the cold container cools your blood…then consuming the drink helps you stay hydrated. As you probably already know, dehydration is a common cause of energy depletion on sweaty days.

Helpful: If a cold sports drink such as Gatorade or Powerade is available, choose that. If you've been sweating, the carbs and electrolytes that it provides truly will help your body restore its hydration and energy levels—that isn't just empty marketing. For people who want to avoid sugar, a good choice is mineral water, which naturally contains electrolytes, instead of sugary drinks. Or you can eat a piece of fruit.

Don't worry about whether you drink caffeinated or noncaffeinated beverages—caffeine ingestion during exercise does not have the diuretic effect commonly believed. But don't overdo it with caffeinated drinks on hot days either. Soda, iced tea and iced coffee can be tempting beverage options, but excessive caffeine consumption after the morning hours can make it hard to fall asleep.

●**Cover up with breathable, sweat-wicking fabrics.** People tend to show skin when it's hot, donning tees, tanks, skirts and shorts that leave their limbs exposed. But even if you use sunscreen responsibly and avoid sunburn, the sun's heat on that exposed skin can drain your energy over the course of the day.

If you're going to be in direct sunlight for a significant amount of time on a hot day, it's better to cover your limbs with loose-fitting, light-colored garments made from sophisticated synthetic fabrics that are designed to allow heat to escape and wick sweat away from the body.

Examples: Under Armour Iso-Chill, Arctic Cool and Nike Dri-FIT make garments for men and women. For professional wear, there's Rhone's Commuter Dress Shirts for men ($118) and Long Sleeve Delta Pique Polo for men ($92). Lululemon offers Everlux garments for women, such as In Movement leggings ($98).

Also, wear a visor or a brimmed hat made from a a breathable, sweat-wicking fabric. This will keep you cool by keeping sunlight off your face and won't trap heat around your head.

Example: Under Armour Airvent Iso-Chill Fish Cap, $28.

• **Exercise inside, using equipment such as a treadmill, elliptical machine or stationary bike…** or with simple exercises you can do anywhere, such as squats, push-ups and planks. But before starting these indoor exercises, set up one or more fans aimed at the spot where you will be doing your workout and set them to high speed. (Be sure to do this even if your home is air-conditioned.) The breeze will allow your sweat to evaporate, which will cool your skin.

If you don't want to skip your outdoor exercise on a hot day, at least schedule it for early in the morning or late evening, when temperatures are cooler.

Warning: If you experience potential symptoms of heat stroke, such as faintness, dizziness, confusion, rapid heartbeat or rapid breathing, seek hydration right away…bring your body temperature down as quickly as possible with ice packs, cold drinks and/or cool showers…and seek medical attention immediately.

How to Choose the Right Athletic Shoes

Vahan Agbabian, clinical instructor and rehabilitation specialist, MedSport sports medicine program, University of Michigan Health System, Ann Arbor.

When you work out or play a sport, your shoes affect your performance—and your risk for injury.

Key: Choose sport-specific footwear.

Examples: Tennis shoes have side support and flexible soles for fast changes in direction…running shoes give maximum shock absorption…walking shoes need low heels that bevel inward so feet roll easily through the stride. *Also…*

• **Learn your foot type.** Ask a podiatrist or athletic trainer…or visit a shoe store that offers computerized foot-type analysis.

Wide feet: A too-narrow shoe leads to shin splints, so if even wide-size women's shoes feel tight, try men's shoes.

High arches: Look for a shoe with a thick, shock-absorbent heel, such as a gel heel or air bladder.

For feet that roll inward: You need a deep heel cup and wide mid-foot base.

For feet that roll outward: Choose a somewhat rigid shoe.

• **Check a shoe's flexibility by bending and twisting it.** It's too flexible (and thus can lead to ankle sprains) if it bends at mid-sole instead of the ball…flattens at the heel cup…or wraps like a towel when twisted. A shoe that's hard to bend or twist is too rigid (except for cycling) and may cause shin splints.

• **Know when to purchase a new pair.** Wear and tear affect a shoe's ability to support and protect. Replace sports shoes after they've taken about 500 miles' worth of steps. If you're a walker or runner, that's easy to calculate. Otherwise, replace shoes when treads and heels are visibly worn.

Do Compression Braces and Sleeves Work for Knee Arthritis?

Barbara Bergin, MD, orthopedic surgeon, Texas Orthopedics, Sports & Rehabilitation Associates, Austin. DrBarbaraBergin.com

I sometimes tell patients to apply any kind of sleeve or brace because it has a *proprioceptive* effect. That refers to your brain's ability to sense where your bones, joints and muscles are—even without looking—and take steps to control their function and position.

In other words, the presence of something around the knee—even a piece of duct tape or Kinesio Tape, a type of therapeutic elastic adhesive tape that can be worn for extended periods of time—can actually send more sensory information to the brain, making it more aware of the extremity. Then the brain can send subconscious, corrective impulses down to that extremity—in essence, increasing awareness of the affected part so that your body unconsciously adjusts muscles and joints to accommodate them as you move about.

I often give the example of a pinky toe. You might think your pinky toe is just sitting there limp, resting inside your shoe. But it's not. Your brain is subconsciously putting it there. It's not sticking it up in the air. It's not shoving it down into the sole of your shoe. Now, tell your brain to stick the pinky up in the air. That's not proprioception.

That's your conscious brain directing your toe to go there. But let's say you have a blister on your pinky. Now you're not going to walk around all day saying "Brain! Bend my toe down away from my shoe." Instead, proprioception will eventually take over. The leather on your shoe will act as a messenger to your brain, much as a brace might for your knee, and your wonderful brain will guide that toe away from the abrasive leather.

Proprioception is one reason why a lot of folks with arthritis like the feel of having a sleeve or brace on their knee or anywhere on the body for that matter, such as an ankle sleeve. It's why athletes like to use compression braces and sleeves, tight clothing and Kinesio Tape.

Wearing a compression brace will not directly prevent your knee from twisting in a way that might injure it. But it may help your brain's awareness of your body in space so that you might avoid moves that could cause further injury and pain.

While compression garments and wraps have no potential to cure disorders of bones and joints for those suffering with arthritis or patients with injuries, they just seem to feel better. That's a good enough reason, if you want to try one of these garments or Kinesio Tape—or even an Ace bandage. See if it helps. And yes, you could even try duct tape, a kind of primitive version of Kinesio Tape. It might work quite nicely—although it's going to hurt like hell and give you a waxing when you take it off!

PART II:
Healing Fitness Strategies

10

Better Balance and Bone Health

Catch Your Balance Problem Before It's Too Late: These Easy Exercises Could Save Your Life…

Jason Jackson, MSPT, a physical therapist in the outpatient rehabilitation department at Mount Sinai Hospital in New York City, where he specializes in balance training, along with prosthetic training, manual therapy and neuromuscular disease.

No one expects to get seriously injured—or even die—from a fall. But it happens all the time. And while older adults are at greatest risk for falls, there are no age requirements for taking a tumble.

Surprising statistic: Even among adults in their 30s, 40s and 50s, falls are the leading cause of nonfatal injuries (more than 3 million each year) that are treated in US hospital emergency departments. For adults age 65 and older, falls are the leading cause of fatal injuries.

Certain "fall hazards" are well known—electrical cords and area rugs…slippery floors…medications such as sleeping pills and blood pressure drugs…vision problems…and even poorly fitting shoes.

What often gets overlooked: Subtle changes in the neuromuscular system (the nervous system and muscles working together), which helps keep us upright. Regardless of your age, exercising and strengthening this system before you get unsteady (or fall) is one of the best steps you can take to protect your health. *Here's how…*

WHY OUR BALANCE SLIPS

Does your foot or ankle feel a little wobbly when you stand on one leg? Some of that is probably due to diminished strength and flexibility. After about age 40, we begin to lose roughly 1% of our muscle mass every year. As we age, we also become more sedentary and less flexible. These factors make the body less able to adapt to and correct a loss of balance.

The nervous system also gets less sensitive with age.

Example: Sensory receptors known as *proprioceptors* are found in the nerve endings of muscles, tendons, joints and the inner ear. These receptors make us aware of our bodies in space (*proprioception*) and can detect even the slightest variations in body positions and movements. But they don't work well in people who don't exercise them (see suggestions on next page)—and these people find it harder to keep their balance.

The other danger: Muscle weakness, even when it's slight, can lead to apprehension about losing your balance. You might then start to avoid physical activities that you feel are risky—walking on uneven pavement, for example. But avoiding such challenges to your balance actually accelerates both muscle and nervous system declines.

ARE YOU STEADY?

If you're afraid of falling or have a history of falls, a professional balance assessment, done by your doctor or a physical therapist, is the best way to find out how steady you are on your feet. *The assessment usually includes tests such as the following (don't try these tests on your own if you feel unsteady)…*

•**Sit-to-stand.** Sit in a straight-backed chair. If your balance and leg strength are good, you'll be able to stand up without pushing off with your hands.

•**Stand with your feet touching.** You should be able to hold this position for 15 seconds without any wobbling.

•**The nudge test.** Ask someone to gently push on your hip while you're in a normal stance. If you stagger or throw out your hands to catch yourself, your balance is questionable. If you start to fall, your balance needs improvement.

BOOST YOUR BALANCE

Balance, like strength and endurance, can be improved with simple workouts. Incorporate the exercises below into your daily routine—while at the grocery store, in the office, while watching TV, etc. Do them for about 15 minutes to 30 minutes a day, three to four days a week (daily if you have the time). *What to do…**

•**One-legged stands.** You don't have to set aside time to do this exercise. You simply stand on one leg as you go about your daily activities—while waiting in line, for example. Lift your foot about six inches to 12 inches off the floor to the front, side and back. Try to hold each position for about 15 seconds, then switch legs. This strengthens the muscles in the ankles, hips and knees—all of which play a key role in one's balance.

*Do these exercises next to a stable object, such as a countertop, if you feel unsteady. Also, they are more easily done while wearing shoes. When you feel comfortable doing these moves, you can perform them barefoot to add difficulty.

•**Heel raises.** This move is good for balance and strength. While standing, rise up on your toes as far as you can. Drop back to the starting position, then do it again. Try for 10 repetitions. You can make this exercise more difficult by holding weights. Start with three-pound weights, gradually increasing weight as you build tolerance.

FOR MORE BENEFITS

Once you have become comfortable with the exercises described earlier, you can up your game with the following to keep you even safer from falling…

•**Balance on a Bosu ball.** It's a rubberlike half-ball (about two feet in diameter) that you can use for dozens of at-home workouts, including balance and abdominal exercises.

Cost: About $100, on Amazon.com and in some sporting-goods stores.

Example: With the flat side on the floor, start by standing with both feet on the ball. Your muscles and joints will make hundreds of small adjustments to keep you balanced. When you get better at it, try to stand on one leg on the ball. When you're really comfortable, have someone toss you a basketball or tennis ball while you maintain your balance.

JUST FOR FUN

You don't always need formal balance exercises. *Try this…*

•**Walk barefoot.** Most of us spend our days in well-padded shoes that minimize the "feedback" between our feet and the ground. Walking without shoes for at least a few minutes each day strengthens the intrinsic muscles in the feet and improves stability. If you prefer to wear socks, be sure to use nonslip varieties that have treads to avoid slipping on wood or tiled floors.

Also helpful: Minimalist walking/running shoes. They're made by most major footwear companies, such as New Balance, Adidas and Nike, as well as by Vivobarefoot. Because they have a minimal amount of heel cushioning and arch support, they give the same benefits as barefoot walking but with a little extra protection.

What's Really to Blame for Your Balance Problems

Victor M. Romano, MD, a board-certified orthopedic surgeon in private practice in River Forest, Illinois, where he specializes in sports medicine. He is also a clinical affiliate faculty member at Midwestern University Chicago College of Osteopathic Medicine and a clinical assistant professor at Loyola University in Chicago. He is author of *Finding the Source: Maximizing Your Results—With and Without Orthopaedic Surgery.* RomanoMD.com

If you feel a little wobbly on your feet, you may chalk it up to the fact that you're simply growing older. After all, when your muscles, joints and vision don't work as well as they once did, it can destabilize you—making a fall more likely.

No one wants to break a hip and end up using a walker or living in a nursing home, so you're probably doing your best to prevent a disabling fall. But are you doing all you can to address the underlying causes of poor balance?

To learn about these hidden culprits, we spoke with Victor M. Romano, MD, a board-certified orthopedic surgeon who diagnoses and repairs ailing bones, joints and muscles. In his practice, he has learned about unexpected issues that can sabotage balance.*

THE MISALIGNMENT PROBLEM

The medical community has almost entirely ignored two scientific papers published just over a decade ago in *Practical Pain Management*, which uncovered a missing link in the role that chronic pain and muscle weakness play in causing poor balance.

The problem: If a joint (where two bones connect) is out of correct alignment, the body unconsciously compensates to restore stability. For example, if one of the joints in the right foot is out of alignment, the body unconsciously overuses the left foot. This "compensation" causes left knee pain, weaker muscles on the right side—and poorer balance. Because there are more than 300 joints in the human body, it can be challenging to find a misalignment—even for an orthopedic surgeon!

*Check with your doctor before starting this—or any new—exercise program.

Dr. Romano's solution: A series of simple stretches that I have developed and successfully used in my practice over the past five years—called the Romano Stretches—prevent or correct nearly every misalignment that can cause balance problems. By doing these stretches, you will help restore your balance, relieve aches and pains, improve strength and flexibility—and, in turn, prevent falls.

THE ROMANO STRETCHES

The following stretches address the most common areas where misalignment occurs in the human body, leading to balance problems. *Do the stretches daily—you can complete them all in just a few minutes...*

●**Pelvic stretch.** Restoring pelvic balance improves your side-to-side balance and range of motion of your shoulders. You will feel this stretch in the lower back and buttocks.

What to do: While lying flat on your back, grab your right knee with your left hand and bring your knee across your body toward the left side 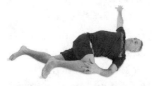 of your chest. At the same time, stretch your right arm and shoulder to the right, keeping them on the floor. (See above.) Turn your head to the right for an additional stretch if you desire. Hold for five to 10 seconds. Next, do the exercise on the other side, grabbing your left knee with your right hand, and stretching your left arm and shoulder to the left while turning your head to the left if you desire. Repeat twice on each side of your body.

●**Hip stretch.** This stretch helps restore alignment in the back and neck—and is excellent for reversing loss of balance and restoring mobility of the 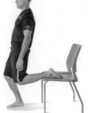 hip. You should feel this stretch in the top of your thigh, particularly toward the hip.

What to do: While standing about six to 12 inches in front of a chair, bend your right leg at the knee so that your foot (toes pointed) and a few inches of your shin rest on the seat of the chair. Lean back to feel a stretch in your right groin. Then slowly bend your left knee slightly to get a deeper stretch. Hold the stretch for five to 10 seconds and return to an upright position. Then do the same stretch with your left leg on the chair behind you, bending your right knee. Repeat twice on each side.

If you feel unstable while doing this stretch: Use a chair with arms and hold onto them as you lean back or stand next to a sturdy counter or desk to steady yourself.

•**Rib stretch.** A misalignment in the ribs can cause pain and weakness in the upper back, neck, shoulders, hands and elbows—all of which can contribute to poor balance. You should feel this stretch in your upper back and ribs.

What to do: While standing, bend your arms to a 90-degree angle and bring your elbows out to your sides, parallel to the ground and just below shoulder level. Forcefully and quickly, pull your elbows backward in two short bursts and repeat two to three times.

•**Back stretch.** This stretch is excellent for relieving upper and lower back pain. Patients with this problem have impaired balance when moving their heads up or down or turning side to side. This stretch should be felt in your lower back.

What to do: While standing, put your fists against the small of your back and arch your back as far as you can for five to 10 seconds. Relax and slowly exhale while stretching. Repeat two to three times.

4 Ways to Build Better Balance

Carol Clements, MA, who has more than 45 years of experience as a personal trainer and teacher of many movement arts, techniques and methods. She is also author of *Better Balance for Life* and works privately with clients in New York City. CarolClements.com

When it comes to health risks, most people can rattle off a list that includes being overweight, eating an unhealthy diet and sitting too much. Few people would think to name poor balance as a serious danger…but they should.

Balance is a crucial but under-recognized element of good health. Unfortunately, loss of muscle strength and other factors cause us to become more wobbly as we age. So it's no surprise that one of every four adults age 65 and older in the US reports falling each year.

The good news is, balance is a skill that you can improve. *Here's how…*

GETTING STARTED

Feeling insecure about your balance can lead to a fear of falling, which will inhibit your daily activities—and actually increase your risk of falling. Practicing your balance will help you gain more confidence and overcome any fear you may have.

Important: Balance problems can be caused by a variety of medical conditions. Some of the most common causes are abnormalities in the vestibular system (the inner ear)…weak muscles or unstable joints…less visual acuity…certain medications…alcohol…and various neurological disorders, including peripheral neuropathy—especially involving nerves of the feet. Your doctor can rule out any medical problems that may make balance practice unsafe or give you the go-ahead to begin the regimen described below.

4 BALANCE BOOSTERS

To improve your balance, a good strategy is to fit a few targeted moves into your everyday activities. Within a matter of days, you'll begin to incorporate them into your daily routine—and without even breaking a sweat. *My favorite everyday balance boosters can be done while…*

•**Watching television.**

What to do: While sitting, take off your shoes and socks, prop one foot up on a coffee table or the couch, and interlace your fingers between your toes. Use your fingers to spread out all five toes so that they are not touching one another. Maintain this position for one minute. Relax. Repeat on your other foot. Then alternate flexing and pointing each foot 10 times. Finally, try to wiggle each toe one at a time. This may be difficult at first, but remember that you will improve with practice. These relaxed micro-movements of the foot are an important part of standing and balancing.

- **Brushing your teeth.**

What to do: Lightly place the fourth (ring) finger of your nonbrushing hand on the edge of the sink or vanity, so as you stand, you have that bit of support from your finger on the counter but are not holding on tightly. (Use this finger, since it is capable of only light touch to steady yourself.) Move one foot slightly behind you and off the floor. This exercise will force you to adjust your center of gravity and recruit more hip and core muscles to stabilize yourself. Alternate feet morning and night, optimally for as long as it takes you to brush your teeth. If you lose your balance at first, touch the nonstanding foot to the floor lightly to steady yourself and calmly resume balancing.

To up your game: Stand on one foot *without* touching the sink…then with your free arm extended overhead.

- **Talking on the phone.**

What to do: Stand up. With your feet hip-width apart and your knees directly over your ankles, imagine yourself squeezing a balloon between your shins. This squeezing motion, called adduction, will strengthen your adductor muscles of the inner thighs and hips to help keep you stable.

- **Walking down a hallway.**

What to do: Find a safe, clear hallway and walk down it backward at least once a day.

This exercise requires coordination of reversed foot mechanics and the transfer of weight in the less familiar backward direction. The first time you do this, look over your shoulder and count the number of steps it takes until you reach the end. After that, you can count out that number of steps in your head while keeping your gaze forward. If you feel unsteady, reach out to the wall on either side of you or have someone with you. Gazing forward is easier on the neck, and you can't use sight to orient yourself in the familiar forward direction.

Most important: In addition to these exercises, find an enjoyable activity that keeps you on your feet. Whether it's dancing, playing table tennis, flying a kite or walking your dog, the more you move, the better your balance!

To Check Your Balance, Start With This Self-Test

Carol Clements, MA, who has more than 45 years of experience as a personal trainer and teacher of many movement arts, techniques and methods. She is also author of *Better Balance for Life* and works privately with clients in New York CIty. CarolClements.com

Balance is a critical element of your overall well-being. But it's not something you can take for granted. It can decline almost imperceptibly, and a dangerous fall can happen in a split second.

A frightening trend: Deaths from falls are on the rise in the US, according to a 2018 report from the Centers for Disease Control and Prevention. The number of people age 65 and older who died as a result of a fall jumped from 18,334 in 2007 to 29,668 in 2016. While the reasons for this steep increase are not fully understood, good balance is undoubtedly among the best defenses against this serious danger.

If you're concerned about your balance, be sure to discuss it with your doctor. There can be a variety of underlying causes. If you think your balance is fine, give yourself the following quick self-test to see just how steady you really feel on your feet.

What to do: Stand upright, with your feet together, behind a sturdy chair. Cross your arms over your chest and slowly close your eyes. If necessary, place one hand on the seat back for support. Do you feel stable? Wobbly? Nervous? Notice how you react to this balance challenge. (By excluding sight, you rely on your body's use of sensory nerve endings and other body-orienting input that contributes to achieving balance.)

It's a good idea to tell your doctor about your results—and to repeat the self-test periodically to informally check on your balance.

Beware of This Hidden Cause of Falls

Maura Cosetti, MD, director of the Cochlear Implant Center at the Ear Institute of the New York Eye and Ear Infirmary of Mount Sinai in New York City, with Rebecca Shanonhouse, editor-in-chief, health content, Bottom Line Inc. Dr. Cosetti is also associate professor of otolaryngology and neurosurgery at Icahn School of Medicine at Mount Sinai in New York City.

If you're hearing isn't as good as it used to be, you already know that just making a simple phone call can sometimes be difficult. Untreated hearing loss also has been linked to more serious dangers—increased risk for dementia, depression and even cardiovascular disease, to name a few.

Here's another risk you might not know about. The sounds that you hear (or don't hear) can strongly affect your risk of falling. Even mild hearing loss—the kind that can make conversations challenging—can nearly triple the risk.

Yet when doctors evaluate patients who have suffered falls, the leading cause of deadly injury for older Americans, they tend to focus on vision, neuropathy in the feet or bone problems, without giving a second thought to hearing, says Maura Cosetti, MD, director of the Cochlear Implant Center at the Ear Institute of the New York Eye and Ear Infirmary of Mount Sinai in New York City. That's a mistake.

We all use sound information to keep ourselves balanced, especially in cases where other senses, such as vision or proprioception (our awareness of the position and movement of the body), are compromised, she explains.

Sadly, even though one in three older adults has some degree of hearing loss, about 85% don't use hearing aids or receive other forms of treatment.

People who notice symptoms of hearing loss—muffled sounds, tinnitus or a sensation that one or both ears are blocked—should get a hearing test. Medicare and most private insurers pay for annual audiologic evaluations, along with some hearing-related tests.

Your hearing is precious...and well worth caring for!

The Secret to Preventing Falls: Don't Wear Thick-Soled Sneakers

Hylton Menz, PhD, professor and National Health and Medical Research Council senior fellow at La Trobe University in Victoria, Australia. He is the author of the textbook *Foot Problems in Older People: Assessment and Management* and a coauthor of *Falls in Older People: Risk Factors and Strategies for Prevention.*

Each year, more than one in every four people over age 65 suffers a fall, a mishap that is far more dangerous than most people realize.

Important research: In a 20-year study of nearly 5,600 women ages 70 and older, breaking a hip doubled the risk for death in the following year. Men who suffer a broken hip after a fall are also at increased risk for an untimely death.

Most people know the standard recommendations to reduce their risk for falls—get medical attention for balance and vision problems...improve the lighting in and around their homes...and eliminate loose carpets, cords and other obstacles.

What often gets overlooked: Painful feet...foot deformities such as bunions...weak foot and ankle muscles...and improper footwear also can significantly increase one's risk for falls.

Scientific evidence: In a study in the *British Medical Journal*, a comprehensive program of foot care reduced falls by one-third among a group of older people with assorted foot problems.

GET A FIRM FOUNDATION

With age, the muscles that support our ankles and feet often become weak—a common problem that contributes to foot pain and reduced activity levels. Structural abnormalities in the feet, such as bunions and hammertoes, undermine stability. And conditions that blunt sensations in the feet, such as nerve damage commonly caused by diabetes, may impair the ability of one's feet to react quickly and adjust to potentially hazardous conditions.

BASIC FALL-PREVENTION WORKOUT

Stretching and strengthening exercises can reduce foot pain—and lower your risk for falls. *Basic exercises to perform daily...*

● **To increase your ankles' range of motion.** Sit in a chair with one knee extended. Rotate your foot in a clockwise, then counterclockwise direction. Repeat 10 times with each foot, in each direction.

● **To strengthen your toe muscles.** Place small stones or marbles on the floor in front of you. While seated, pick up the stones with your bare toes and place them in a box, one by one. Pick up 20 stones with each foot, then repeat.

● **To stretch your calf muscles.** Stand about two feet from a wall, then lean into it with one leg slightly bent at the knee about three inches in front of the other. Then reverse the position of your feet and lean forward to stretch the muscles of the other calf. Hold the stretch for 20 seconds, three times for each leg.

PROPER FOOTWEAR

The right shoes are essential for everyone, but especially those with problem feet.

Most women know to avoid high heels, which make it more difficult to maintain balance. But many people opt for flimsy slip-on footwear, such as flip-flops, which may be comfortable but often become loose or come off the foot altogether, creating a balance hazard. It's far better to wear shoes that fasten to your feet with laces, Velcro or buckled straps.

Surprising fact: Most people assume that thick, cushiony soles, such as those found on most sneakers, help prevent falls because they tend to provide good support for your feet. But thinner, harder soles, such as those on some walking shoes, are safer because thin-soled shoes allow your feet to feel the sensations that help you maintain balance. A trade-off between comfort and safety may be necessary—you may have to wear less cushiony shoes that optimize balance.

Also, be sure that your shoes are the right size. Your feet may slide around in shoes that are too loose, while tight footwear won't allow your toes to respond to variations in the ground to help maintain stability while walking.

Remember: Shoe size often changes with age, as feet swell and spread. So have your feet measured every time you buy shoes.

Slightly more falls occur indoors than outdoors, and the proportion increases with age. Therefore, even when you're at home, proper footwear is crucial.

Important recent finding: When researchers at Harvard's Institute for Aging Research followed a group of older adults for more than two years, they found that more than half of those who fell indoors were barefoot, in their stocking feet or wearing slippers. These injuries tended to be more serious than those of people who were wearing shoes when they fell.

Best to wear at home: Sturdy, thin-soled shoes that have more structural integrity than the average slipper.

DO YOU NEED ORTHOTICS?

Many adults over age 65 could benefit from wearing orthotics—inserts that fit inside the shoe—to help prevent falls by providing additional support.

Properly made orthotics may improve the way your feet move as you walk, distribute your weight more broadly to reduce pressure on sensitive spots and help convey sensory information to your feet, all of which may lessen the risk for falls.

If you have structural foot problems due to diabetes or rheumatoid arthritis, you may need customized orthotics from a podiatrist.

Typical cost: About $400. Insurance coverage varies. But over-the-counter versions (made with firm material, not just a soft cushion) may work as well if your feet are relatively normal and your foot pain is fairly mild. Good brands include Vasyli and Langer. Usually, you will be able to transfer orthotics between shoes.

Most people find that full-length orthotics are less likely to slip inside the shoe than the half-length variety. Full-length orthotics also may feel more comfortable, especially if you have corns or calluses under the toes or on the ball of your foot.

GETTING HELP

If you have foot problems, seek care from a podiatrist or other health professional—and be sure to mention any concerns about falling. Also ask for exercises, in addition to the ones described here, to address your specific foot issues.

Agility Exercises That Prevent Falling

Michelle Gray, PhD, assistant professor of kinesiology, department of health, human performance and recreation, University of Arkansas, Fayetteville, and codirector, Office for Studies on Aging, College of Education and Health Professions, also at University of Arkansas.

Agility, meaning the ability to quickly change speed and/or direction, decreases with age. That, in turn, increases the odds of falling—for instance, when someone darts out in front of you unexpectedly—setting the stage for the bone fractures that can rob you of your mobility, your independence and even your life.

Self-defense: Safeguard your agility with an easy and fun workout that you can do at home using an inexpensive type of exercise equipment called agility cones. And if you think you're too young or too fit to benefit from agility cones, think again. Pro football players do versions of this workout all the time—and they know what works!

Agility cones look like those orange traffic cones you see on the highway, but smaller. They are typically six to 12 inches high and can be purchased at sporting-goods stores or online for as little as $2 apiece. You'll need four cones—but if you want to give this agility workout a try right now, you can start out by using overturned plastic drinking cups or empty plastic jugs. Then if you like the workout and want to stick with it, go ahead and invest a few dollars in the cones—with their bright color and stabilizing base, they'll be easier to see and less likely to topple than a cup or jug.

Michelle Gray, PhD, assistant professor of kinesiology at the University of Arkansas, recommends the following workout. The movements promote agility because they require the vestibular (balance) system of the inner ear to work in concert with the muscular systems, especially the very fast-twitch "type IIx" muscle fibers that allow you to move suddenly.

Do the workout at least twice a week. Use a long hallway or large room indoors…or go outdoors.

Make sure that you're on a surface free of any objects you could trip over.

Throughout: Move as quickly as you can while still maintaining control—don't push any faster than you can safely go. Try not to knock over any cones, since object avoidance is part of being agile. For each exercise, complete two or three sets, taking a brief rest between sets.

If you have a history of falls: Stick with just the first easy exercise until your agility improves and you feel confident about moving on to the intermediate and advanced exercises…and check with your doctor each step of the way.

●**Easy: Up-and-Go.**

Setup: Place one agility cone eight feet in front of a sturdy chair. Sit in the chair.

Move: Rise from your seated position, walk quickly to the cone, maneuver around it in a clockwise direction, return to the chair and sit back down. Repeat 10 to 15 times—that's one set. For the next set, maneuver around the cone in a counterclockwise direction.

●**Intermediate: Weave In/Weave Out.**

Setup: Arrange four cones in a straight line, each about eight feet apart. Stand next to the first cone in the line.

Move: Walking quickly, weave in a zigzag pattern between the cones. When you reach the last cone in the line, walk around it and return, again weaving between the cones, to your starting position. Repeat two or three times—that's one set.

●**Advanced: Square Drill.**

Setup: Arrange four cones in a square, with each side of the square measuring 10 to 15 feet. Stand to the outside of any cone, with the cone next to your right foot (we'll call this cone number one).

Move: Facing forward and moving around the square clockwise, walk quickly toward the outside of cone number two. When you reach it, switch to a sideways walk or shuffle, moving to your right toward cone number three. When you reach it, turn your body and walk or shuffle sideways to your left toward cone number four.

When you reach it, turn your body and carefully walk backwards toward cone number one. Repeat two or three times—that's one set. For the next set, start with your left foot at the outside of cone number one and move around the square counterclockwise.

After you've mastered these moves: Work on safely increasing your speed…try the drills with one eye closed, then the other…get creative and invent your own agility exercises…or watch a football team practice to learn some new agility drills you can try.

Best Exercise to Prevent Falls: Tai Chi

Study titled "Effectiveness of a Therapeutic Tai Ji Quan Intervention vs a Multimodal Exercise Intervention to Prevent Falls Among Older Adults at High Risk of Falling," by researchers at Oregon Research Institute, Eugene, published in *JAMA Internal Medicine*.

While plenty of research shows that exercise is effective at preventing falls among seniors, there is not much scientific consensus as to what kind of exercise is the safest and most effective. So researchers at Oregon Research Institute compared the fall-preventive effects of different kinds of exercise in 670 adults age 70 and older who had had a fall during the previous year or were at increased risk for falling because of impaired mobility.

The participants were randomly assigned to one of three exercise programs—stretching (the control)…a multimodal program of aerobic, strength and flexibility exercises…or a popular tai chi program for seniors called *Tai Ji Quan: Moving for Better Balance* (TJQMBB). Each group exercised for 60 minutes twice a week for 24 weeks.

Results: Compared with the multimodal exercise, TJQMBB reduced falls by 31%…and compared with the control (stretching), TJQMBB reduced falls by 58%. During the course of the study 733 falls were reported among 324 of the participants—363 falls in the stretching group…218 falls in the multimodal group…and 152 in the TJQMBB group. Also, fewer participants had falls in the TJQMBB group compared with the other groups—85 participants in the TJQMBB group reported falls, compared with 127 in the stretching group and 112 in the multimodal group.

There were no injuries related to any of the exercises and all the exercise programs were deemed equally safe. The researchers concluded that TJQMBB offers a significant reduction in fall risk for older people compared with traditional exercise programs.

Tai Ji Quan: Moving for Better Balance is based on the ancient Chinese martial art of tai chi and incorporates eight movements that have been modified into exercises that synchronize movement, balance and breathing. TJQMBB is being promoted for older adults by the National Council on Aging. You can find additional details about the program on its site NCOA.org. Search "Tai Ji Quan." If you want to try TJQMBB, classes are offered at many YMCAs.

Lose the Belly Fat for Better Bone Health

Miriam Bredella, MD, assistant professor of radiology, Massachusetts General Hospital, Boston.

When researchers studied the bones of 50 overweight women, those with more deep fat around the belly had significantly lower bone mineral density, and therefore higher osteoporosis risk, than those with more fat around the buttocks and hips.

Theory: Visceral (belly) fat leads to lower levels of growth hormone and insulin-like growth factor, both of which promote bone health.

If you are a woman with a waist circumference greater than 34.6 inches: Eat a healthful diet, and exercise to bring your waist size down.

4 Balance Exercises to Keep You Steady on Your Feet

Caroline DeGroot, MPT, a physical therapist at AthletiCo Physical Therapy in Bannockburn, Illinois. DeGroot founded AthletiCo's Vestibular Program, which focuses on helping people with dizziness, balance disorders and concussions.

When you are young, you can walk confidently just about anywhere without much thought—such as on an uneven sidewalk—or while chatting at the same time. As you get older, just glancing sideways at a store window while strolling can make you wobble—and fall. *Here's what's going on…and some moves that will keep you steadier on your feet…*

WHY FALLS OCCUR

One in four Americans over age 65 falls each year. One reason is that older people are more prone to medical conditions that compromise balance—such as vertigo, dizziness, arthritis-related stiffness and weakness, stroke and loss of sensation in the feet from vascular diseases. But even without major health issues, normal physical and vision changes can affect balance.

Your eyes signal the brain where you are in space relative to other objects, which helps keep you stable. Wearing bifocals or progressive lenses requires your focus to change back and forth between lenses, making it harder to notice a loose rug, sidewalk crack or pet.

The natural age-related decline in muscle strength and flexibility also makes it harder to right yourself once your center of gravity is thrown off. That's why the key to staying on your feet is to build your muscle strength and improve your flexibility and agility. *Here's how—work up to doing each move daily to get the most benefit…*

FOOT TAPS

As we age, our pace typically slows, our step length shortens and our stance widens as shifting from one leg to the other feels less secure. To keep your strides long and confident and avert a shuffling gait, you can do foot taps—an exercise that trains your body to safely shift your center of gravity left and right.

How to do it: Stand in front of a step that is four-to-six-inches high (such as a footstool), feet hip-width apart. Slowly raise one foot to tap the step. Return that foot to the ground and then tap with the other foot. Movement should be slow and controlled. Work up to 20 taps for each foot in a session. As your stability improves, try a higher step (six-to-eight inches)…or try tapping the step as lightly as possible to further improve balance and increase muscle control.

Safety note: If needed, you can hold a railing or counter for support. If you use a cane for general walking assistance, hold it in the hand you usually use to hold it throughout the exercise, regardless of which foot you're tapping. If you're using a cane only while recovering from an injury or for a condition that affects your gait, such as arthritis, hold the cane on the side opposite to the injury or painful extremity.

HEAD TURNS

When you turn your head, a response called the vestibular spinal reflex (VSR) causes your brain to send messages to adjust postural muscles to keep you from being pulled in the direction your head turns. Your VSR can become less effective as you age, causing you to often stumble while turning your head. The following exercise helps train your VSR.

How to do it: Stand with your feet hip-width apart. If you need to, you can hold on to a railing, wall, sturdy piece of furniture or counter for support. Now slowly turn your head as far as you comfortably can to the right and then to the left, while maintaining upright posture. Repeat as a continuous movement for 10 repetitions.

Make sure to stay upright without leaning to one side. If you feel dizzy, pause, then continue at a slower pace.

For additional challenge: If you held on to a support, try doing the exercise without holding on to anything. Or try it with your feet only a few inches apart…or with your feet together…or with one foot in front of the other, heel-to-toe. Don't overextend your ability, though—safety first!

OVER-THE-SHOULDER WALKS

Try this exercise once you feel comfortable with standing head turns. You will look left and right as you walk—similar to what you might do when scanning shelves while grocery shopping or walking down a hallway while searching for an apartment number.

How to do it: Stand at one end of a long hallway, feet hip-width apart. Turn your head to look over your right shoulder. Maintaining that gaze, take three or four steps forward. Now turn your head to look over your left shoulder while you continue to walk forward another three or four steps. Repeat for a total of five times per side. If you feel dizzy or unsteady, stop turning your head and gaze straight ahead for a few steps. To increase the challenge, increase how quickly you turn your head.

Variation: Try head turns in a store or library. Having a stationary visual target—the items on the shelves—recruits your vision while challenging your VSR.

BALL HANDOFF

People who worry about falling often are self-conscious about walking—which is counterproductive. The more attention you pay to how you're walking, the more shuffled and fractured your gait becomes. Natural gait needs to be reflexive. This exercise uses a ball for distraction to help your gait become more fluid, increase your walking speed and improve your ability to shift weight left and right.

Safety note: This exercise is not recommended if you need to use a cane to walk.

How to do it: You'll need a partner who is comfortable walking backward and a small ball, such as a tennis ball. Start at one end of a long hallway with your partner facing you and a few feet in front of you, holding the ball. Walk forward while your partner walks backward—handing off or gently tossing the ball back and forth to each other as you go. Perform this exercise for two to three minutes or until you feel tired.

Solo variation: Stand in front of a wall, and march in place while you toss the ball at the wall and catch it as it bounces back. Repeat for 30 seconds at a time, for a total of three times.

Unsteady on Your Feet? A Video Game Can Help

Colin Milner, CEO of the International Council on Active Aging, an organization dedicated to improving fitness and quality-of-life issues in older adults, Vancouver, British Columbia, Canada.

Fact: One in four Americans age 65 and older falls each year, and falls are the leading cause of injuries—both fatal and nonfatal—in this age group.

Staying fit and strong, engaging in exercises that target your "core" abdominal muscles and practicing balance-oriented regimens, such as yoga and tai chi, are key to preventing falls. But another solution may be as near as your TV—active video games that get you on your feet and moving. Dubbed "exergames," they're great for everyone—from healthy older adults who want to stay that way to those challenged by chronic conditions that impair balance.

BEFORE THE FALL

Changes that often come with aging can make you more wobbly on your feet. The biggest contributor for otherwise healthy people is general physical decline—loss of strength and power, poor balance and slower reaction time. Vision problems, foot-health issues, such as peripheral neuropathy, and medication side effects also can contribute to balance issues, as can certain medical conditions, such as Parkinson's disease.

Staying active and fit is the best way to maintain the muscle strength and quick reaction time needed for good balance. But even if you haven't been particularly active, exergames can help you improve balance in a short period of time.

GET IN THE GAME

Exergames are video games that involve "whole-body motion." You can see an animated version of yourself (your "avatar") on screen, which makes it easier to make the right moves. When it comes to balance research, most of the studies use the Nintendo Wii Balance Board, which you stand on for some of the games in Nintendo Wii Fit. It relays your movements to the screen and lets you adjust your stance in real time. *Exergames…*

●**Help healthy older people who live independently improve balance.**

Example: One 2015 study of retired Australian men and women published in *Journal of Aging and Physical Activity* found that 30-minute unsupervised sessions of Wii balance gaming three times a week over six weeks significantly improved balance as measured by tasks such as standing on one leg…compared with a similar group that was encouraged to simply keep exercising in their normal way. Their enjoyment in playing also increased over the six weeks.

●**Are safe.** A recent review of 60 studies looking at the effectiveness of gaming technology for adults age 65 and older published in *International Journal of Medical Informatics* concluded that "exergames show promise as an intervention to improve physical function in older adults, with few reported adverse events."

●**Are great for people with chronic conditions that affect mobility and balance.**

Example: A Northwestern University study of patients with Parkinson's disease found that eight weeks of playing Wii Balance Board (the games included marble tracking, skiing and bubble rafting) three times per week significantly improved measures of gait and balance. Other research has found that exergames help stroke patients recover muscle function and balance.

Ready to play, but not sure where to start? Exergames range from light activity to a real workout. It's definitely an investment—you'll need to buy a Nintendo Wii, which is no longer manufactured by Nintendo. Prices for a refurbished or used console, available online, range from $100 to $600 and a Wii Balance Board costs about $45. Nintendo's current gaming console, Switch, has a popular Ring Fit Adventure game that involves role playing and defeating enemies using real-life exercises such as yoga and strength training. Between fights, you may encounter some unusual methods of transportation such as squat-powered launch pads and waterfalls for paddling. The Switch also features

---

Fabulous Foot Stretches

By strengthening and stretching your feet, you can improve coordination, balance and stability.

What to do: Without shoes, move your foot in circles, first one way and then the other, then side to side, moving only your foot and ankle, not your leg…do toe curls—flex toes as much as possible and then uncurl them…with your foot flat on the floor, lift your big toe without lifting the other toes, then try lifting the others without lifting the big toe…use your feet to pick up items such as marbles or pencils…spread your toes apart like a fan…roll a small rubber ball or golf ball under the sole of your foot to massage it.

University of California, Berkeley Wellness Letter. BerkeleyWellness.com

---

minigames that include balance exercises (but be sure to review the system carefully, especially if you have a chronic condition that affects physical balance). *Once you're set up, here are some other popular games to try…*

●**DanceDanceRevolution, which has you two-stepping on a sensored pad to match the dance moves shown on a screen.** It features 30 dance tracks and three levels of fitness. ($49)

●**Wii Ski.** Use the balance board to hit the slopes on any of 14 breath-taking courses including races, freestyle, moguls and slaloms at beginner, intermediate and black diamond levels. ($23)

●**Wii Sports.** This suite of games uses a hand-held remote to let you play tennis, baseball, golf, bowling and boxing. ($55)

If you haven't been active for a while, or have physical limitations or a chronic health condition, talk with your doctor before trying exergaming. Research from University of Washington also finds that combining exergaming with regular sessions with a physical therapist is a particularly effective way to improve balance quickly.

Your Bones Are in Danger— and Osteoporosis Isn't the Only Threat

Neil Binkley, MD, professor in the divisions of geriatrics and endocrinology at University of Wisconsin (UW) School of Medicine and Public Health, Madison. He is director of the UW Osteoporosis Clinical Research Program and associate director of the UW Institute on Aging. Aging.wisc.edu

We've been told that the best way to prevent fractures is to prevent or treat osteoporosis—diet, exercise and, if needed, medications. But that approach has not been successful.

For people with osteoporosis, medications do prevent many spinal fractures—but fewer than half of hip and other fractures, according to a major study published in *The New England Journal of Medicine*. And many people who fall and break bones don't even have osteoporosis.

Example: An overweight or obese person may have good bone density (from carrying that extra weight) but still get fractures. Unless he/she has the muscle strength to carry that extra weight, mobility issues—such as difficulty getting up off the toilet or climbing stairs—can lead to falls that cause fractures. Rather than hip fractures due to weakened bones, they tend to get ankle or lower-leg fractures.

In the end, it's preventing fractures—from any cause—that really matters. Many of us think that if we break a bone, our friendly orthopedic surgeon will put it back together and life will go on as usual. But after age 50—and especially after age 65—a fractured bone can threaten independence and quality of life. And that's what we fear most about aging—losing independence…not being able to drive…and winding up in a nursing home. The classic example is a hip fracture, which often sends people to nursing homes and is linked to a shorter life span. But breaking an ankle, an arm or even a wrist can make daily life harder at home…and make it tougher to be mobile.

To find out what is really needed to prevent fractures, we spoke with geriatrician and endocrinologist Neil Binkley, MD. He started with a simple question—"What causes most fractures in older people?"

The answer: *Falling.*

Here's how to prevent falls—and the fractures that could end your independence…

●**Eat for muscle strength, not just bones.** Getting enough calcium and vitamin D—standard elements of osteoporosis prevention—still is important. But pay close attention to calories and protein, too. These are essential to maintaining muscle strength—and that's as important as strong bones in preventing fractures. After all, when our muscle strength declines, we fall. And when we fall on weak bones, guess what? They break.

Protein needs are based on your body weight. To calculate your individual needs, multiply your body weight by 0.45. For a 150-pound woman, that's 67 grams a day…for a 185-pound man, 83 grams. To get a sense of what that looks like, a three-ounce serving of tuna or salmon contains about 22 grams of protein and an egg contains six grams, on average. Aim to include good sources of protein—seafood, lean meat, poultry, eggs, nuts, seeds, soy and legumes such as beans and peas—at every meal.

For some older people, a waning appetite also can mean that they just don't eat enough calories. If you're not eating enough, a registered dietitian can help find practical ways to help you get enough protein and calories each day.

●**Get strong—and balanced.** Now that you're nourishing muscles, make them work. Exercise helps keep your bones and muscles strong, so it's vital for lowering your fracture risk. The best exercise is the one that you'll actually do, whether it's walking, biking, swimming or team sports. Beyond general fitness, exercises that improve core strength and balance are key to fall prevention. *Suggestions*…

●Join a tai chi class. This ancient Chinese set of gentle, slow-moving exercises strengthens lower limbs and improves balance. Several studies have found that practicing tai chi regularly significantly reduces fall risk in older adults.

●Yoga may help, too. It can strengthen bones, and while it is less well-studied for fall prevention, it has been shown to improve balance and mobility in older people.

●**Take fall-prevention classes.** One popular, evidence-based program is Stepping On, a seven-week, two-hours-per-week workshop, first developed in Australia, that now is offered in 20 US states. It is geared to healthy adults over age 65. One study, published in *Journal of the American Geriatrics Society*, reported that people who participated in Stepping On had 31% fewer falls over the next 14 months, compared with a similar group of people who didn't go through the program. To find programs like this in your area, check with the National Council on Aging's Fall Prevention website (NCOA.org/healthy-aging/falls-prevention).

●**Consider physical therapy.** If you've fallen and have been injured—even if you didn't break a bone—you're waving a red flag that a fracture could be in your future. A physical therapist can do a formal strength-and-balance assessment...show you exercises to strengthen muscles, bones, walking posture and balance...and help you find classes in your community.

●**Make your home safer.** *A key part of fall prevention is taking a look at what you can do to make it less likely that you'll trip and fall...*

●Do you have night-lights in your home? Consider putting a night-light in your bathroom for those middle-of-the-night trips.

●Are there throw rugs that you might slip on? Get rid of them!

●Is there clutter on the floor or stairs that you could stumble on? Declutter!

●Do you need to get on a chair or step stool to reach things on high shelves? Put everyday items on lower shelves that are easy to reach.

●Is it hard to get in and out of your bathtub without slipping? Consider installing grab bars or replacing your tub with a walk-in shower.

Some of your safety changes may need to be in your own behavior—such as drinking less alcohol. That's a fall risk that many older people don't con-sider. And don't forget to get your vision checked regularly. If you can't see it, you can trip on it.

●**Review your medications.** Some medications (prescription or over-the-counter) or medication interactions can cause dizziness, light-headedness or low blood pressure, which can increase the risk of falling. Key medications to be aware of include antihistamines, sleep aids, pain pills, antidepressants and antianxiety medications. In addition, some medications, such as glucocorticoids (steroids taken for inflammatory and autoimmune conditions) contribute to bone loss. If you are taking medications that increase your fall risk, talk to your doctor to see if you can reduce the dose, find an alternative—or modify how you take it, such as only at bedtime.

It's not that strong bones aren't important—they're a key part of a fracture-prevention plan... but only one part. If your doctor has prescribed a diet, exercise program or medication for you to prevent or treat osteoporosis, continue following those instructions. Osteoporosis medications often are prescribed based on an individual's estimated risk for fracture. For individuals at high fracture risk, the benefits of reducing that risk far outweigh the risk of side effects. But just taking medications is not enough.

Now you know what else you need to do to protect yourself.

THIS EXERCISE PREVENTS FALLS

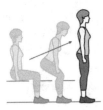

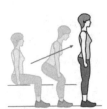

One of the simplest and most effective exercises—and one that you can do almost anywhere—is the Chair Rise. *Do this daily to strengthen the muscles in your thighs and buttocks, which can help keep you steady on your feet and prevent falls...*

●**Sit toward the front of a sturdy chair,** with your knees bent and feet flat on the floor, shoulder-width apart.

●**Rest your hands lightly on the seat on either side of you,** keeping your back and neck straight and chest slightly forward.

- **Breathe in slowly.** Lean forward and exhale as you stand up—feel your weight on the front of your feet.

- **Pause for a full breath in and out.**

- **Breathe in as you slowly sit down.** Try not to collapse down into the chair. Rather, control your lowering as much as possible.

- **Breathe out.**

Repeat for a total of 10 to 15 stand/sits. Rest and breathe for a minute, then do another set of 10 to 15. You may need to work up to this level over several days or a few weeks. The goal is to get to the point where you can complete two sets without using your hands at all.

How You Exercise May Be Weakening Your Bones!

Oddbjørn Klomsten Andersen, MSc, doctoral candidate, Norwegian School of Sport Sciences, Oslo, Norway. He is lead author of the study titled "Bone health in elite Norwegian endurance cyclists and runners: a cross-sectional study," published in *BMJ Open Sport & Exercise Medicine*.

Cycling is great exercise—especially for your heart and muscles. But research has found that cycling and other low-impact activities don't do your bones any favor. There's no need to abandon your favorite sports! Just make sure to add these other activities to your fitness regimen so your bones stay strong and healthy.

Of course, any exercise is better than no exercise. It's well accepted that high-impact activities—such as running, volleyball, basketball and tennis—are good for your bones, particularly by helping to prevent osteoporosis and fractures as we age. It's thought that the repeated pounding against the ground minutely bends bones in the legs, hips and spine...triggering an increase in bone cells that strengthens those bones to withstand future impacts.

Researchers from the Norwegian School of Sport Sciences wanted to look at the effect of low-impact exercise on bones. For their study, they compared the bone mineral density (BMD) of 21 healthy male and female elite runners, ages 18 to 35, with the BMD of a similar group of 19 elite cyclists. Most of the cyclists and five of the runners also did heavy resistance training. The researchers measured BMD for total body, femoral neck (thighbone) and lumbar spine using dual-energy X-ray absorptiometry (DXA). Both groups also consumed adequate amounts of calcium according to current recommendations.

Results: The cyclists had much lower BMD than the runners.

If most of your exercises are the low-impact sort, it might be a good idea to take some additional steps to keep your bones healthy. *The National Osteoporosis Foundation recommends...*

- **Get enough calcium and vitamin D.** It's best to get calcium from diet—foods such as milk, cheese, yogurt, collard greens and sardines (with bones) are good sources. Aim for 1,200 mg of calcium daily for women age 51 and older...and 1,000 mg/day for men until age 71, and 1,200 mg/day thereafter. Both men and women age 50 and older should also get 800 IU to 1,000 IU of vitamin D daily. Salmon, oysters, egg yolks and mushrooms are good food sources. Sunlight is another source of vitamin D. You can also get both calcium and vitamin D from fortified foods, such as orange juice. If you don't get enough of these nutrients from diet, talk to your doctor about supplements.

- **Do weight-bearing exercise and resistance training.** While the Norwegian study was not designed to see if weight-bearing exercise helped protect bone (for instance, the cyclists might have had even worse bone health if they hadn't done resistance training), other research has shown that it does benefit bones. The theory is that resistance training—including using free weights, a weighted vest, exercise bands and weight machines—causes muscles to pull on bones, which stimulates them to increase their density. In fact, the National Osteoporosis Foundation suggests that everyone do muscle-strengthening exercises two to three days per week and weight-bearing exercises for 30 minutes most days of the week.

•**Do balance exercises.** Yoga and Pilates can also help protect bones by improving strength and flexibility. But since some positions can put you at risk for fractures if you already have low bone density, be sure to check with a trained therapist to learn which exercises are safe for you.

•**Jump around.** As little as 10 minutes of jumping exercises—such as jumping jacks, jump rope or jump squats—three times a week has been shown to increase bone mass in children and adolescents. Adults may need more jumps to reap these benefits. If high-impact jumping is not an option, perhaps because of arthritis or other joint issues, low-impact weight-bearing exercises such as using an elliptical or stair-step machine will provide some benefit. Aim for 30 minutes on most days of the week.

•**Know your BMD.** A bone mineral density scan lets you and your doctor know what shape your bones are in and what's your risk for future fractures is. The US Preventive Services Task Force recommends screening for osteoporosis with bone measurement testing (such as a DXA scan) for all women over age 65…and women under age 65 who are at high risk for fracture. The National Osteoporosis Foundation recommends a bone density test for men ages 70 and older…and for men ages 50 to 69 with risk factors. Discuss with your doctor how often to schedule additional scans.

The Surprising Reason Why People Fall

Julie Wetherell, PhD, a board-certified geropsychologist at the VA San Diego Healthcare System and professor of psychiatry at the University of California, San Diego.

A loose rug…a tottering gait…a powerful drug …and poor eyesight are all well-known causes of falls. But there's a hidden risk that few people would ever guess.

Recent development: Researchers are now discovering that, paradoxically, the fear of falling significantly increases one's risk of falling. In fact,

if you're very afraid of falling, you are 34% more likely to fall than someone with the same level of health and fitness who isn't as afraid. Why the difference? It's probably because you slow your walking speed, widen your stance and stiffen your body—changes that worsen balance. *What you need to know about this dangerous risk…*

WHY THE FEAR?

Make no mistake, falls are scary. In adults age 65 and older, falls are the number-one cause of injury-related visits to emergency departments. Studies show that two out of five older adults are afraid of falling, including many who are reasonably fit and have never taken a spill. In fact, research shows that more seniors are afraid of falling than of robbery, financial troubles or even ill health!

Here's a quick rule of thumb: If you've had two or fewer minor falls in the past year…if you don't walk more slowly than other people your age… and if you can stand up from a chair without using your arms, you probably don't need to limit your activities dramatically due to concern about falling. However, if you are more afraid of falling than you need to be, it's important to take steps to reduce your fear.

It helps to see a physical therapist for an evaluation. He/she can assess your need for an assistive device such as a cane or walker and, if needed, give you exercises to improve your balance and strength.

WHAT ELSE HELPS

My colleagues and I conducted a small, preliminary study that reduced fear of falling in eight seniors. Each participant received eight one-hour sessions in his/her home conducted by a physical therapist and psychologist. *Among the approaches we used…*

•**Exposure therapy.** With this type of therapy, you're exposed to what you fear, little by little, in a safe environment, until you're comfortable encountering or doing the thing you fear. In this study, exposure was the most effective technique for reducing fear of falling.

Example: If you avoid taking baths, perhaps because a friend fell in the tub and you think it will happen to you, start by sitting on the side of the tub. When this is no longer fear-provoking, put your legs in the tub. After that, put your legs in the tub with a little bit of water in the bottom. Then do so with four inches of water.

You may need to repeat each of these actions 20 to 30 times over a few weeks until you are certain you can do each one without fear. The final action would be taking a bath.

If you are very concerned about doing this, you might want to start by having a person present while you do these activities—perhaps for a week in the same room, then for a week in the next room, then on a different floor. Eventually, doing these activities alone will reinforce the sense that you can bathe safely.

Note: The risk of falling and fear of falling are two different things. Precautions that reduce the risk of falling can sometimes make fear of falling worse. In the example above, if there's always another person present, it could foster fear, sending you the message that bathing alone is very dangerous.

Caution: If your doctor or physical therapist says that it isn't safe for you to do an activity alone, then your fear is not unwarranted or excessive and you should not do exposure therapy.

What you can do: Gradually expose yourself to the specific situations you fear, or ask a psychologist or physical therapist to help you do so. A friend or family member can do this as well if he gets some training from a psychologist or physical therapist.

•**Home safety.** If you make your home more fall-proof, you'll be less afraid of falling. For example, replace loose floor coverings with mats that have slip-resistant backing…make sure no cords or cables are in walkways…install grab bars in the bathroom…and put a slip-resistant mat in the tub or shower stall. Also, use brighter lights.

•**Cognitive restructuring.** This technique replaces counterproductive, fearful thoughts with helpful, fear-reducing thoughts. To get started, identify thoughts that are unhelpful. Next, when you have such a thought, substitute a helpful thought. For example…

You think: "If I walk on the grass, I'm likely to fall."

Substitute: "I have walked on the grass many times and didn't fall."

•**Exercise.** *Balance-improving exercises that the people in my study found enjoyable and effective…*

•Walking backward. This strengthens legs, improves balance and builds confidence.

What to do: Find a place where you can walk backward for 10 to 20 feet without looking over your shoulder to avoid obstacles, then reverse direction and walk backward the other way. Try to do this two to three times per day.

Helpful: See how it's done at Eldergym.com/backward-walking-for-increased-balance.

If you are very concerned about doing this exercise, start by doing it with someone else in the room and gradually work up, over a month or so, to doing it alone.

•Sit down in a chair and stand up without using your hands. This exercise is easy to do, builds leg strength and improves balance and confidence. Repeat at least 10 times, once a day.

The Best Bone-Building Exercises

Raymond E. Cole, DO, clinical assistant professor, Department of Internal Medicine, Michigan State University College of Osteopathic Medicine, East Lansing. He is author of *Best Body, Best Bones: Your Doctor's Exercise Rx for Lifelong Fitness.*

Women (and men) whose bones are fragile and porous—due to the severe loss of bone density that characterizes osteoporosis—often avoid exercise for fear that jarring or twisting motions could cause fractures.

Done properly, however, exercise is not only safe for people with osteoporosis or its milder form, osteopenia, it actually can reduce or even reverse bone loss. For people whose bones are still healthy, exercise helps ensure that osteoporosis never develops.

Reason: When a muscle exerts tension on a bone, it stimulates specialized cells that increase new bone formation. Also, when muscles that contribute to balance are strengthened, falls (and resulting fractures) are less likely.

Keys: Doing the types of workouts that build bone most effectively...and modifying techniques as necessary to avoid overstressing already weakened bones.

What to do: Start by exercising for 10 to 20 minutes several times a week, gradually building up to 30 minutes a day six days per week. Alternate between a strength-training workout one day and an aerobic activity the next.

Important: Before beginning the exercise program below, ask your doctor which instructions you should follow—the ones labeled "If you have healthy bones" or the ones labeled "If you already have bone loss."

STRENGTH TRAINING FOR BONES

The only equipment you need are hand weights (dumbbells) and ankle weights (pads that strap around the ankles), $20 and up per pair at sports equipment stores.

For each exercise, begin with one set of eight repetitions ("reps"). If you cannot do eight reps using the suggested starting weights, use lighter weights. Over several weeks, gradually increase to 10, then 12, then 15 reps. Then try two sets of eight reps, resting for one minute between sets...and again gradually increase the reps. When you can do two sets of 15 reps, increase the weight by one to two pounds and start again with one set of eight reps.

Keep your shoulders back and abdominal muscles pulled in. With each rep, exhale during the initial move...hold the position for two seconds... inhale as you return to the starting position. Move slowly, using muscles rather than momentum. Do not lock elbow or knee joints.

•**UPPER BODY.** These exercises build bone density in the shoulders, arms and spine.

If you have healthy bones: Stand during the exercises. Start by holding a five-pound weight in each hand...over time, try to work up to eight, then 10, then 12 pounds.

If you already have bone loss: To guard against falls, sit in a straight-backed chair while exercising. At first, use no weights or use one- or two-pound weights...gradually work up to three-, then five-, then a maximum of eight-pound weights if you can. Avoid heavier weights—they could increase the risk for vertebral compression fractures.

•**Arms forward.**

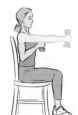

To start: Bend elbows, arms close to your body, hands at chest-height, palms facing each other.

One rep: Straighten elbows until both arms are extended in front of you, parallel to the floor...hold...return to starting position.

•**Arm overhead.**

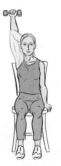

To start: Raise right arm straight overhead, palm facing forward.

One rep: Bend right elbow, bringing right hand down behind your head...hold...return to starting position. Do a set with the right arm, then with the left.

•**Arms up-and-down.**

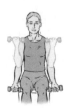

To start: Have arms down at your sides, palms forward.

One rep: Keeping elbows close to your sides, bend arms to raise hands toward shoulders until palms face you...hold...lower to starting position.

•**MIDBODY.** This strengthens and stabilizes "core" muscles (abdomen, back, pelvic area). By improving body alignment, it helps prevent falls and reduces pressure on the vertebrae, protecting against compression fractures of the spine. No weights are used.

If you have healthy bones: Do this exercise while standing...or try it while lying on your back, with knees bent and feet flat on the floor.

If you already have bone loss: Done while standing, this is a good option for osteoporosis patients who are uncomfortable exercising on

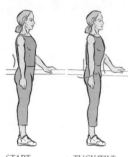

START   TUCK/TILT

the floor. If you have balance problems, hold onto a counter…or sit in a chair.

•Tummy tuck/pelvic tilt.

To start: Have arms at sides, feet hip-width apart.

One rep: Simultaneously contract abdominal muscles to draw your tummy toward your spine, tighten buttocks muscles, and tilt the bottom of your pelvis forward to flatten the arch of your back…hold… return to starting position.

•LOWER BODY. These moves increase bone density in the legs and feet. For each rep, raise the leg as high as possible without leaning…hold for two seconds…return to starting position.

Advanced option: Try not to touch your foot to the ground between reps.

If you have healthy bones: Start by wearing a two-pound ankle weight on each leg…gradually increase to 10 pounds per ankle.

If you already have bone loss: Hold onto a counter for balance. To begin, use no weights…build up, one pound at a time, to five pounds per ankle.

•Leg forward-and-back.

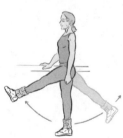

To start: Stand on your right foot.

One rep: Keeping both legs straight, slowly swing left leg forward and up…hold… swing leg down through the starting position and up behind you…hold…return to starting position. After one set, repeat with the other leg.

•Leg out.

To start: Stand on your right foot.

One rep: Keeping both legs straight, slowly lift left leg out to the side…hold…

Illustrations by Shawn Banner

return to starting position. After one set, repeat with the other leg.

BONE-BENEFITING AEROBICS

Biking, stationary cycling, swimming and rowing are good for heart health—but they do not protect against osteoporosis.

Better: Weight-bearing aerobic activities in which you're on your feet, bones working against gravity, build bone mass in the hips and legs.

If you have healthy bones: Good choices include jogging, dancing, stair climbing, step aerobics, jumping rope, racket sports and interactive video games, such as Wii Fit and Dance Dance Revolution. If you enjoy walking, you can boost intensity by wearing a two- to 20-pound weighted vest ($50 and up at sports equipment stores).

Warning: Do not wear ankle weights during aerobic workouts—this could stress your joints.

If you already have bone loss: Refrain from high-impact activities (running, jumping) and those that require twisting or bending (racket sports, golf). Do not wear a weighted vest.

Safe low-impact options: Walking, using an elliptical machine (available at most gyms), qigong and tai chi.

Yoga for Bone Health

Carol Krucoff, C-IAYT, E-RYT, a yoga therapist and codirector of the Integrated Yoga for Seniors Professional Training at Duke Integrative Medicine, Durham, North Carolina. She is the coauthor of *Relax into Yoga for Seniors: A Six-Week Program for Strength, Balance, Flexibility and Pain Relief.* HealingMoves.com

I f yoga makes you think of only stretching and improving your flexibility, think again. Many yoga poses require you to hold your body weight, which puts pressure on your bones, stimulating new bone to form. So, if you need to do weight-bearing exercises to protect your bones, consider yoga—especially if you don't have access to weights or want a form of exercise that's easier on your joints than an activity like running. Here are some of the yoga positions that can improve bone health…

One of the benefits of yoga for bone health: Many yoga positions require that you support your body weight with your legs and/or arms. In some positions, such as downward dog or plank, both your arms and legs support your body weight. These postures provide a boost to bones in both the upper and lower body, a claim that can't be made by activities such as running or walking, which just involve the lower body. A study by researchers at University of California, Los Angeles found that yoga reduced the curvature of the spine in adults with *hyperkyphosis* (also known as "dowager's hump"), a condition that often is caused by bone loss.

Here are a few simple yoga poses that help to build bones. For best results, do each pose three times a week. (For details on how long to hold each pose, see below.)

Bone-building yoga poses…

CHAIR POSE

What it does: Strengthens the bones of the legs and hips.

How to do it: Stand with feet hip-distance apart. Extend your arms forward at shoulder height. (To make the move more difficult, you can put your arms over your head with your upper arms parallel to your ears.) Bend your knees, bow forward at the hips, stick your bottom out and lower it down as if you were going to sit in an invisible chair. Make sure that your back is straight, not rounded, and that your knees are not in front of your toes. Hold the position for two or three slow, deep breaths, then return to standing. Repeat five times, working your way up to 10 times.

SPINAL BALANCE

What it does: Strengthens bones in the arms, shoulders and thighs.

How to do it: Come onto all fours—with your knees directly under your hips and your wrists directly under your shoulders. Moving slowly, extend the left leg out behind you and raise it to hip height, toes toward the floor. Next, extend your right arm forward and raise it to shoulder height. Hold for one full, easy breath. Then return to the starting position and switch sides. Repeat three times on each side, working up to holding the pose each time for three breaths.

WARRIOR II

What it does: Strengthens bones of the lower body.

How to do it: Step your feet about three to four feet apart. Extend your arms out to both sides and parallel to the floor, palms facing down. Turn your left foot 90 degrees to the left and angle the toes of your right foot toward the left. Bend your left knee (make sure that your left knee is over your left ankle) and align the arch of your right foot with the heel of your left foot. Straighten your right leg, pressing the outer heel into the floor. Gaze out over the left fingertips. Hold for three to five breaths, then switch sides and repeat.

PLANK

What it does: Strengthens bones in the arms, shoulders and legs.

How to do it: Come onto all fours with your palms flat against the floor under your shoulders, fingers spread wide. Extend your right leg out behind you, toes tucked under. Next, extend your left leg out behind you, toes tucked under, so that your body forms a straight line from the top of your head to your heels. Stay here, balanced on your hands and toes, for three full breaths. If you can't breathe easily with your legs straight, bring your knees to the floor and perform the pose with your knees on the floor. This version of the pose is easier to do but still strengthens the arm bones.

To learn the postures accurately, you can take a class with a registered teacher. The Yoga Alliance (YogaAlliance.org), a national yoga education organization, which maintains a national registry of teachers who have completed at least 200 hours of yoga teacher training, can help you find a teacher in your area.

11

Better Breathing for Health and Fitness

Just Breathe...the Right Way

Rebecca Dennis, a breath coach and founder of BreathingTree.co.uk, a website that's dedicated to health-promoting breathing strategies. Based in London, she is author of *And Breathe: The Complete Guide to Conscious Breathing for Health and Happiness.*

It's the first and last thing we do in this world—take a breath. But somewhere in between, far too many of us lose touch with how to breathe naturally, fully...and correctly. Though we inhale and exhale about 20,000 times each day, most of the time we take short, shallow breaths that I call "stress breaths."

Why does our innate sense of how to breathe properly slip away from us? Whether we're fighting traffic or multitasking, our fast-paced lives often throw us into a stress-driven spiral that interferes with our ability to optimally fuel our bodies with life-sustaining oxygen. People who are suppressing feelings such as anger or emotional pain tend to hold their breath. *Fortunately, a few simple strategies can help us reclaim our breathing skills...*

MORE THAN "BELLY BREATHING"

We have all heard the term "belly breathing," but the real key to proper breathing is not so much your belly but your diaphragm. Deeply breathing from this dome-shaped sheet of muscle at the bottom of the rib cage is vital for respiratory function.

True diaphragmatic breathing uses the entire respiratory system—starting with the belly, then moving on to the midsection and into the chest.

Try it: Inhale through your nose, directing your breath into your stomach. Allow your diaphragm to drop downward and the rib cage to expand, thus creating space for the lungs to inflate. Pause for a moment, then exhale through your mouth and feel the rib cage contract. The motion of breath should go in and out like a wave. To adopt this healthier way of breathing, practice for a minute or two several times a day until it feels natural.

This form of breathing stimulates the parasympathetic nervous system (PNS), which slows your heart rate and breathing, lowers blood pressure and diverts blood toward the digestive system.

THE HEALING EFFECTS

Proper breathing offers a number of powerful health benefits, including...

• **Reduced anxiety and depression.** Deep breathing is believed to help elevate levels of serotonin and endorphins, naturally occurring "feel-good" chemicals. A study by Harvard Medical School psychiatrists showed that those who meditated daily for four years—a practice that relies heavily on conscious breathing—had longer telomeres, the protective "caps" on the ends of chromosomes that serve as biomarkers of longevity and slower aging.

●**Protection against viruses.** Our lymphatic system, which moves cleansing, vital fluids through our muscles and tissues, relies on breathing, movement and gravity to continue flowing. By promoting a healthy lymphatic system, deep breathing can play a crucial role in protecting the body from viruses, bacteria and other health threats.

●**Less constipation.** Deeper breathing (and the stress reduction that goes along with it) promotes intestinal action and stimulates overall digestion. This can improve conditions such as constipation and irritable bowel syndrome.

●**Improved sleep.** The relaxation that occurs with deep breathing is likely responsible for its positive effect on sleep quality.

BEST BREATHING FIXES

Targeted breathing exercises can help you deal more effectively with stress...and day-to-day health challenges such as indigestion, insomnia and fatigue. The best part is that you can do these exercises anywhere. *Among my favorite quick breathing fixes—they can also help with respiratory conditions such as asthma and chronic obstructive pulmonary disease (COPD)...*

●**Alternate nostril breathing.** This breathing exercise helps put you in a calm and centered state.

What to do: Breathe in deeply through your right nostril while pressing the left nostril closed with your right index finger...then exhale through the left nostril while pressing the right nostril closed with your right thumb. Next, inhale through the left nostril (right nostril still closed)...then close the left nostril and exhale through the right. The exhalations should take about twice as long as the inhalations. Repeat the cycle 10 times.

●**4-7-8 breathing.** If you are plagued by insomnia, this breathing exercise can put you to sleep within minutes.

What to do: Exhale completely through your mouth, making a "whoosh" sound. Close your mouth and inhale quietly through your nose to a count of four. Hold your breath for a count of seven. Exhale completely through your mouth, making

a "whoosh" sound, to a count of eight. This is one breath.

Now inhale again and repeat the cycle three more times. Do this exercise when you need help going to sleep or if you awaken and want to get back to sleep.

Why Sucking in Your Stomach Harms Your Health

Steven Weiniger, DC, a chiropractor in private practice in Atlanta and author of *Stand Taller, Live Longer: An Anti-Aging Strategy.* He has served on the White House Conference on Aging.

Many people mistakenly believe that holding their stomach muscles tight not only makes them look more trim and fit, but also helps them stand straight and tall. But constantly sucking in your stomach muscles makes it impossible to breathe correctly which in turn prevents you from having good posture. Poor posture leads to a host of other problems, including a sore neck and shoulder muscles, poor balance, arthritis and injuries. Indirectly, the shallow breathing that results from such a stance also can lead to anxiety and even lowered self-esteem.

Most people believe that they are breathing correctly, but in reality, they are not. So here is a three-step program to get you on your way to stronger posture and better health.

STEP 1: PICTURE THIS!

Before we get to proper breathing, you first need a realistic idea about the current state of your posture.

Here's an easy way to evaluate your posture: Have someone take full-length pictures of you standing, facing front and facing sideways...and don't try to stand "right" for this photo session. You may be quite surprised by what your photos reveal. For example, many people lean to one side, a common problem that creates asymmetry and misalignment in the body.

What to look for: On the front view, draw a line from the center of your forehead to directly between your feet to see whether there is a difference from one side to the other. On the side view, look to see if your cheekbones are further forward than your chest, which indicates a forward head thrust. Moving through your day with misaligned posture changes everything. When you do this, your nervous system adjusts and adapts to your bad-posture habits, so that your crooked body begins to feel symmetric and normal to you—but it isn't.

STEP 2: FINE-TUNE YOUR BREATHING

Now that you have a better idea of your true posture, we can move on to breathing. After years of holding in their tummies, many people have a tendency toward chest breathing. If you're not sure whether or not this describes you, you can consider achy muscles in your neck and shoulders a good clue. Chest breathing requires muscles in these areas to do work that they are not designed for, so it's not all that surprising that they're sore by the end of the day.

Some good ways to evaluate your own breathing: Place one hand on your belly and the other on your chest as you breathe to see which moves more, belly or chest—that's your default breathing mode. Your goal is to have belly breathing be your natural style. Another approach is to ask someone else to watch you breathe and report on what he/she sees. Ask someone to observe your breathing while you are lying down to see whether your chest and/or belly moves out when you breathe in.

What belly breathing feels like: Try this to get familiar with the sensation of proper belly breathing. Lie on your stomach, cradle your forehead on your crossed arms and slowly breathe. This position locks the chest, thereby forcing breath into the abdomen—note how this feels because this is what you want to learn to do naturally.

STEP 3: REPROGRAM YOUR POSTURE

Now that you have learned about your posture and breathing tendencies…and you have experienced the sensation of belly breathing…perform the following exercises to help reprogram yourself to breathe deep into your belly throughout the day. If you make it a point to spend a few minutes on these exercises several times during the day, belly breathing—and stronger posture—will become instinctive.

Breathing Technique Exercise: In a seated or standing position, pull your shoulders back to expand your chest (lifting it toward the ceiling, keeping your head level and shoulders down) while holding your back straight. Now breathe deeply into your belly—place one hand on it to feel the subtle movement. Take five breaths as slowly as you can. With practice, you will eventually begin to breathe this way without having to think about it.

Breathing Focus Exercise: A good way to learn how it feels when your belly expands with your breath is to use a long scarf or stretchy resistance exercise band (such as TheraBand, available at sporting-goods stores and online). Grasp the ends of the scarf or band, elbows bent at your sides, and wrap it around your waist tightly enough so that it squeezes just a bit. Now take five breaths, consciously, pushing your belly out with each breath.

Breathing for Alignment and Balance: Using your best posture, stand on one leg and raise the other so that it barely touches or is slightly off the ground. Take five deep, controlled breaths while striving to remain still. Observe how your body must readjust to maintain control of your balance, realigning and shifting your center of gravity with each breath. This is not easy to do—you may find yourself flailing to stay upright, especially if your posture is off-center. If so, try placing a finger on a wall for support, but touch the wall only as much as is necessary. Now repeat with the other leg off the floor. Doing "balance breathing" two or three times a day helps improve balance and alignment, and over a few weeks, most people find that they can balance with greater stability.

So if you feel like your stomach sticks out, consider doing sit-ups to strengthen your abdominal muscles…or perhaps think about losing weight, because sucking it in isn't the solution.

Easiest Exercise Ever: Breathe for Better Performance

Richard Firshein, DO, director and founder of the Firshein Center for Integrative Medicine in New York City and author of several books, including *Reversing Asthma: Breathe Easier with This Revolutionary New Program.* FirsheinCenter.com

What if you could practice a simple form of exercise that would benefit your heart… strengthen your lungs…help modulate stress…and, if you are an athlete and interested in optimum fitness, take your performance to a higher level…and you could get all these benefits without even getting out of your chair? And without breaking a sweat. How great would that be?

It's not too good to be true, and though you can buy inexpensive devices to help you do this, you don't need any fancy equipment for the following breathing exercises.

TAKE A DEEP BREATH…

A recent study at Indiana University demonstrated that doing simple breathing exercises can bring big health benefits for many types of people, including athletes, seniors and people who are ill with respiratory diseases, among others.

The study was small, but results were impressive. The test subjects were 16 male bicyclists—not professionals, but avid amateurs. Twice a day, half the cyclists took 30 breaths through a device known as an inspiratory muscle trainer (IMT) that made them work harder to bring air into their lungs. Another eight cyclists used the same type of device but set to a low level that required only a slight additional effort to breathe.

Researchers discovered that after six weeks of these daily exercises, the cyclists who worked hard to breathe now required about 1% less oxygen during low-intensity exercise and 3% to 4% less oxygen during high-intensity exercise—which indicated that their bodies were functioning more efficiently. The control group experienced virtually no change in their oxygen requirements during exercise.

So how important are these results? And who exactly can benefit from breathing exercises? To find the answers, we spoke with Richard Firshein, DO, director of the Firshein Center for Integrative Medicine in New York City, where patients (including those with asthma) are taught better breathing techniques through a program he developed called "Breath of Life." Dr. Firshein, a former asthma sufferer himself, is author of *Reversing Asthma.*

WHO NEEDS BREATH TRAINING?

When we draw air into our lungs, we use not only the powerful muscles at the bottom of the rib cage (the diaphragm), but also the intercostal muscles that run between the ribs. Though we use these muscles with every breath, they only rarely get additional exercise (like the kind that arm muscles get when we lift weights) to strengthen them further.

But that's a shame, he said, because exercising our breathing muscles more vigorously helps in two ways. First, stronger muscles are able to draw more air into the lungs, which then have more oxygen to utilize…and second, exercising enables these muscles to use oxygen more efficiently, delivering more oxygen to the rest of the body.

That's especially important to…

• **Athletes, whose performance is boosted by every bit of additional energy.**

• **People with asthma and other respiratory ailments.**

• **Older people, especially those over 50.** Like other muscles, our breathing muscles atrophy with age so that they're unable to draw as much air into the lungs—unless they're strengthened by exercise.

DO-IT-YOURSELF BREATH TRAINING

This type of exercise can be done very efficiently at home. If you want to follow the same plan as in the study, you'll need to purchase an IMT, which is an inexpensive plastic device used by athletes and people with asthma and other respiratory conditions to strengthen their breathing muscles. Virtually everyone can benefit from using one.

Though IMTs can cost up to $225, most people don't need complex features and options and will do fine with the less expensive models, said Dr. Firshein. He likes one made by Expand-A-Lung ($29.95) and said that PowerLung is another good brand. Both are available online.

To use an IMT: Following the instructions on your device, start with the low resistance setting. Insert it in your mouth and breathe through it for two to five minutes, twice a day. Over a month or two, gradually increase the resistance level, working up to a total of 15 or 20 minutes per session.

Note: Discuss this with your doctor first if you have a breathing condition such as asthma or COPD.

THE NO-TECH BREATHING PLAN

You also can strengthen your breathing muscles without equipment. *Here are two exercises to try…*

Breathing exercise #1: Twice a day, spend about five minutes breathing in slowly through your nose, letting your belly expand as far as is comfortable. Then, while exhaling, consciously push the air from your belly, up through your lungs and out through your mouth. Now, after you've exhaled (but not after you've inhaled), hold your breath for a few seconds—this increases the carbon dioxide level in your body. This is thought to be helpful in relaxing the muscles around the lungs to reduce strain and muscle spasm, both of which contribute to the pressure people with asthma often feel during exercise and even at rest. For the same reason, count slowly to five as you breathe in and to seven as you breathe out.

Breathing exercise #2: Now, to exercise the upper breathing muscles, again breathe slowly in and out—but this time through your mouth, expanding and contracting your chest instead of your stomach. Purse your lips to make it slightly more difficult for the air to get in and out. And again, count to about five as you breathe in and to seven as you breathe out, and hold your breath for a few seconds after you exhale.

If you slowly increase the resistance by adjusting how tightly you purse your lips when you exhale,
you will strengthen the muscles important to respiration and mimic the benefits of using an IMT.

Build to doing both of these exercises for a total of 15 to 20 minutes per day, taking about a month to get there.

Dr. Firshein said that it's not necessary to consult your doctor before starting breathing exercises unless you have asthma or another medical condition that affects your breathing or stamina.

Regardless of which exercise method you choose, he said that the result will be an overall increase in strength and endurance. That's an advantage not just in sports but in everyday life.

Remember to Breathe

Cedric X. Bryant, PhD, chief science officer, American Council of Exercise, San Diego.

At the gym, personal trainers repeatedly tell clients to remember to breathe. Why?

Efficient breathing not only enhances exercise performance and improves how you feel while training, but it also helps prevent workout injuries and problems (such as hernia, spotty vision, dizziness and fainting) that can result from the natural tendency to hold your breath while exerting yourself. Focus overall on taking deep, full breaths instead of shallow ones. But match your breathing strategy to the exercise.

During flexibility workouts: Exhale while you stretch and lengthen…inhale deeply at least a few times while holding each pose.

During strength workouts: Inhale at the rest phase of the exercise…exhale at the difficult, effort phase.

During cardio workouts: Use a comfortable, flowing breathing pattern to match your movements (while walking briskly, try inhaling for three steps, exhaling for two).

How to Breathe to Reduce Stress

HealthLetter.MayoClinic.com

Deep breathing, which uses the diaphragm rather than chest muscles, pulls oxygen in more effectively than shallower breathing.

To practice it, sit straight in a comfortable chair with feet flat on the floor or lie down flat…close your eyes, and place one hand on your stomach…breathe deeply through your nose, into the back of your throat and down to your belly, letting your chest expand…let your abdomen slowly deflate as you breathe out…repeat several times, increasing the amount of time for inhalation and exhalation…direct your breath into your upper back, letting your ribs spread and relax with each breath in and out…don't force it—let your breath flow naturally.

Breathing Technique Can Lower Blood Pressure

Daniel Craighead, PhD, postdoctoral researcher, integrative physiology department, University of Colorado at Boulder and leader of a study of 50 people, presented at the Experimental Biology 2019 conference in Orlando, Florida.

Inspiratory Muscle Strength Training (IMST) involves breathing in vigorously through a special handheld device originally developed to help critically ill people breathe without ventilators. This technique also has been shown effective in helping develop the weak breathing muscles of people with obstructive sleep apnea. Now early results of a new study show that regular use of IMST can lower systolic blood pressure (the top number) nearly twice as much as aerobic exercise does. IMST users also had better large-artery function and lower heart rate and oxygen consumption during exercise than study subjects not using the technique. Inspiratory muscle trainers already are commercially available—ask your doctor if you should consider IMST.

Deep Breathing for GERD Relief

Study titled "Diaphragmatic Breathing Reduces Belching and Proton Pump Inhibitor Refractory Gastroesophageal Reflux Symptoms," by researchers at Singapore General Hospital, published in *Clinical Gastroenterology and Hepatology.*

Between the heartburn and acid reflux—that sour taste in your mouth—GERD, or gastroesophageal reflux disease, is a challenging condition, and options to treat it leave a lot to be desired.

Wouldn't it be great if you could reduce your GERD symptoms and perhaps eliminate drugs just by breathing?

You can, according to a study done in Singapore—we'll tell you how.

Background: Drugs called proton pump inhibitors, or PPIs, the most commonly taken GERD medications, are designed to limit how much acid your stomach makes, but they don't help everyone. And even when they do provide some relief, you can't rely on them long-term because of the risk for serious side effects. Over-the-counter PPIs such as *lansoprazole* (Prevacid 24hr), *esomeprazole* (Nexium 24h) or *omeprazole magnesium* (Prilosec) should be used for only 14 days at a time and only three times a year, according to the FDA.

While prescription-strength PPIs can be used for longer periods under a doctor's supervision, various studies have raised concerns about possible links to everything from nutritional deficiencies to kidney disease to dementia.

A different class of drugs called H2 blockers—including *famotidine* (Pepcid), *cimetidine* (Tagamet) and *ranitidine* (Zantac)—are considered safer than PPIs, but neither class of drug is cleared for use beyond two weeks or helps with the problem of excessive belching, a distressing symptom that affects up to half of GERD sufferers. Most of these burps come from air trapped in the esophagus, created by fermentation in the stomach and heartburn meds simply aren't designed to address "supragastric" (above the stomach) belches. Besides being its own problem, excessive belching can bring on more reflux episodes and worsen GERD.

The study: Researchers knew that the type of belching suffered by GERD patients stems from involuntary contractions of the diaphragm, the main muscle that facilitates breathing and contains acid in the stomach. Therefore, they reasoned, purposely focusing one's breathing on the diaphragm might help GERD patients with the belching and lessen the occurrence of GERD.

They recruited 36 people with GERD who had been on PPI therapy without getting relief from belching and split them into two groups. The people in one group had four one-on-one sessions of diaphragmatic breathing therapy (DBT) with a therapist over a period of four weeks…while those in the other group were put on a waiting list for the training.

The results: After the month of therapy, the number of belches was cut in half in 60% of the deep breathers, whereas no one in the control group had any reduction. Even better, participants' other GERD symptoms and their overall quality of life improved, too. They continued to be followed for four months and said they maintained better control of their belching and their GERD through the breathing…and had less need for PPI medication for other symptoms.

TRY IT YOURSELF

Strengthening the diaphragm does lessen reflux. The breathing technique practiced by these GERD patients isn't complicated—all it takes is some focus.

Here's how to breathe from your diaphragm…

- **Get comfortable in a chair.**

- **Place one hand over your abdomen below your rib cage and the other on your chest.**

- **Breathe in deeply through your nose on a slow count of four to fill your lungs.** Then slowly let out the breath through your lips, again on a slow count of four. This allows your diaphragm to go through its full range of motion, dropping down as you inhale and rising up as you exhale. If you're doing it right, the hand on your belly should move up and down with each breath, but the one on your chest should remain almost still. As you gain practice, keep inhalation to a slow count of four, while extending exhalation to a slow count of eight.

Practice diaphragmatic breathing for five to 10 minutes at a time, three times day.

Bonus tips: If you have GERD, lifestyle changes like not drinking alcohol and avoiding food within three hours of bedtime may soothe the burn as well. Try out some safe home remedies, too.

Yoga Breathing: The Surprising Secrets to Its Benefits

Sundar Balasubramanian, PhD, C-IAYT, a cell biologist and assistant professor of research in the department of radiation oncology at Medical University of South Carolina in Charleston. He is also founding director of Prana Science Institute, PranaScience.com, a website dedicated to research and education on yoga breathing. His research has been published in *International Psychogeriatrics, Evidence-Based Complementary and Alternative Medicine* and other professional journals.

Most health-savvy people know that deep breathing has a wide range of mind-body benefits backed by loads of scientific evidence.

But cell biologist and certified yoga therapist Sundar Balasubramanian, PhD, C-IAYT, was inspired to investigate further after a realization that he produced an abundance of saliva while practicing controlled yoga breathing exercises collectively known as pranayama. He has since conducted pioneering research into the role that spittle (aka "spit") plays in the healing effects of deep breathing.

HIDDEN POWERS OF SALIVA

Hundreds of studies have demonstrated the benefits of yoga breathing—ranging from lower blood pressure and less depression to better concentration and improved lung function—but it's not known why saliva is produced so abundantly during pranayama.

191

Recognized mainly for its role in promoting healthy digestion, saliva is comprised of about 98% water and various other substances, such as enzymes that help break down food. When people go about their daily activities, they produce about 25 to 50 ounces of saliva daily. However, if you're stressed, your mouth becomes dry. So it makes sense that when your body is extremely relaxed—as occurs during yoga breathing—you produce more saliva than you ordinarily would.

But how does that boost in saliva production contribute to pranayama's benefits? It's been established that saliva contains more than 1,000 proteins along with other crucial molecules, such as neurohormones. And it's been shown that the specific makeup of each person's saliva is unique, and it can change from day to day—even moment to moment based on one's emotional and physiological responses. *Saliva is believed to contribute to the healing effects of yoga breathing by…*

•**Increasing brain-boosting proteins.** Through our research published in *International Psychogeriatrics,* we discovered that a protein called nerve growth factor (NGF) increased 10 times more in the saliva of people practicing pranayama for a single 20-minute session compared with study participants who quietly read an article for the same length of time. This is significant because NGF goes straight to the brain, where it encourages brain cell growth. NGF levels are substantially lower in Alzheimer's patients.

•**Elevating cancer-suppressing proteins.** With a study published in *Evidence-Based Complementary and Alternative Medicine,* we confirmed that pranayama not only stimulates saliva production but also elevates levels of proteins with immunity-building and cancer-suppressing properties.

•**Reducing inflammatory markers.** Pranayama also reduces production of inflammatory biomarkers in saliva that are linked to such conditions as pain, depression and diseases, such as scleroderma and post-traumatic stress disorder (PTSD), according to research we published in *BMC Complementary and Alternative Medicine.*

TWO EXERCISES TO GET STARTED

With such varied health benefits—and a new understanding of saliva's crucial role in delivering them—you may be eager to try pranayama.

If you're just starting out with yoga breathing, it's common to worry that you'll "do it wrong." But the truth is, all you have to do is breathe, count and pay attention to how you're feeling. If you don't force an uncomfortable breathing practice or hold your breath for too long, there's nothing about pranayama that you can do wrong.

Important: If you have a respiratory disorder, such as emphysema or chronic obstructive pulmonary disease (COPD), consult your physician and/or a yoga therapist on the right exercises for your condition.

Even though there are numerous approaches to yoga breathing, here are two simple exercises to get you started—for best results, sit up straight, close your eyes and do one or both of the following throughout the day…

•**Beginner humming breath.** Also called "bee breath" because of the buzzing sound you make, this exercise is a good introduction to yoga breathing. It's quick, easy and doesn't require you to hold your breath.

What to do: Breathe deeply and inhale as much as you can comfortably. Then hum as you slowly exhale at a rate that is comfortable for you. Repeat this exercise for a minute or two when you wake up…and before eating breakfast and your other meals or snacks throughout the day to stimulate your saliva flow.

•**Cooling breath.** This exercise promotes copious saliva production by stimulating the glands in your oral cavity.

What to do: Roll your tongue in a U-shape. Inhale slowly through your tongue, then exhale through your nostrils. Repeat for five to 10 minutes. If you can't roll your tongue, inhale through your mouth while smiling and exhale through your nostrils.

To learn more about yoga breathing, go to PranaScience.com.

Can't Catch Your Breath? The Problem May Have Nothing to Do With Your Lungs…

Len Horovitz, MD, an internist and pulmonary specialist at Carnegie Medical PC, a private practice, and clinical instructor in medicine, Weill Cornell medicine, both in New York City. *New York Magazine* has included him among "The Best Doctors in New York" for both pulmonary and internal medicine. He is a contributor to the medical anthology *The Singer's Guide to Complete Health*.

Perhaps climbing a flight or two of stairs has never really affected your breathing—until now. Or maybe you notice that it's harder to breathe even when you're simply watching television. What's going on?

You might wonder whether you are developing a common lung problem such as asthma or chronic obstructive pulmonary disease (COPD)—especially if you're over age 40…you have a history of allergies…are a current or former smoker…or have been exposed for long periods to secondhand smoke, heavy dust or chemical fumes.

But don't be too quick to make assumptions. There's a chance that your lungs have nothing to do with your shortness of breath.

WHEN BREATHING IS A STRUGGLE

Breathing allows us to bring oxygen into the body and expel carbon dioxide. When your body doesn't have enough oxygen or has too much carbon dioxide, you automatically breathe faster. You'll perceive this as breathlessness, a condition known as dyspnea.

What you may not realize: Dyspnea can be caused by dozens of different problems. *Among the most common…**

●**Anemia.** It occurs when you do not have enough red blood cells or hemoglobin, a substance in blood that transports oxygen to tissues throughout the body. Various forms of anemia—such as iron-deficiency anemia or pernicious (low levels of vitamin B-12) anemia—can cause breathlessness.

*If you experience a degree and/or frequency of breathlessness that is new to you, see your doctor.

Anemia may be accompanied by: Fatigue, rapid heartbeat, leg cramps or difficulty concentrating.

Next steps: Anemia can readily be detected by blood tests, such as a complete blood count (CBC) and blood analyses to examine the size/shape of red blood cells.

Treatment: Your breathing will improve once the underlying cause of the anemia is identified and treated—with supplemental iron or vitamin B-12, for example, or with antibiotics for an ulcer (internal bleeding from an ulcer is a common cause of anemia). Iron-deficiency anemia also can occur with some cases of colon cancer due to a slow loss of blood from the colon.

●**Anxiety.** It is a common cause of breathlessness. When you are stressed or anxious, you tend to take short, shallow and rapid breaths. This breathing pattern, known as hyperventilation, is inefficient and causes changes in the normal balance of oxygen and carbon dioxide.

Anxiety may be accompanied by: A rapid heartbeat, numbness or tingling in the hands or feet and sometimes a feeling of faintness.

Next steps: Your doctor will first check for possible physical causes of breathlessness, such as asthma or a lung infection. You might be given a chest X-ray and spirometry, a test that's administered in your doctor's office and involves blowing into a device to measure lung capacity.

Treatment: If tests show that you are physically healthy, your doctor may refer you to a psychiatrist or other anxiety-treatment specialist. You might benefit from counseling or an antianxiety medication, such as *lorazepam* (Ativan) or *clonazepam* (Klonopin).

Also helpful: Abdominal breathing, which involves inhaling deeply through the nose for about 10 seconds, then slowly exhaling for about 10 seconds. But don't make the mistake of performing this technique only when you're feeling anxious. If you do it for about five minutes a few times a day, you'll slowly begin to naturally breathe more deeply all the time, including during times of stress. If you feel light-headed while practicing abdominal breathing, stop for 20 seconds, then start again.

●**Side effect of beta-blockers.** These drugs are prescribed for high blood pressure, angina, heart failure and mild anxiety. Drugs in this class often cause shortness of breath because they affect beta-adrenergic receptors in the lungs as well as in the heart and arteries.

Use of beta-blockers may be accompanied by: Wheezing, changes in heartbeat or dizziness.

Next steps: Suspect that the beta-blocker may be to blame if your symptoms began within two weeks of starting the drug. When you see your doctor, bring a list of all the medications that you take. Breathlessness also can be caused by an allergic reaction to a medication, such as an antibiotic.

Treatment: If the breathlessness is too uncomfortable, ask your doctor about switching to a different class of blood pressure medication. Or he/she might prescribe one of the newer selective beta-blockers, such as *metoprolol* (Lopressor) or *acebutolol* (Sectral), which are somewhat less likely to affect the lungs than older beta-blockers.

●**Heart failure.** It often causes shortness of breath because the heart can't supply the body with adequate amounts of oxygen. What usually happens is that the heart's pumping chambers, or ventricles, don't fill with enough blood, so less blood is circulated with each heartbeat. Or the chambers don't generate enough force to circulate blood efficiently.

Heart failure may be accompanied by: Fatigue, a persistent cough or swelling of the feet, ankles and legs.

Next steps: Among other tests, your doctor will probably order an EKG, a chest X-ray to determine whether the heart is enlarged or there's fluid in the lungs, and a blood test for the hormone BNP (levels increase in patients with heart failure).

Treatment: You'll probably be given medications that lower blood pressure and reduce the heart's workload. You also might need surgically implanted electrodes to correct heartbeat irregularities (arrhythmias) or increase the force of the heartbeat.

Important: Shortness of breath also is a classic sign of a heart attack. If you're suddenly breathless and it's a new symptom, get to an emergency room right away or call 911.

●**Pulmonary embolism.** You should suspect that you have this condition, which occurs when a blood clot enters a lung, if you have sudden shortness of breath. What usually happens is that a blood clot from a leg vein travels to an artery in a lung and blocks circulation. About 30% of patients with a pulmonary embolism will die if they don't get emergency treatment.

Pulmonary embolism may be accompanied by: Chest pain and/or coughing (with or without blood). Some patients will notice pain, swelling or discoloration on part of one leg—a sign that blood clots have formed.

Next steps: Call 911. An ultrasound or CT scan will be used to detect clots. Your doctor might order a lung ventilation/perfusion scan to show how well blood is flowing through the lungs.

Treatment: You will be hospitalized if you have (or are suspected of having) a pulmonary embolism. You'll probably be given intravenous heparin, a fast-acting blood thinner, along with oral *warfarin* (Coumadin) to prevent additional clots from forming. Most patients will continue anticoagulant therapy for at least six months.

MORE FROM DR. HOROVITZ...

Is It Pneumonia?

Even a slight cold or the flu can take your breath away, but don't assume that a cold or the flu is all you have.

Many people who think they have a cold actually have pneumonia, a lung infection that kills about 50,000 Americans every year.

Walking pneumonia, the term for mild cases, usually clears up on its own within a week to 10 days.

More serious cases of pneumonia, however, often require hospitalization and treatment with antibiotics. Serious cases of pneumonia usually are caused by bacteria rather than viruses.

Red flags: Fever, cough, discolored or bloody mucus, chest pain and chills—especially when accompanied by shortness of breath—warrant a visit to your doctor right away.

Also important: Get vaccinated for pneumonia if you're age 65 or older…or if you have pneumonia risk factors such as smoking or a history of heart/lung disease, diabetes or liver disease.

Acute bronchitis, inflammation of the main air passages to the lungs, is less serious than pneumonia but also can cause shortness of breath. Check with your doctor.

Play the Harmonica to Strengthen Your Lungs

Vivian Low, MPH, RN-BC, FPCNA, clinical manager of the cardiovascular and pulmonary rehabilitation program, El Camino Hospital, Mountain View, California.

Missy Von Luehrte, RN, pulmonary rehabilitation nurse, El Camino Hospital, Mountain View, California.

John Schamen, MD, Ontario Aerobics Center, Canada.

Blowing the blues is good for your lungs. So is just about anything else you play on a harmonica. Whether your tastes run to "Love Me Do," "Sweet Home Chicago" or that 19th-century nonsense ditty "Oh! Susanna," as little as 10 minutes a day playing a harmonica may give you better breathing. In fact, what they're calling "harmonica therapy" is gaining steam in pulmonary-rehabilitation programs across the country for people with asthma, COPD and even lung transplants. But don't let the word "therapy" put you off. Playing the harmonica is a ton of fun, and it's good exercise for healthy lungs, too.

Whether your lungs are compromised or in good shape, you should try it—here's why…

TOE-TAPPING MUSIC-MAKING CLINICAL THERAPY

How does harmonica playing strengthen the lungs? Experts say that it mimics the inspiratory (inhaling) and expiratory (exhaling) breathing exercises taught by pulmonary rehabilitation staff.

When you play a harmonica, you create sounds by the resistance of your breath against the instrument's reeds. Unlike, say, the clarinet, you're working against that reed resistance when you're exhaling and when you're inhaling. That strengthens the diaphragm (the largest muscle of the respiratory system), encourages deep breathing, and may help clear mucus from the lungs. While scientific studies haven't specifically validated therapeutic harmonica playing, it mimics…and encourages… the breathing exercises that have been shown to improve lung function.

Lung specialists around the country believe in it. "We use harmonicas for all patients with pulmonary disease," says Missy Von Luehrte, RN, pulmonary rehabilitation nurse at El Camino Hospital in Mountain View, California. It's not only effective but fun and relaxing, easy to learn and an inexpensive, easy-to-carry instrument, she says. Patients like it, too. Says Vivian Low, MPH, RN-BC, clinical manager of the pulmonary-rehabilitation program at El Camino Hospital, "Anecdotally, in all the programs across the United States that have used harmonica with lung patients, the patients feel that they are strengthening their breathing."

FOR PEOPLE WITH HEALTHY LUNGS, TOO, IT'S INTERNAL POWER LIFTING

Some experts believe that playing a wind instrument such as the harmonica can benefit everyone, especially as we age. After about the age of 30, most people begin to lose lung function. By age 50, even people with healthy lungs may lose 50% of their younger capacity, says John Schaman, MD, Ontario Aerobics Centre, a cardiac rehabilitation center in Ontario, Canada. "There is considerable anecdotal evidence that those who use their lungs in more extraordinary ways have less decline," he says.

Sure, you can get deep breathing in other ways, such as meditation practice and yoga, and that's great. What harmonica adds is resistance, says Von Luehrte. "It's like lifting weights for your lungs."

DO YOU NEED A SPECIAL TYPE OF HARMONICA?

Some experts recommend harmonicas specifically developed for lung therapy. The Pulmonica, (Pulmonica.com) for example, is designed to create more resistance than a standard harmonica, promoting the clearance of secretions. It makes a pleasant sound, but you can't as easily use it to play songs. The Seydel Medical Harmonica, which Dr.

Schaman helped develop, uses chords rather than single notes, so it may be easier for some people to learn than a standard harmonica.

Others prefer everyday harmonicas. Pulmonary nurse Von Luehrte thinks devices such as the Pulmonica and the Seydel can take the fun out of a simple, joyful musical experience, making harmonica play more like other physical therapy exercises and less of a relaxing, social activity. And while playing chords may be easier and create more resistance, it hasn't been shown that one way of playing is better, healthwise, than another.

So go play…a minimum of 10 minutes a day—more is better. Many pulmonary centers across the country have harmonica therapy groups, which can make it a more social—and musical—experience. Plus the instructors can teach patients the basics of proper breathing and playing. Some senior centers are getting into the act, too. The most important skill to learn is to breathe with your diaphragm to help your lungs expand, according to nurse Low. If you want to explore a musical approach, check out the book and CD "Harmonica for Fun and Health" (available at MelBay.com) to get you started. Or you can Google "harmonica therapy" or "learn to play harmonica" to find a number of instructional sites.

4 Secrets to Easier Breathing

Gerard J. Criner, MD, a professor of medicine and director of pulmonary and critical care medicine at Temple Lung Center at Temple University School of Medicine in Philadelphia. He is codirector of the Center for Inflammation, Translational and Clinical Lung Research.

Simple ways to help yourself when you just can't catch your breath…

If you can't catch your breath, walking, climbing stairs or simply carrying on a conversation can be a challenge.

When breathing is a struggle, you wouldn't think that exercise is the answer. But it can be a solution for people with chronic obstructive pulmonary disease (COPD) or heart failure or even for healthy people who occasionally become short of breath.*

Four better-breathing techniques that really help…

PURSED-LIP BREATHING

When you're feeling short of breath, inhale through your nose for two seconds, then pucker your lips as if you were going to whistle or blow out a candle. Exhale through pursed lips for four seconds.

How it helps: It prolongs the respiratory cycle and gives you more time to empty your lungs. This is particularly important if you have emphysema. With emphysema, air gets trapped in the lungs. The trapped air causes the lungs to overinflate, which reduces the amount of force that they're able to generate. This results in a buildup of carbon dioxide that makes it difficult to breathe.

You may need to do this only when you're more active than usual and short of breath. Or you may breathe better when you do it often.

CHANGING POSITIONS

Simply changing how you stand or sit can improve breathing when you're feeling winded.

How it helps: Certain positions help muscles around the diaphragm work more efficiently to promote easier breathing.

Examples: While sitting, lean your chest forward…rest your elbows on your knees…and relax your upper-body muscles. When standing, bend forward at the waist and rest your hands on a table or the back of a chair. Or back up to a wall…support yourself with your hips…and lean forward and put your hands on your thighs.

CONTROLLED COUGHING

Your lungs produce excessive mucus when you have COPD. The congestion makes it harder to breathe. It also increases the risk for pneumonia and other lung infections. A normal, explosive cough is not effective at removing mucus. In fact, out-of-control coughing can cause airways to collapse and

*If you don't have COPD, you should see a doctor if you have shortness of breath after only slight activity or while resting, or if shortness of breath wakes you up at night or requires you to sleep propped up to breathe.

trap even more mucus. A controlled cough is more effective (and requires less oxygen and energy). You also can use this technique to help clear mucus from your lungs when you have a cold.

How to do it: Sit on a chair or the edge of your bed with both feet on the floor. Fold your arms around your midsection…breathe in slowly through your nose…then lean forward while pressing your arms against your abdomen. Lightly cough two or three times. Repeat as needed.

Important: Taking slow, gentle breaths through your nose while using this technique will prevent mucus from moving back into the airways.

COLD-AIR ASSISTANCE

This is a quick way to breathe better. When you are short of breath—or doing an activity that you know will lead to breathlessness, such as walking on a treadmill—position a fan so that it blows cool air on your face. You also can splash your face with cold water if you become short of breath.

How it helps: Cool air and water stimulate the trigeminal nerve in the face, which slows respiration and helps ease shortness of breath. That's why the treadmills and exercise bikes used in respiratory-rehabilitation facilities often are equipped with small fans.

WHEN TO GET BREATHING HELP FROM A PROFESSIONAL

You can do many breathing exercises on your own without the help of a health professional. For the techniques below, however, it's best to first consult a respiratory therapist (ask your doctor for a referral) to ensure that you know how to do the exercise properly. You can then continue on your own.

•**Paced breathing for endurance.** This technique is useful for people who have COPD and/or heart failure, since it improves lung capacity and heart function.

How it helps: With practice, this technique can increase your cardio-respiratory endurance by 30% to 40%. To perform the exercise, a metronome is set at a rate that's faster than your usual respiratory rate. Your therapist will encourage you to breathe as hard and as fast as you can for, say,

about 15 minutes. (Beginners might do it for only a few minutes at a time.)

Example: The metronome may be set for 20 breaths per minute to start, and you may eventually work up to 40 breaths per minute.

You'll notice that breathing becomes easier when you're doing various activities—for instance, when you're exercising, climbing stairs or taking brisk walks.

•**Inspiratory muscle training.** Think of this as a workout for your breathing muscles. It is especially helpful for people with COPD or other lung diseases and those recovering from respiratory failure. People who strengthen these muscles can improve their breathing efficiency by 25% to 30%.

How it helps: For this breathing exercise, you'll use a device known as an inspiratory muscle trainer, which includes a mouthpiece, a one-way valve and resistance settings. When you inhale, the one-way valve closes. You're forced to use effort to breathe against resistance. Then the valve opens so that you can exhale normally. This breathing exercise is typically performed for 15 minutes twice a day. You can buy these devices online.

Good choice: The Threshold Inspiratory Muscle Trainer, available at FitnessMart.com for $59.95.

Lung Fitness for Flu Season

Andrew L. Rubman, ND, medical director, Southbury Clinic for Traditional Medicines, Southbury, Connecticut. SouthburyClinic.com

Everyone dreads getting sick in the wintertime, but some people find themselves unusually vulnerable to respiratory infections…most particularly those who have asthma or a history of bronchitis. We all know about flu shots and washing hands and avoiding crowds, but there's lots more you can do to fortify yourself—and your respiratory system in particular—even before the sick season kicks in.

First and foremost, remember that the better shape you and your respiratory system are in, the more you'll be able to tolerate exposure to germs without falling ill. Anything that weakens your immune system—such as eating poorly, stress or not getting enough sleep—increases your vulnerability to whatever is going around. And previous illness makes it worse. Not only does illness deplete energy, but with severe respiratory infections (and other diseases, too), there may be scarring and some tissue damage in your lungs that leaves you weaker and more vulnerable. More often than we realize, an illness may not be fully resolved, even after you feel better. There may be underlying colonization with mold organisms in the respiratory tract as well. When researchers at the Mayo Clinic cultured patients with chronic rhinosinusitis, over 90% showed positive culture for fungus, including mold. Mold infestation in respiratory tissues weakens the structure and capability of the lungs, allowing easier colonization of potentially infectious bacteria.

STRENGTHEN YOUR IMMUNE SYSTEM

The following supplements can be helpful in supporting lung health and immune health...work with your own doctor for specific dosing.

INDIAN TOBACCO

This botanical remedy has a history of use for conditions such as asthma, pneumonia and bronchitis. I may prescribe Indian tobacco (also called lobelia, it's not really tobacco at all—the leaves have a tobacco-like taste) as a preventive to strengthen lungs and a treatment for respiratory ailments.

Note: Lobelia is potentially toxic in large doses and should be taken only under the guidance of a health-care provider with experience in botanical medicines.

SELENIUM: NATURE'S INFLAMMATION FIGHTER

This essential trace mineral has potent antioxidant properties to protect the body from inflammation and damage caused by free radicals. It fortifies the immune system to do battle with microorganisms. Research even suggests that a high intake of selenium is associated with a reduced risk of death from colorectal, prostate and lung cancers. While the usual dose is 200 mcg a day, I frequently go further, prescribing a daily dosage as high as 400

mcg to 500 mcg, taken in three doses, as a preventive during flu season.

VITAMIN C: THE ANTIOXIDANT VITAMIN

This antioxidant-packed nutrient remains a major player in immune system maintenance. Research demonstrates that vitamin C can significantly boost antimicrobial activity, including the activity of natural killer cells that hunt down and vanquish germs. Supplementation with up to one gram (1,000 mg) daily can be helpful and is usually well-tolerated.

Note: Some studies suggest that vitamin C may not be safe for patients undergoing chemotherapy.

FISH OIL: A RICH SOURCE OF OMEGA-3 FATTY ACIDS

Tuna and salmon (preferably wild) are rich sources of omega-3 fatty acids. Eat these three times a week. Look for fish oil supplements with the highest levels of docosahexaenoic acid (DHA) and eicosapentaenoic acid (EPA), which ideally should make up more than 50% of the total dosage. (*Caution:* If you take a blood-thinning medication such as warfarin, speak with your doctor before taking fish oil supplements.)

MULLEIN: A VELVETY SMOOTH THROAT SOOTHER

When patients complain of a scratchy throat or congestion and sense a respiratory problem coming on, I often prescribes mullein. This herb contains mucilage, a substance that soothes irritated respiratory passages, along with saponins that help loosen mucus. Laboratory studies have shown that mullein can kill many viruses on contact. To make a cup of mullein tea, add one to two teaspoons of dried leaves and flowers to boiling water and steep for 10 minutes. Strain before drinking.

N-ACETYL CYSTEINE AND L-THEANINE

New and emerging research supports using n-acetyl cysteine and L-theanine to strengthen lung function. Discuss with your doctor whether either or both are appropriate for you, and, if they are, what the dosage should be.

AVOID POLLUTANTS

Respiratory disorders of all kinds, including flu and pneumonia, are more apt to develop when foreign particles are or inhaled into the lungs, including from chimneys, wood stoves and fireplaces. This causes inflammation, which leads the delicate mucous membranes lining the respiratory system to become swollen, irritated and more susceptible to infection.

It's important to make an effort to protect your lungs from this environmental assault, especially during the winter months when flu season is in full force. Consider, with your physician's oversight, taking antioxidant supplements for protection. In one study, children with asthma who took vitamins C and E were less likely to experience breathing problems from air pollution than children who did not.

MAKE YOUR LUNGS STRONG

Exercising the lungs may help fend off disease as well. Many tend toward "shallow breathing," failing to fully inflate the lungs with air or clear them completely. This limits the exchange of gases. Use the intentional breathing of Pranayama yoga to strengthen your lungs. *Here's how...*

•**Sit up straight, with your spine, neck and head in a straight line.** Do so cross-legged on a floor mat, small pillow or rug, or—if you find that uncomfortable—just use a chair.

•**Close your eyes and relax.** Meditate, or visualize yourself in a peaceful environment—for example, lying on the beach, listening to the sound of the waves.

•**Take a full, deep, intentional breath, filling lungs from the bottom up.** To make sure you are doing this correctly, place your hand on your stomach and feel this area (which is above and behind the diaphragm, a vital muscle for respiration) expand before air fills the upper chest.

•**Inhale for a count of three**...exhale for a count of six. As time goes on, with practice you will be able to gradually increase these counts (ideally, at the same one-to-two ratio).

•**Do this for 10 minutes once or twice a day.**

Note: I believe that unless you have ongoing respiratory issues, the various breathing and blowing devices that promise to increase respiratory capacity are a waste of money. Deep breathing achieves the same results, and for free.

DRINK UP

It is important to remain well-hydrated, drinking plenty of water and other fluids all year, but especially during flu season since fluids moisturize the mucous membranes and help keep nasal discharge thin. Dehydration can lead to dizziness, disorientation and even vulnerability to shock. Decaffeinated herbal teas, broth, diluted fruit juice and sparkling water are all good choices.

RECOVERY AFTER ILLNESS

Recovery should focus not only on resting so you will feel better, but also on improving your underlying function to better resist the next challenges. A professional nutritional consultant or physician formally trained in nutrition can be helpful in making certain you are completely over the illness and ensuring you get strong for the future.

RESPECT THE ENEMY

You can't reduce your risk of illness to zero, even with all these precautions. Recognize that flu and pneumonia can be serious and their complications potentially life-threatening, especially in older people. If you suspect something is wrong—for example, if you have chronic chest pain, a persistent cough, shortness of breath or green or yellow sputum—see your physician promptly for proper diagnosis and treatment.

12

Routines That Heal Pain

How to Exercise Despite Pain in Your Knees and Back

Marilyn Moffat, PT, DPT, PhD, a practicing physical therapist and professor of physical therapy at New York University, New York City. She is coauthor of *Age Defying Fitness: Making the Most of Your Body for the Rest of Your Life*.

Exercise is the magic elixir. It protects the heart, strengthens bones, lifts mood, increases energy, improves memory, boosts metabolism and prevents disease. But how can you get these benefits if your body hurts?

That is the problem for millions of Americans with chronic pain, especially knee pain or back pain. You want to exercise, but getting over that "pain hump" while you exercise is just too tough.

The irony is that pain not only makes regular exercise tougher—it also makes it more important. Why? It's a path toward less pain and a greater ability to do everyday tasks.

Here are exercises that almost everyone can do. But no single exercise is perfect for everybody, and your unique limitations and physical condition will dictate your ideal activity. Many people with chronic joint or back pain benefit from a detailed individual plan developed with a physical therapist. Ask your health-care provider for a recommendation or go to the website of the American Physical Therapy Association (MoveForwardPT.com), and click on "Find a PT" at the top of the page. It's always a good idea to check with your doctor before beginning a new exercise program.

When trying these exercises, start slowly, be cautious and pay attention to doing them correctly.

Important: Many people may need to build up to the "hold" times. For example, if an exercise calls for you to hold a pose for 30 seconds and that's too hard, try doing it for 10 seconds. If even that's too hard, just hold it as long as you can. You'll get stronger over time.

Stop immediately if any particular movement causes sharp pain, especially in a joint area. On the other hand, muscle fatigue (even burn) should be expected, especially with strengthening exercises. It's a good thing! *Let's get moving…*

IF YOU HAVE KNEE PAIN

The best way to reduce knee pain is to increase the strength and flexibility in the muscles that support your knee. The key is to find exercises that permit pain-free range of motion. That means taking the load off the joint as much as possible. Walking in waist-deep water is a great way to do this—but not everyone has regular access to a pool. *Alternatives…*

•**Seated straight-leg raises build up the quadriceps, which help support the knees.**

What to do: Sit on the floor with your back against a wall. With one knee bent and the other leg straight out in front of you, wrap your hands around your bent leg, then slowly raise the straight leg up, keeping the knee as straight as possible— hold for 30 seconds. Then slowly lower the straight leg back to the floor. Do the exercise two or three times on each side.

•**Bridges strengthen the hamstrings and quadriceps (key knee muscles),** as well as the glutes and both the front and back of your body's core.

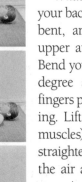

What to do: Lie on your back with your knees bent, and your feet and upper arms on the floor. Bend your elbows to a 90-degree angle, with your fingers pointing to the ceiling. Lift your glutes (butt muscles) off the floor, then straighten one leg out in the air at the level of the opposite knee and hold for 30 seconds. Bend the knee down, put your foot back on the floor and lower your butt. Alternate legs. Do this exercise two or three times per leg.

IF YOU HAVE BACK PAIN

People with spinal stenosis (narrowing of the spaces within the spine) or other degenerative changes in the low back have a hard time with many exercises. Even walking can be difficult with spinal stenosis because each step slightly extends the spine, which narrows the spinal canal, exacerbating the pain.

What helps: Increasing flexibility and core strength. Yoga planks with the spine straight or slightly rounded are especially beneficial—they strengthen the core muscles that support the back as well as the arm and leg muscles. Pay attention to good form.

•**Basic front plank.** Start on your hands and knees with your hands directly under your shoulders and your knees directly under your hips. Straighten one leg all the way back, then the other leg, and you should be in perfect position. (If weight

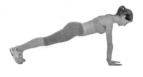

bearing on straight arms is too difficult, do a plank on your forearms.) Tuck your chin in so that your neck is straight and you are looking at the floor. Your spine should be in a straight line and not arched. Maintain as straight a line as is comfortable from your head through to your ankles. Hold for 30 seconds. Do two or three times.

•**Side plank also strengthens the core muscles and the arms and legs.** Start by lying on your left side and with your left hand directly under your left shoulder. Ideally your feet should be stacked

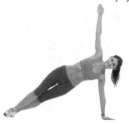

one on top of the other, but it's fine to start with the bottom knee bent. Lift your hips off the floor, and keep a straight line from your head through your shoulder, hips and feet. As you lift your hips, push your left hand into the floor. (Again, if weight bearing on a straight arm is too difficult, do the side plank on your forearm.) Hold for 30 seconds. Alternate sides. Do two or three times on each side.

AEROBIC FITNESS FOR ANYONE WITH PAIN

Whether you have pain in your knees or back (or hips or somewhere else), getting aerobic activity to improve your circulation and protect your heart can be challenging. But it's vital! *Here are ways to do it…*

•**Recumbent exercise bikes** (the kind where you are seated against a backrest) and seated stepper machines allow you to build your aerobic capacity. Being seated while doing aerobic exercise usually is easier for your back and reduces the forces on your knees that would occur if you were using a treadmill. The seated stepper, which resembles a recumbent elliptical machine, engages your arms as well as your legs. Many gyms have these machines.

Photo credit: GettyImages

What about walking? It's great if you can do it comfortably.

Tip: To absorb impact, wear sneakers that have good cushioned bottoms, add gel inserts into the sneakers and wear padded socks.

•**When walking on a treadmill,** use the handrails for support and to off-load some of the force of the body weight on your back and knees.

•**When walking outside,** choose school tracks or nature paths if possible—they're a little easier than paved sidewalks and roads—and you might consider walking poles. They help to absorb some impact, engage your upper body, help intensify your workout and improve stability. They are available at sporting-goods stores and online. Be sure to use two poles for the best balance and posture.

RX for Pain in the Back… Neck…Shoulders…More— A Simple Exercise Can Do the Trick

Joel Harper, a personal trainer in New York City who designs workouts for Olympic athletes, celebrities, musicians and business executives. He created the workout chapters for the best-selling YOU series of books by Michael Roizen, MD, and Mehmet Oz, MD. He is creator of the PBS best-selling DVDs *Firming After 50* and *Slim & Fit.* JoelHarperFitness.com

Before you turn to surgery or drugs for back or neck pain or carpal tunnel syndrome, try a simple exercise instead. Many of the most common injuries and disorders affecting joints, muscles, tendons, ligaments and/or nerves can be prevented, and often relieved, with targeted exercises and stretches. These work as massage for your muscles. (If the exercise or stretch starts to hurt, ease up.)

CARPAL TUNNEL PAIN

Carpal tunnel syndrome is caused by pressure on the median nerve that passes through a narrow "tunnel" in the wrist. Even a small amount of swelling or inflammation in this area can cause numbness, tingling and weakness. People who perform repetitive motions of the hand and wrist—such as assembly-line workers and those who often use computers, smartphones and the like—have a high risk of getting it. *Exercises that help…*

•**Wrist twists.** Get down on your hands and knees. Rotate your hands so that your middle fingers on each hand are facing directly toward the same knee, thumbs on the outside. Keep your elbows soft and your head down. Maintain this position for about five deep inhales. It helps to gently relax into the position. Gradually walk your knees away from your fingers to increase your stretch.

•**Wrist circles.** This movement "opens up" the wrist and reduces tightness. With your elbows bent, hold both hands in front of your torso, with the palms facing up. Rotate your hands/wrists in a complete circle five times. Then do five more circles in the opposite direction.

Important: It's normal for one wrist to be tighter than the other. Rotating both wrists simultaneously a few times a day will help keep the muscles balanced.

NECK PAIN

This is another malady of the computer age. People who work on computers often spend hours in the same hunched-over position without taking breaks to stretch.

Fact: Neck pain usually is caused by shoulder tension. Exercises that target the neck aren't the most effective, because they don't address shoulder tightness. *Exercises that help…*

•**Shoulder rolls.** Stand straight, with your arms relaxed at your sides. Roll your shoulders in a backward circle slowly five times. Then roll them forward five times.

•**Chicken wing.** Place the back of your right hand on your right hip, with your palm facing out. Your elbow should jut out like a chicken wing. With your left hand on your right elbow, gently pull the right elbow toward your belly button. Keep your left and right shoulders at the same height. Hold the stretch for five deep inhales with your chest lifted, then repeat on the other side.

LOW BACK PAIN

The back stretches recommended by most trainers temporarily will relieve tightness and pain, but they don't affect muscles in the hips. Tightness in the hips pulls the spine out of alignment, which can cause painful contractions in muscles in the lower back. *Exercises that help…*

•**Hip rolls.** Stand up straight with your hands on your hips and your feet perfectly together. Make a complete circle with your hips, rotating to the right. Do this five times. Repeat in the other direction.

•**Wall hammock.** Sit on the floor with your back against a wall, your left foot flat on the floor and your left knee bent. Cross your right ankle over your left knee. From this position, slide your tailbone toward the base of the wall to cause a stretch. Hold the position for about 20 seconds, then relax. Switch legs, and do the stretch again.

PLANTAR FASCIITIS

This is a painful inflammation of the plantar fascia, the band of connective tissue that runs from the heel bone along the bottom of the foot toward the toes. *Exercise that helps…*

•**Toe rolls.** Stand up straight with your hands on your waist. Keeping the toes of your right foot on the floor, raise the right heel. Rotate your right knee in a circle, keeping the toes as motionless as possible on the floor. Repeat five times clockwise and five times counterclockwise. Repeat with the other foot.

SHOULDER PAIN

Shoulders often hurt because of inflammation or a small tear in the ligaments that make up the rotator cuff, the four major muscles and tendons in the shoulder.

Start by doing shoulder rolls, described above. *Another exercise that helps…*

•**Shoulder squeezer.** Lie on the floor on your right side, with your knees slightly bent. Prop your right arm up on your tricep, with the back of the upper part of your arm flat on the floor and the fingers of your hand pointing up. Place your left hand on the back of your right wrist, and very gently press until your right palm is going toward the floor. Hold for three deep inhales, relax and then repeat once. Then switch sides.

SHIN SPLINTS

They're common in runners and those who engage in stop-and-start sports, such as tennis, soccer and basketball. Repetitive and excessive force on the muscle on top of the shinbone (the same muscle that lifts the toes) can cause inflammation and/or "micro-tears" in the muscle fibers. *Exercise that helps…*

•**Knee lifts.** This is among the best exercises for reducing tightness in the muscle and, in some cases, helping shin splints heal more quickly. Do this exercise very slowly and only if you don't have knee problems. (If you have knee problems, talk with your doctor or physical therapist.)

Kneel on the floor so that you're sitting on your heels, with your shins flat on the floor. Lean back slightly, and put your palms on the floor next to each heel and your thumbs on the arches of the bottoms of your feet. Using your hands for support, press down with your arms to raise your shins slightly off the floor. At this point, you will be balancing on your hands and toes. Hold the stretch for five to 10 deep inhales, then repeat five times.

No More Neck Pain! 4 Simple Stretches

Robert Turner, PT, OCS, a board-certified orthopedic clinical specialist and clinical supervisor at the Hospital for Special Surgery's Spine Therapy Center in New York City. Turner is also a licensed acupuncturist and certified Pilates instructor.

Neck pain can be agonizing. But there's more at stake than the discomfort itself. This common complaint also can lead to collateral damage that you'd never expect—by contributing to anxiety or depression.

Problem: Far too many people live with this painful condition for years because they don't really get to the root of the problem.

What's the cause of all this pain? Much of it boils down to poor posture—we sit at computers or in cars for hours at a time…our heads leaning forward to help us see the screen or the road. With our arms extended in front of us, we naturally round forward and our chests tighten, weakening the back muscles—a significant but under-appreciated cause of neck pain.

If you hold a phone between your ear and shoulder or carry a heavy bag over one shoulder, you're only making matters worse. Or you may awaken with a "crick" in your neck from sleeping in an awkward position. And if you lie on the couch for hours at a time, you're speeding the muscle atrophy and inflexibility that will keep you in misery.

But there is hope! Doing the right type of stretching is incredibly effective at relieving neck pain.

What gets overlooked: While you might be tempted to target only the neck itself in these stretches, it's crucial to also do chest and back stretches to help correct musculoskeletal system imbalances and restore flexibility.

Here are four great stretches for neck pain—the entire routine can be performed in about 10 minutes.* (If you're short on time, just do the first two stretches when you start to feel neck discomfort or after you've been sitting for 90 minutes.)

●**Chicken wings.** This move opens the chest and strengthens the shoulder blades, which helps relieve pressure on the neck.

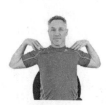

What to do: While sitting up straight on a chair, extend your arms out to the sides and touch your fingertips to your shoulders. Roll both shoulders back and down. You should feel the muscles between your blades contract. The key is not working too hard—give it 50% of your effort, not 100%—or you'll end up straining your neck. Hold for one breath in and one breath out, then relax. Repeat 10 times. Perform this series twice a day.

●**Triple neck stretch.** These exercises stretch the larger muscles that attach the head and neck to the shoulders.

*These exercises are safe for most people. If you experience pain, numbness or tingling in the hand or arm that does not go away after exercise or becomes worse, don't do the exercise again and tell your doctor.

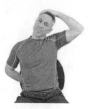

What to do: While sitting on the edge of a chair, lightly press the back of your right hand against the middle of your lower back, with your right elbow pointing directly out to the side. While looking straight ahead, tilt your head to the left, being careful not to rotate your neck. (You can use your left hand to gently pull your head down, intensifying the stretch.) Hold for five to 10 breaths.

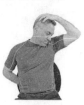

For the second step, with your right hand still on your back and your head still tilted to the left, rotate your chin down so that your nose is pointing toward your left armpit. You'll start to feel a deeper stretch in the back of your neck and chest. (Keep sitting tall, and don't let your right shoulder hunch forward.) Hold for five to 10 breaths.

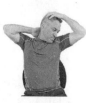

Lastly, with your nose still pointing toward your armpit, place the palm of your right hand behind your neck, keeping your shoulder blades down, and hold for five to 10 breaths. Repeat the three-step series on the other side of your body, and you have just completed one round. Try to do one or two more rounds throughout the day...or whenever pain crops up.

●**Prone extension.** This move strengthens your back muscles so that your neck does not have to work so hard to maintain proper posture.

Note: If you have low-back pain, put a pillow under your hips when doing this stretch and the next one to avoid straining this part of your back.

What to do: Lie on your stomach on a padded mat or carpet with your hands stacked beneath your forehead, legs straight and your knees and ankles together.

Pull your navel in toward your spine to help support your lower back, and push both shoulder blades down toward your feet as you inhale and

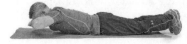

arch your upper back at least two to three inches off

the floor (your hands and arms should rise with your upper body). Exhale on the way back down. Repeat for a total of 10 lifts. Take a brief break, then repeat two more sets, eventually progressing to three sets of 15.

•**Shoulder blade lift.** This stretch will strengthen the back and shoulder muscles that help maintain correct head and neck alignment.

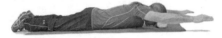

What to do: Lie on your stomach on a padded mat or carpet with a rolled-up towel placed beneath your forehead, nose pointing toward the floor to keep your neck in a straight line and your arms pointed forward in a Y formation.

While keeping your head down and neck relaxed, inhale as you lift your arms, hands and upper chest a few inches off the floor…hold for a beat, and exhale as your arms lower back down. Repeat 10 times. You will feel the muscles around the shoulder blades and middle back engage to lift the arms.

Caution: If you experience shoulder pain, modify the stretch by bending your elbows into a wide goalpost position. People who have had rotator cuff surgery or a shoulder injury can try this move while lying facedown on a bed, raising the arms off the edge of the bed toward the ceiling.

Simple Stretches That Really Do Relieve Pain in Shoulders and Neck

Ben Benjamin, PhD, a sports medicine and muscular therapy practitioner since 1963. The founder of The Benjamin Institute in Cambridge, Massachusetts, he conducts seminars and workshops on Active Isolated Stretching across the US and is the author of several books, including *Listen to Your Pain: The Active Person's Guide to Understanding, Identifying, and Treating Pain and Injury.* BenBenjamin.com

I f you suffer from pain or stiffness due to an injury, arthritis or even a neurological disorder, such as Parkinson's disease or multiple sclerosis, a type of bodywork known as Active Isolated Stretching (AIS) may give you more relief than you ever thought possible.

What makes AIS different: While most other stretching techniques recommend doing each stretch for 30 seconds or longer, AIS uses brief, two-second stretches that are done eight to 10 times each.

What's the advantage of quick, repeated stretches? This approach gives the muscle a full stretch without triggering its stretch reflex—an automatic defense mechanism that causes the muscle to contract and ultimately undo many of the stretch's benefits. The result is that muscles stretch more efficiently and avoid the buildup of waste products that lead to muscle soreness.

Developed by American kinesiologist Aaron Mattes about 35 years ago, AIS also stretches each muscle group at a variety of different angles, thus stretching all muscle fibers equally.

A MINI REGIMEN

To get a sense of AIS, try the stretches in this article. While doing each one, slowly count to yourself "one-one thousand, two-one thousand"—never any longer than two seconds. Always exhale while performing the stretch and inhale as you return to the starting position.

The first repetition of each stretch should be gentle…the second should go up to the point where you begin to feel resistance. Subsequent repetitions should push just beyond this point (with the help of your hands, a rope or other aid, if necessary) to go a few degrees further each time, thus providing a maximum stretch. If you feel discomfort during a stretch, stop the stretch at that point. If a stretch feels painful from the start, then skip it.

Daily AIS exercises that help relieve common types of pain…*

SHOULDER STRETCHES

Purpose: To help prevent muscle strain and joint sprain by increasing flexibility.

1. With your right elbow bent, position your right arm at a 90° angle in front of your body. Place your right palm on the back of your right

*Check with your doctor before performing these movements.

shoulder. Exhale and extend your flexed arm upward as far as possible. Gently assist the stretch with your left hand. Repeat eight to 10 times on each side.

2. With your right elbow bent and your right arm positioned at a 90° angle in front of your body, place your right palm on the back of your right shoulder. Drop a two- to three-foot rope over your right shoulder and grasp the bottom of it with your left hand. Gently pull the rope to move your right arm upward behind your neck at a 45° angle for a maximum stretch. Return to the starting position after each repetition. Repeat eight to 10 times on each side.

NECK STRETCHES

Purpose: To help prevent neck injuries, relieve stiffness and improve range of motion.

1. Tuck your chin as close to your neck as possible. Put both your hands on the back of your head and, while keeping your back straight, gently bend your neck forward, bringing your chin as close to your chest as you can. Return to starting position. Repeat 10 times.

2. Gently bend your head to the right side, moving your right ear as close as possible to the top of your right shoulder. Exhale and place your right hand on the left side of your head to gently extend the stretch. Keep your left shoulder down. Focus your eyes on a point directly in front of your body to keep your head in an aligned position. Repeat 10 times on both sides.

GETTING STARTED

For people who are new to AIS, I advise working with an AIS practitioner for hands-on instruction. If the movements are done incorrectly, you will get no benefits and could even hurt yourself. To find a practitioner near you, go to StretchingUSA.com and click on the "Practitioner Directory" link. Sessions are not typically covered by insurance and usually range from $50 to $150 per session. The site also offers books, including *Specific Stretching for Everyone*, and DVDs if you prefer to learn a complete AIS regimen on your own.

How to Relieve Shoulder Pain Without Surgery

Beth E. Shubin Stein, MD, associate attending orthopedic surgeon and a member of the Sports Medicine Service at Hospital for Special Surgery in New York City.

The shoulder is the most movable and complex joint in the human body. And it's basically unstable.

Imagine a golf ball perched on a tee. That's your shoulder. The humerus (upper arm bone) is the ball and the scapula (shoulder blade) is the tee. It doesn't take much to knock them apart.

So it's no wonder that as you get older, normal wear and tear often leads to shoulder pain. You might notice the discomfort while serving a tennis ball, reaching for a jar on a shelf, carrying a heavy suitcase or simply putting on a sweater or fastening a bra. *The most likely culprits…*

● **Impingement.** The rotator cuff, a collection of muscles and tendons surrounding the humerus, gets pinched between that bone and the scapula.

● **Frozen shoulder.** Tissue around the shoulder joint gets inflamed and stiff.

● **Tendinitis.** Rotator cuff tendons become inflamed or irritated.

● **Bursitis.** Tiny fluid-filled sacs (called bursa) that act as a gliding surface to reduce friction between shoulder tissues become inflamed.

Each condition is caused by inflammation, often as a response to tiny injuries that you didn't notice when they happened. Each can get so painful that surgery seems like a good idea. But why go through that discomfort, recuperation and expense if you can avoid it?

Surprising truth: With pain management and physical therapy, two-thirds of patients get better on their own.

But if your shoulder is bothering you, that doesn't mean you can just do nothing. Your pain will continue and even may intensify the next time you overstress the shoulder. Worse yet, you could get a rotator cuff tear, which definitely requires surgery and then four to six months of recovery.

To learn the best way to avoid shoulder surgery, we interviewed orthopedic surgeon Beth E. Shubin Stein, MD. *Her advice…*

If you feel pain in a shoulder and your movement is restricted, see an orthopedist right away to rule out a rotator cuff tear. As long as your rotator cuff is intact, you have a very good chance of making your shoulder feel better and avoiding surgery if you, in consultation with your doctor, follow these steps.

MANAGE YOUR PAIN

The first step is to manage your pain so that you can start physical therapy. Ice your shoulder for 20 minutes at a time, two or three times a day. Also, take a nonsteroidal anti-inflammatory drug (NSAID), either over-the-counter or prescription, to reduce inflammation and pain (don't exceed the recommended dosage).

If that's not enough to ease pain and allow exercise, your doctor can give you a cortisone shot. It's a potent anti-inflammatory, but repeated shots can limit a tendon's healing ability.

My protocol: If a first cortisone shot works for two months or more and you can exercise, I typically recommend a second shot and continuing physical therapy.

But if the first cortisone shot doesn't ease pain and allow exercise, I offer patients platelet-rich plasma (PRP) injections ($1,000 to $2,500). It's experimental and generally not covered by insurance. If PRP doesn't work, another option is to use donor stem cells from amniotic membranes to help regenerate tendon tissues. This can be about twice as expensive as PRP, and insurance most likely won't cover it either. These treatments don't work for everyone, but if they do, shoulder discomfort should subside within three days to a week.

Tip: You also may want to consider acupuncture as a complement to any of the above approaches.

Once pain isn't holding you back, it's time to get your shoulder moving. You can complete this stretching/strengthening program in 15 minutes. Do it twice a week. It's also great for anyone who wants to avoid shoulder problems.

Important: You should never feel pain when doing either stretching or strengthening exercises.

These exercises might sound like a lot of work, especially if you've become accustomed to avoiding using your shoulder because of pain. But take it from someone who both performs necessary shoulder surgery and does my best to help patients avoid it—it's well worth the effort to avoid the knife. I do these exercises myself two or three times a week—I've had shoulder pain in the past, but these exercises let me stay strong and pain-free.

STEP 1: GET LIMBER

Much of the work of supporting the shoulder falls to the rotator cuff. *These stretches improve rotator cuff flexibility and support normal range of motion…*

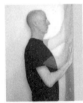

• **Wall crawl.** Stand facing a wall. Place the palm of one hand in front of your chest and "walk" it upward along the wall. Go as high as you can without feeling pain, hold for three to five seconds, and walk your hand back down. Do five to 10 repetitions. Switch hands and repeat.

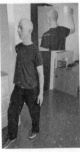

• **Doorway stretch.** Stand in an open doorway, and place your right hand flat against the wall next to the right side of the doorway frame at shoulder height, with your elbow bent. Keeping your right hand in place, step forward with your right foot, bending your right knee (as in a lunge), with your left leg stretched behind you. You should feel a stretch in your shoulder but not any pain. Hold for three to five seconds, and do five to 10 repetitions. Repeat with the left arm on the left side of the doorway and left foot stepping forward.

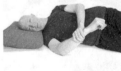
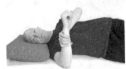

• **Side stretch.** Lie on your side on the floor (on an exercise mat or rug), your painful shoulder on the floor and your head supported on a pillow or bolster so that your spine is in a straight line. Bend the arm that's on the floor at the elbow, with the forearm and hand raised and palm facing your feet. Now use your other hand to gently push the wrist of the bent arm toward the floor. Hold for three seconds and release. Do a total of 10 reps. Repeat with your other arm.

STEP 2: STRENGTHEN THE RIGHT MUSCLES

While impingement, frozen shoulder, tendinitis, and bursitis often are referred to as overuse issues, I prefer to call them "understrength" issues. The problem isn't the 100 times you serve during a typical tennis match—it's that your muscles aren't strong enough to handle the stress you're placing on them. Even people who lift weights often focus on the biceps and triceps and ignore the rotator cuff.

Caution: Stay away from military presses and other exercises that require you to lift weights overhead—that can injure your shoulder. Skip kettlebells, too—they require swinging that can inflame your shoulder.

My recommendation: To build the strength of your rotator cuffs, use resistance bands, which do the job and are safer. *Try these three stability builders…*

•**External rotation.** Loop a resistance band at waist height around a secure anchor such as the base of equipment at a gym or a strong door handle of a locked door at home. Standing sideways

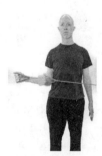

to the anchor, grab both ends of the band with one hand so it's taut. Keep your elbow bent and against your side and your hand near your stomach. Now pull the band away from your stomach, keeping your elbow against your side, until you feel light tension on the outside of the shoulder.

Hint: Your shoulder blade should move toward your spine. Hold for one second. Do a total of 10 reps. Repeat with your other arm.

•**Internal rotation.** This is the reverse of the external rotation. Keep the resistance band looped around a secure anchor, and stand in the same position as above. But this time, grab the band with the hand that is closest to where it's anchored. Keeping your elbow bent and at or near your side, pull the band across your torso toward your belly button. Hold for one second. Do a total of 10 reps. Repeat with your other arm.

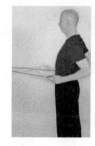

•**Rowing.** With the elastic band securely anchored as above, grab one end of the band in each hand so it's taut. Pull both arms back, bending your elbows and keeping them close to your sides. Hold for one second. Do a total of 10 reps. Repeat with your other arm.

Keep Your Hands Young and Strong–7 Simple Exercises Reduce Pain and Stiffness

Anjum Lone, OTR/L, CHT, an occupational and certified hand therapist and chief of the department of occupational therapy at Phelps Hospital in Sleepy Hollow, New York.

Most patients with arthritis do not recognize the importance of simple daily hand exercises, which can improve joint lubrication…increase your range of motion and hand strength…and maintain or restore function. These exercises also are helpful for people who have a hand injury or who heavily use their hands.

SAVE YOUR HANDS WITH EXERCISE

Most hand and wrist exercises can be done at home without equipment. But don't exercise during flare-ups, particularly if you have rheumatoid arthritis. Patients who ignore the pain and overuse their hands and wrists are more likely to suffer long-term damage, including joint deformity.

Important: Warm the joints before doing these exercises—this helps prevent microtears that can occur when stretching cold tissue. Simply run warm water over your hands in the sink for a few minutes right before the exercises. Or you can warm them with a heating pad.

Before doing the hand exercises here, it also helps to use the fingers of the other hand to rub and knead the area you'll be exercising. This self-massage improves circulation to the area and reduces swelling.

Do the following exercises five times on each hand and work up to 10 times, if possible. The entire sequence should take no more than five minutes. Perform the sequence two to three times a day.*

#1: Tendon glides.

Purpose: Keeps the tendons functioning well to help move all the finger joints through their full range of motion.

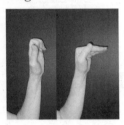

What to do: Rest your elbow on a table with your forearm and hand raised (fingertips pointed to the ceiling). Bend the fingers at the middle joint (form a hook with your fingers), and hold this position for a moment. Then bend the fingers into a fist, hiding your nails. Don't clench—just fold your fingers gently while keeping the wrist in a neutral position. Now make a modified fist with your nails showing. Next, raise your fingers so that they are bent at a 90-degree angle and your thumb is resting against your index finger (your hand will look similar to a birds beak). Hold each position for three seconds.

#2: Thumb active range of motion.

Purpose: Improves your ability to move your thumb in all directions. Do the movements gently so that you dont feel any pain.

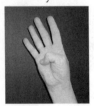

What to do: Rest your elbow on a table with your forearm and hand in the air. Touch the tip of the thumb to the tip of each finger (or get as close as you can). Then, flex the tip of your thumb toward the palm. Hold each of these positions for three seconds.

#3: Web-space massage.

Purpose: Using one hand to massage the other hand strengthens muscles in the active hand while increasing circulation in the passive hand.

What to do: Clasp your left hand with your right hand as if you are shaking hands. With firm but

*For more exercises, see an occupational therapist. To find one, consult the American Occupational Therapy Association, AOTA.org.

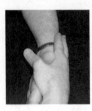

gentle pressure, use the length of your left thumb to massage the web (space between the thumb and the index finger) next to your right thumb. Then, reverse the position and massage the web next to your left thumb. Massage each web for 30 seconds.

#4: Wrist active range of motion.

Purpose: To maintain proper positioning of the wrist, which helps keep the fingers in correct alignment.

What to do: Rest your right forearm on a table with your wrist hanging off the edge and your palm pointing downward—you'll only be moving

your wrist. Then place your left hand on top of your right forearm to keep it stable. With the fingers on your right hand held together gently, raise the wrist as high as it will comfortably go. Hold for three seconds.

Next, make a fist and raise it so the knuckles point upward. Now, lower the fist toward the floor. Hold each position for three seconds.

#5: Digit extension.

Purpose: Strengthens the muscles that pull the fingers straight—the movement prevents chronic contractions that can lead to joint deformity.

What to do: Warm up by placing the palms and fingers of both hands together and pressing the hands gently for five seconds. Then place your palms flat on a table. One at a time, raise each finger. Then lift all the fingers on one hand simultaneously while keeping your palm flat on the table. Hold each movement for five seconds.

#6: Wrist flexion/extension.

Purpose: Stretches and promotes muscle length in the forearm. Forearm muscles move the wrist and fingers. Flexion (bending your wrist so that your palm approaches the forearm) and extension (bending your wrist in the opposite direction) help maintain wrist strength and range of motion.

What to do: Hold your right hand in the air, palm down. Bend the wrist upward so that the tips of your fingers are pointed toward the ceiling. Place your left hand against the fingers (on the palm side) and gently push so that the back of your right hand moves toward the top of your right forearm. Hold for 15 seconds. Switch hands and repeat.

Now, bend your right wrist downward so that the fingers are pointed at the floor. Place your left hand against the back of your right hand and gently push so your palm moves toward the bottom of the forearm. Hold 15 seconds. Switch and repeat.

#7: Finger-walking exercises.

Purpose: Strengthens fingers in the opposite direction of a deformity. This exercise is particularly helpful for rheumatoid arthritis patients.

What to do: Put one hand on a flat surface. Lift the index finger up and move it toward the thumb, then place the finger down. Next, lift the

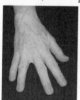

middle finger and move it toward the index finger. Lift the ring finger and move it toward the middle finger. Finally, lift the little finger and move it toward the ring finger. Repeat on your other hand.

Photos: Anjum Lone.

Back Pain Mystery Solved: This Little-Known Joint Could Be the Cause

Jo Ann Staugaard-Jones, MA, an advanced Pilates and Hatha yoga instructor and trainer based in Andover, New Jersey. She is a former professor of kinesiology, exercise science and dance at County College of Morris in Randolph, New Jersey, and the author of *The Vital Psoas Muscle* and *The Concise Book of Yoga Anatomy.* Move-Live.com

I t's easy to blame nagging low-back pain on a muscle strain or even a disk problem. But that's not always the real cause.

A surprising culprit: Up to one-third of chronic low-back pain can actually be traced to pelvic instability. The sacroiliac (pronounced *sak-ro-il-ee-ak*) joints, commonly called the SI joints, are located on both sides of the pelvis, connecting it to the lower part of the spine (sacrum).

If this little area of the body gets out of whack, that is when the trouble begins. Unlike other joints throughout the body, a healthy SI joint doesn't flex and extend. Instead, it's considered a "gliding" joint, meaning that the ligaments holding it together can shift, but that shifting is ideally kept to a minimum. The SI joint's main job is to hold the lower spine and pelvis together to increase stability.

Certain life events can cause excess movement in the SI joint, however. Pregnancy is a big one—the SI joints can be affected when ligaments and joints in the pelvic area loosen before giving birth.

For women who are years beyond childbearing age—and men, too—SI joint pain is slightly different. Usually affecting only one side of the pelvis, this type of SI joint trouble leads to a chronic, nagging pain in the lower back, which typically worsens when bending over from a standing position. Sitting, which the average American does for up to 13 hours per day, is another risk factor for SI joint pain—it weakens these joints and promotes inflammation.

EASY STEPS THAT HELP

If you have SI joint pain (marked by a consistent ache on either side of the base of your spine) or suspect that your SI joints may be contributing to low-back pain, see an orthopedic specialist to confirm your diagnosis. Movement tests and an X-ray or a CT scan will be performed.

A clue to watch for: If your pain improves when lying down, this is a sign that the SI joints may be involved. (This can also be a sign of spine degeneration, which can affect the SI area.)

In addition to the following exercises, most doctors recommend the following to help relieve pain due to one or both SI joints...

•**Ice.** It reduces inflammation and produces a brief numbing effect that temporarily relieves pain. Ideally, ice the affected area for 15 minutes three times a day.

What to do: Lie on your belly with an ice bag on the painful area. You can alternate ice packs with a heating pad after the first 24 hours of treatment, when inflammation has subsided, to increase blood flow to the area.

●**Massage.** For some people, this helps…for others, it can aggravate the problem. If you would like to try massage, ask the therapist to use gentle pressure to promote circulation but avoid deep tissue work.

●**SI belt.** It is designed to relieve overtaxed ligaments by decreasing motion in and around the pelvis. The research on these belts is mixed. One study reported significant pain reduction in those wearing the belt, while other research found no such benefit or a worsening of pain for a small number of people.

If you want to try an SI belt, a good product is the Serola Sacroiliac Hip Belt (about $45, depending on size). But if pain seems to worsen with a belt, stop using it.

●**Pain-relief medication.** If the therapies described above and exercise routine below don't give you adequate relief, you may need to add pain medication such as *ibuprofen* (Advil) or topical arnica gel.

EXERCISE FOR YOUR SI JOINTS

The main goal of a workout to relieve SI pain is to balance the strength of the muscles and tendons surrounding the joints so they can provide stability. Exercises that work the transverse abdominis (the deep ab muscles that support internal organs)…the deep external hip rotators that connect the sacrum to the thighbone…and the gluteus muscles will also help the SI joints remain strong yet supple. If you're in pain, relax the muscles and do these exercises when pain has lessened. *Try the following 10-minute routine three times a week—you should get relief within three to six weeks…*

●**Squats.**

What to do: While holding a light weight (five pounds to start, working up to 10) or a 10-pound bar overhead (keep your shoulders down), stand in front of a mirror with a chair behind you to assist with the exercise.

(Holding a bar or weights overhead helps keep the body in correct alignment.) Engage your ab-

*As with any exercise program, check with your doctor first.

dominal and back muscles as you bend your knees, lowering yourself toward a sitting position. (If your lower back begins to sway, you have gone far enough and need to pull your naval in toward your spine.) Allow your hips to fall back toward the chair until your buttocks lightly touch the chair, but do not sit down. Aim for your upper thighs to be parallel to the floor. Hold the squat for 10 to 20 seconds, while breathing deeply, then slowly return to a standing position. Repeat three to five times.

●**Hand/knee balance.**

What to do: Get down on all fours in a tabletop position with your back as level and flat as possible. Your hands should be directly under your shoulders and your knees under your hips. Begin by stretching your right leg back and lifting it to hip height, then slowly lift your left arm forward in line with your ear. Keep your pelvis stable and centered and your core muscles tight. Hold for 10 seconds. Then return to the tabletop position and repeat on the other side. Alternate sides for one minute.

●**SI stretch.**

What to do: Lie on your back on an exercise mat or carpeted floor with your legs straight and your arms outstretched to your sides. Bend your right knee toward your chest, then let it fall across your body to the left, letting your hips roll with it. (Keep both your shoulders on the floor.) Relax and breathe in and out for a minute before repeating on the other side.

Ahhhhhh Stretch for a Stiff Back

Arthur H. White, MD, is a retired orthopedic spine surgeon based in Walnut Creek, California, and author of *The Posture Prescription: The Doctor's Rx for Eliminating Back, Muscle, and Joint Pain.*

It's the end of the day and your back feels stiff and hunched over from sitting at a desk for hours. *Here's a simple move for fast relief…*

The draping stretch feels great—and promotes good posture—because it pulls the shoulders back and stretches the chest muscles. It requires a large inflated exercise ball, available at sporting-goods stores for about $20.

Your goal is to lie backward over the ball so that your back is somewhat arched yet fully supported. To get into position, sit on the floor with your knees bent and the ball nestled against your rear end and lower back. Carefully raise your hips and step your feet away little by little until your mid-back, upper back and the back of your head are resting on the ball. Your feet should be flat on the floor, shoulder-width apart…knees bent at about 90 degrees…neck relaxed and tilted back (not too far)…and arms hanging out to the sides. Allow your body to relax as you drape over the ball in this position, enjoying the stretch along your spine. Hold for a minute or two…repeat daily.

Yoga for Low Back Pain

Beryl Bender Birch, founder of the Hard & the Soft Yoga Institue and the nonprofit Give Back Yoga Foundation, GiveBackYoga.org, both based in East Hampton, New York. She is the author of *Power Yoga, Beyond Power Yoga* and *Boomer Yoga.*

In a recent study, people with chronic low back pain who practiced yoga (two 90-minute sessions weekly for six months) reported less pain and disability than those receiving conventional treatment, such as medication and surgery.

Recommendation: Do the Locust Posture.

What to do: Lie on your stomach with your legs and feet together, arms back at your sides, facedown and chin on the floor. Inhale, then exhale while raising your head, shoulders and legs into the air. Press your hands into the floor for balance.

Get Rid of Back Pain in Just 7 Minutes a Day

Gerard Girasole, MD, an orthopedic spine surgeon at The Orthopaedic & Sports Medicine Center in Trumbull, Connecticut. He is coauthor, with Cara Hartman, CPT, a Fairfield, Connecticut–based certified personal trainer, of *The 7-Minute Back Pain Solution: 7 Simple Exercises to Heal Your Back without Drugs or Surgery in Just Minutes a Day.*

Of the 30 million Americans who suffer from low back pain, only about 10% of the cases are caused by conditions that require surgery, such as pinched nerves or a slipped disk.

For the overwhelming majority of back pain sufferers, the culprit is tight, inflamed muscles.

Surprising: This inflammation usually is not caused by strain on the back muscles themselves, but rather a strain or injury to the spine—in particular, to one of five "motion segments" in the lower back.

Each segment, which is constructed to bend forward and back and side to side, consists of a disk (the spongy cushion between each pair of spinal vertebrae)…the two vertebrae directly above and below it…and the facets (joints) connecting the vertebrae to the disk.

Unfortunately, the segments' disks or facets can be injured in a variety of ways—by lifting something the wrong way, twisting too far, sitting too long or even sneezing too hard—causing the surrounding muscles to contract in order to protect the spine from further damage.

This contraction and the muscle inflammation that it produces is what causes the intense lower back pain that so many Americans are familiar with.

WHEN BACK PAIN STRIKES

Low back pain caused by inflammation usually subsides on its own within three to six weeks. However, the healing process can be accelerated significantly by taking over-the-counter *ibuprofen* (Motrin) for several days after injury to reduce inflammation if you don't have an ulcer (follow label instructions)…and getting massage therapy to help loosen knotted muscles and increase healing blood flow to them.

Also important: Perform the simple stretching routine described in this article. In my more than 16 years of practice as an orthopedic spine surgeon, it is the closest thing I've found to act as a "silver bullet" for back pain.

How it works: All of the muscles stretched in this routine attach to the pelvis and work in concert to stabilize the spine. Stretching increases blood flow to these specific muscles, thereby reducing the inflammation that leads to painful, tightened back muscles.

GETTING STARTED

In preparation for the back stretch routine described here, it's important to learn a simple approach that systematically stimulates and strengthens your core (abdominal, back and pelvic muscles). This is one of the best ways to protect your spine. Although there are many types of exercises that strengthen the core, abdominal contractions are the easiest to perform.

What to do: Pretend that you have to urinate and then stop the flow—a movement known as a Kegel exercise. Then while lying on your back, place your hands on your pelvis just above your genitals. Now imagine that someone is about to punch you in the stomach, and feel how your lower abdomen tightens protectively.

To do a full abdominal contraction, combine these two movements, holding the Kegel movement while tightening your lower abdomen. Then, continuously hold the full abdominal contraction during all of the stretches described on this page.

7-MINUTE STRETCHING ROUTINE

Do the following routine daily until your back pain eases (start out slowly and gently if you're still in acute pain). Then continue doing it several times a week to prevent recurrences. Regularly stretching these muscles makes them stronger, leaving your lower spine less prone to painful, back-tightening strains.

1. Hamstring wall stretch. Lie face-up on a carpeted floor (or on a folded blanket for padding), positioning your body perpendicular inside a door-frame. Bend your right leg and place it through the door opening. Bring your buttocks as close to

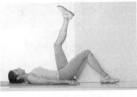
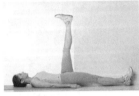
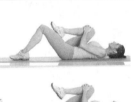
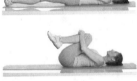

the wall as possible and place the heel of your left foot up against the wall until it is nearly straight. Next, slide your right leg forward on the floor until it's straight, feeling a stretch in the back of your left leg. Hold for 30 seconds. Repeat twice on each side.

2. Knees to chest stretch. Lie on your back with your feet flat on the floor and your knees bent. Use your hands to pull your right knee to your chest. Next, try to straighten your left leg on the floor. While keeping your right knee held to your chest, continue the stretch for 20 seconds, then switch sides and repeat. Finally, do the stretch by holding both knees to your chest for 10 seconds.

3. Spinal stretch. While on the floor with your left leg extended straight, pull your right knee to

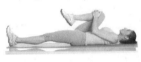
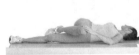

your chest (as in stretch #2), then put your right arm out to the side. Next, use your left hand to slowly pull your right knee toward your left side so that your right foot rests on the back of your left knee. Finally, turn your head toward your right side. Hold for 20 seconds, then reverse the movements and repeat.

4. Gluteal (buttocks) stretch. Lie on your back with your feet flat on the floor and your knees bent. Cross your right leg over your left, resting your

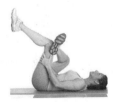

right ankle on your left knee. Next, grab your left thigh with both hands and bring both legs toward your body. Hold for 30 seconds, then switch sides and repeat.

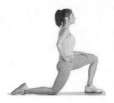

5. Hip flexor stretch. Kneel on your right knee (use a thin pillow for comfort) with your left leg bent 90° in front of you and your foot flat on the floor. Place your right hand on your waist and your left hand on top of your left leg. Inhale and then, on the exhale, lean forward into your right hip, feeling a stretch in the front of your right hip. Hold for 30 seconds, then switch sides and repeat.

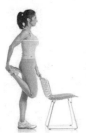

6. Quadriceps stretch. While standing, hold on to the back of a sturdy chair with your left hand for balance. Grasp your right foot with your right hand and gently pull your right leg back and up, with your toes pointing upward. Be sure to keep your right knee close to your left leg. Hold for 30 seconds, then switch sides and repeat.

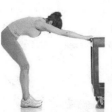

7. Total back stretch. Stand arm's length in front of a table or other sturdy object and lean forward with knees slightly bent so that you can grasp the table edge with both hands. Keep your arms straight and your head level with your shoulders. Hold for 10 seconds.

Next, stand up straight with your left hand in front of you. Bring your right arm over your head with elbow bent, then bend your upper body gently to the left. Hold for 10 seconds, then switch sides and repeat.

Photos: Scott Wynn

Morning Back Stretch

To relieve hip/back tightness—lie in bed with your hands interwoven behind your head and your knees up…drop both knees to one side… hold for three deep breaths…then do the other side.

Fitness trainer Joel Harper, author of *Mind Your Body,* writes the "Your Personal Mind-Body Coach" blog at BottomLineInc.com.

Strengthen Your Hidden Core to End Your Back Pain…for Good

Patrick A. Roth, MD, FACS, chairman of the department of neurosurgery and director of the neurosurgical residency training program at Hackensack University Medical Center in Hackensack, New Jersey. He is also the founder of the North Jersey Brain & Spine Center in Oradell, New Jersey, and author of *The End of Back Pain.*

You're lucky if you haven't suffered a backache recently. It's common…make that very common.

In any three-month period, 25% of adults will suffer at least one day of back pain. Over the course of a lifetime, about 85% of us will experience back pain at some point.

My story: As a spinal surgeon and a former back pain sufferer, I've examined this malady from all angles. What I have discovered is that contrary to our culture of "pop a pill" or "go under the knife," the best course of action starts with discovering your "hidden" core.

FINDING YOUR HIDDEN CORE

If I told you that you needed to strengthen your core, you might assume that means doing crunches to work on your abdominal muscles, or abs. While washboard abs are the most visible and easily trained part of your core, they are only part of a larger muscle group that makes up the core.

In fact, strengthening your abs without also working on your hidden core can make back pain worse. That's because unbalanced core muscles cause an unstable spine.

The muscles you don't see: Your core is a group of muscles that encircles your midsection—front, sides and back. And most of the muscles lie deep inside your body—hidden from view. Taken together, these muscles form an internal brace around your spine, holding it erect, protecting it from damage. In order to reduce or limit back pain, you need to strengthen all your core muscles equally.

THE HIDDEN CORE WORKOUT

The workout I've developed targets all the inner muscles that make up your body's natural support system. Don't worry—even if you're not in great shape, you can start by doing the exercises at your own pace. However, do each of the exercises below so that you'll strengthen all the muscles equally to keep your spine in balance.

Here's the drill: Perform the exercises three times a week...and focus on maintaining proper form. Even if your back is aching, do the exercises if you can—they often give some immediate relief and help prevent future flare-ups.

Give it time: It may take three to four weeks before you notice significant pain reduction.

Important: These exercises can be safely done by most people, but check with your doctor first. See your doctor right away if you have back pain and severe leg pain (a sign of sciatica) or you have a history of cancer (back pain could be a sign that cancer has spread).

EXERCISE 1: Front plank. This exercise focuses on the muscles at the front of the core—the rectus abdominis (the abs) and the transverse abdominis—and the obliques, which are on the sides of the core.

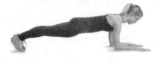

What to do: Start by lying on your stomach on a carpet or mat. Place your hands on the floor at about the level of your ears, with your elbows bent and close to your sides.

Slowly lift your body off the floor using just your forearms and rising up on your toes. Your elbows and hands should remain on the floor. Keep your back straight by contracting your front abdominal muscles. (If you cannot lift your body as described, try supporting your lower body from your knees rather than your toes.)

Breathe normally...and hold the position for 10 seconds. As you are able, increase the amount of time you hold the position. A minute is a good goal for most people.

EXERCISE 2: Side plank. This strengthens the sides of your core—the internal and external obliques.

What to do: Start by lying on the floor on your left side, with your feet together. Prop yourself

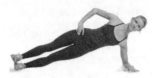

up on your left elbow, with your left hand and forearm flat on the ground and your forearm perpendicular to your body. Put your right hand on your right hip. Contract your abdominal muscles, and raise your hips off the floor until your back is straight.

Breathe normally, and hold the raised position for 10 seconds. As you are able, increase the amount of time you hold the position to 60 seconds. Repeat on your left side.

EXERCISE 3: Birddog. This exercise strengthens the back muscles that support your spine, including the *multifidus* muscles and the *erector spinae* muscles.

What to do: Start on your hands and knees, with your wrists below your shoulders (hands facing forward) and your knees below your hips. Stabilize your spine by tightening your abdominal muscles.

Simultaneously extend your left arm straight forward and your right leg straight back until both

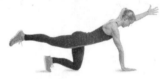

are parallel to the ground. Remember to keep your back and neck straight, without sagging or arching.

Hold this position for two seconds, then return to the starting position. Repeat, using the other arm and leg. Do the cycle five times. As you are able, increase the amount of time you hold the position each time for up to 10 seconds.

START RUNNING

If you have back pain, you've likely been advised to do only low-impact aerobic exercises and avoid running. I disagree. After years of examining runners, I noticed that their disks (and spines) tend to be healthier than those of nonrunners. Unexpected, right? But it makes sense.

All weight-bearing exercises stimulate bone cells so that the bones themselves become stronger. Similarly, disks also improve with high-impact exercise—the cells that make up the gel of a disk proliferate, retaining more water and becoming "fuller," which cushions the bones of the spine, reducing pain.

If you want to try running (and it doesn't cause you knee or hip pain), start slowly. Walk for one mile—and three times during that walk, run for 20 to 30 seconds. Thereafter, double the number of times you run until you're running more than walking. Try to work up to at least 30 minutes, three times a week.

Stretch Away Your Pain: It Takes Only Minutes a Day!

Joseph Tieri, DO, an osteopathic physician, adjunct professor at Touro College of Osteopathic Medicine in Middletown, New York, and co-owner of Stone Ridge Healing Arts in Stone Ridge, New York. Dr. Tieri is also author of *End Everyday Pain for 50+: A 10-Minute-a-Day Program of Stretching, Strengthening and Movement to Break the Grip of Pain.* EndEverydayPain.com.

Those everyday aches and pains that we all experience are commonly chalked up to arthritis. But that condition is the true cause far less often than most people realize.

While your doctor may order an MRI, discover arthritis or a bulging disk, and blame your musculoskeletal pain on that, studies reveal that arthritis and other degenerative conditions often can be detected on the films of *pain-free* middle-aged and older people. Age-related musculoskeletal aches and pains that result from tension and misalignment are far more common than arthritis but don't show up on film. As a result, many patients resort to medicine or even surgery for arthritis or herniated disks when that's not the real source of their pain.

Instead, it's poor posture combined with the inactivity of everyday living and underused joints that leads to stiffness and pain, whether it's shoulder pain, hip pain, back pain, etc.

Good news: Doing strategic stretching, strengthening and range of motion exercises for *just a few minutes a day is enough* to keep your muscles supple, your joints lubricated and everyday aches and pains at bay. Incorporate each of these moves into your daily routine to prevent various types of pain and to help relieve it.

Note: Hold each stretch for 30 seconds if you're younger than age 65…and for 60 seconds if you're 65 or older.

Most of the benefit comes from the first stretch, so one repetition is sufficient. *However, you can repeat these stretches throughout the day whenever your back, neck, hips and/or shoulders feel tight or stiff…*

•**Shoulder and chest stretch.** This is one of the most important—and simplest—moves you can do to reverse the rounded-shoulder posture that affects so many people.

What to do: Lie on the floor (on an exercise mat, if you like), face up, arms straight out to the sides in a "T" position with palms up. That's it! Believe it or not, this very simple stretch helps loosen the tight, shortened muscles in the front of your neck, shoulders and chest.

•**Neck stretch.** This stretch reverses the tension caused when one's head juts forward—common when driving or typing. It also elongates and aligns the neck, creating space for disks between the vertebrae, which lessens the odds of a bulging or herniated disk.

What to do: Begin by lying flat on your back on a bed or a mat on the floor (a wedge mat as shown in the photo below may be more comfortable for older individuals). Allow your head to relax for a 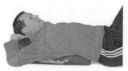 few seconds. Then reach up and place the fingers of both hands in the space beneath your neck. With fingertips touching, move them to the bottom of your head. Now move your fingers up, pushing or sliding the back of your head upwards, feeling the back of your neck elongating. Then hold.

Note: This movement may tilt your head down a bit, but the back of your head should stay in contact with the bed or mat at all times.

•**Psoas stretch.** The psoas (pronounced "SO-az") is the most important muscle you've never heard of—it's the main muscle connecting the spine to the legs, and it works with other muscles to stabilize the lower spine and promote proper body alignment. The psoas often weakens with age and inactivity, leading to lower back and hip pain and poor posture.

What to do: Start by lying flat on your belly (on an exercise mat, if you wish) with your forehead resting on the backs of your crossed hands. Allow your stomach to relax and notice the natural curve of your lower back. For many older patients, this provides enough of a stretch—if so, continue doing this daily for a week or two until you no longer feel the stretch in your lower back, which means you're ready for the next step—slowly press up onto your forearms (Sphinx) or your palms (Cobra). Remember, keeping your belly relaxed as your lower back gently stretches is more important than trying to lift higher.

• **Piriformis stretch.** The piriformis is a small muscle that runs diagonally from the bottom part of the spine to the upper thighbone on each side of the body. Asymmetry can develop after years of driving with your right foot on the gas pedal, crossing your legs the same way or sleeping in the same position, which can cause pain in the hips and lower back.

What to do: Sit in a chair with both feet on the floor. Rest your right ankle on top of your left thigh, just above the knee. Keeping your back straight, gently bend forward at the waist until you feel a stretch in your right thigh and glute. Then repeat on the other side.

The Secret Muscles That Can Cause Chronic Pain

Jo Ann Staugaard-Jones, MA, an advanced Pilates and Hatha yoga instructor based in Andover, New Jersey. She is a former professor of kinesiology, exercise science and dance at County College of Morris in Randolph, New Jersey, and the author of *The Anatomy of Exercise & Movement* and *The Vital Psoas Muscle*. Move-Live.com

Most people have heard plenty about the core—that band of muscles in the abdomen, low back, hips and pelvis. But what if there were some far less well-known muscles that could be causing all your trouble? Say hello to the *psoas* (pronounced SO-as) muscles! Ignoring these crucial muscles can lead to low-back pain and poor posture.

What you need to know…

WHERE ARE THEY?

Located deep within the center of the body, the psoas major muscles are the only muscles that connect the upper and lower extremities of your body. As a pair of muscles on both the right and left sides, they run from the lower spine, past the front of the pelvis, through either side of the groin and attach to the inside of the femurs (thighbones).

So what exactly do these muscles do? The psoas muscles help with the transfer of weight when you're walking or running. When you extend your leg back, for example, the psoas on that side lengthens…when you lift your knee, it contracts. The psoas muscles also act as stabilizers of the lower spine, the pelvis and the legs, aiding body alignment and posture.

What goes wrong: If the psoas muscles are shortened for long periods of time—as occurs when sitting, for example—they can tighten on one or both sides. If the psoas on one side of the body is tighter than the other (from leaning to one side while sitting, for instance), it can also torque the spine, affecting your posture and gait. An imbalance on one or both sides can lead to inflammation and pain while walking.

Unlike toned abs, you can't see the psoas muscles. Because you can't touch your psoas muscles either, it can be difficult to tell if they're the cause of your back pain and poor posture.

There are some clues, however, that may indicate that these muscles are tight or weak—for example, you may also feel discomfort in the hip sockets, the glutes or even the sacroiliac joints, which are in the back of the pelvis. The pain can be in one spot or travel throughout the path of the muscle.

KEEPING YOUR PSOAS MUSCLES IN SHAPE

The first step to keeping the psoas muscles in top shape is to stand up. Instead of sitting for long periods of time, get up and move around at least every hour. To help prevent or relieve psoas-related pain, also do these three exercises every other day (as with any exercise program, check with your doctor first)...

***EXERCISE #1:* Lunge.** Also known as the "runner's stretch," the lunge strengthens and stretches the psoas and thigh muscles.

What to do: Stand with your right foot forward and left leg back (about three to four feet apart). 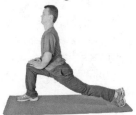 Bend your front knee until it's directly over your toes, at about a 90-degree angle. Slide your left leg straight back until it is almost parallel to the floor. Keep your feet facing forward, and don't let your front knee extend beyond your toes. Your spine should be straight, and you can rest your hands on the floor or the front of one thigh. Hold for up to 30 seconds, then repeat on the other side.

***EXERCISE #2:* Teaser or Boat pose.** This position, used in both Pilates and yoga, works the psoas muscles and several other core muscles.

What to do: Sit on the floor with your legs extended out in front. While keeping your hands on 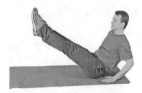 the floor behind your hips, lean back slightly and balance just behind your "sits" bones (beneath your buttocks). Then gently raise one leg and then the other as high as possible, so that your body is in a "V" position. Hold for 10 seconds while keeping your chest lifted and your torso long. If you're able, extend your arms forward for added challenge. Repeat three times, or hold longer.

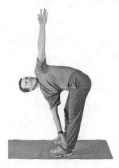

***EXERCISE #3:* Windmill.** This exercise strengthens and stretches the psoas muscles and oblique (side abdominal) muscles.

What to do: While standing with your arms extended out to each side and your knees slightly bent, lean for-ward and touch your left hand to your right ankle as you extend your right arm upward and look up toward the ceiling. Return to the original standing position and repeat on the other side. Do five reps, without rushing, for maximum benefit.

A Fun and Easy Way to Get Stronger and Ease Pain

Karl Knopf, EdD, director of fitness therapy and senior fitness for the International Sports Sciences Association and retired director of adaptive fitness at Foothill College in Los Altos Hills, California. He is author of many fitness books, including *Stretching for 50+* and a board member of Sit and Be Fit, a nonprofit organization dedicated to healthy aging.

I f you've ever been in physical therapy, you've likely used a stretchy latex tube or flat strip called a resistance band. It is incredibly effective at building strength and endurance...easing lower back pain and arthritic discomfort...and improving balance.

What you may not know: Resistance bands are a safe way to build strength on your own if you have a bad back, joint pain or other problems that can make weight-lifting off-limits. Once your health-care provider gives you the green light, first try whatever moves below are right for your condition *without* a band—to make sure you can do the motion without pain or discomfort before adding resistance. (If there is discomfort, check in again with your doctor for advice.) Ideally, these exercises should be done three to four times a week.

If you have low-back pain: It is often due to weak abdominal muscles...tight hamstrings and quadriceps...and/or tight hip flexors (the muscles that connect the legs to the torso). Your goal is to strengthen the abdominals, the lower back muscles and the glutes while reducing hip flexor tension. *What helps...*

•**Pelvic lifts.** While lying on your back, place a band across your hips and grab each end, placing your fists on the floor. Slowly lift your hips to a comfortable height (a 45-degree angle from hips to shoulders is ideal), engaging your glutes (the muscles in your buttocks). Count to one, then return to

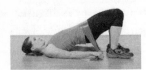

start position. Repeat 15 times.

If you have hip pain or hip arthritis: Years of overuse or being overweight can turn good hips bad. The moves below help promote the stability and mobility that healthy hips need.

Note: If you've had a hip replacement or have severe hip issues, consult your doctor for specific exercises.

•**Seated leg press.** This works the quadriceps (the stronger the leg muscles are, the less stress is placed on painful joints). Sit in a chair, both hands gripping either end of a band so that you can loop 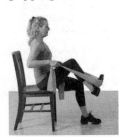 the band around your right foot. Keeping your left foot on the floor, lift the right leg up, gently resting the right foot in the middle of the band. Extend your right leg out in front nearly all the way, then crisscross the band once to keep your foot from slipping off. Pull elbows back to the waist. Slowly bring the right knee in toward your chest, stopping when knees reach a 90-degree angle, and press back out, without locking your knee. Switch sides. Start with just a few reps and gradually build up.

•**Hip extension.** Attach a flat band or tubular band,* see photo, to a door using a door anchor strap (available online or in sporting goods stores). Facing the door, attach the other end of 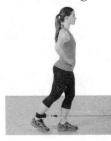 the band to your right ankle. Move far enough away from the door to place some tension on the band. Keeping a slight bend in the left leg, slowly extend your right leg backward, engaging the glutes. You can grasp a chair for balance. Hold for one to two seconds before returning to the start position. Repeat 10 to 15 times. Switch sides.

*People who have had pain or arthritis often like to use a tubular band. It is less likely to tear or snap—and comes with easy-to-grip handles.

If you have a knee injury: Knees are meant to straighten and bend. Any other movement, such as twisting and pivoting, places them at risk. Healthy knees demand strong quadriceps, which provide stability and support. *What to do...*

•**Forward lunge.** Stand with your left foot in the middle of your band and grab the ends with each hand at a location that provides adequate resistance. Typically, your elbows will be waist-high, 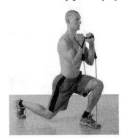 arms bent. Slide your right foot backward, attempting to lower your right knee as low as you comfortably can—to the floor if possible. Now transfer your weight back to your left leg as you push up through your left quad and glutes until standing. You should feel an increase in resistance in your left leg as you rise up. Repeat three to five times. Switch sides.

What to look for...

Resistance bands are available online or in sporting goods stores for about $20 or less. They come in a rainbow of colors, each representing a different intensity. They also come in different lengths—the longer the length, the less resistance. For most beginners, I advise starting with a three- to six-foot flat band. To increase the intensity, you can "choke up" on the band before moving up to a band with a higher level of resistance.

Exercise photos: Courtesy of Ulysses Press/Rapt Productions

Keep Your Hips Forever!

Mitchell Yass, DPT, a specialist in diagnosing and resolving pain and creator of the Yass Method for treating chronic pain. He is the author of *Overpower Pain: The Strength-Training Program That Stops Pain Without Drugs or Surgery.*

Does a diagnosis of arthritis at the hip joint mean that you need surgery? Not necessarily. Most hip and groin pain is caused by muscle weakness or a muscle imbalance. People who correctly exercise these muscles can often eliminate—or at least greatly reduce—their discomfort. Strengthening these muscles also can help ease pain in those who have already had hip replacements… and improve balance.

THE BEST WORKOUTS

The following exercises are ideal for hip or groin pain. After getting your doctor's OK, start by trying to repeat each one 10 times. Take a one-minute break, then repeat two more sets. The whole routine, which should be done two or three times a week, takes about 20 minutes.

•**Hamstring curl.** The hamstrings (in the back of the thigh) play a key role in the functioning of the hip joints. However, the hamstrings are weak in most people—mainly because these muscles aren't used much in normal daily movements.

How this exercise helps: It strengthens hamstrings and helps prevent the opposing muscles (the quadriceps, in the front of the thigh) from shortening and causing muscle strain and/or spasms.

How to do it: Attach one end of a piece of elastic exercise tubing (available in sporting-goods stores and online) to your left ankle. Stand on the other end with your right foot. Leaving more slack will reduce resistance…taking up the slack will increase it.

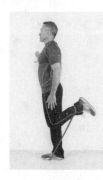

With your feet a few inches apart and knees slightly bent, raise your left foot and curl it backward toward your buttocks as far as you comfortably can. Then return to the starting position. If you feel unsteady, put one hand (on the side opposite the leg you're working) on a wall. Switch legs and repeat.

•**Hip abduction.** This is great for hip or groin pain because the abductor muscles (on the outer thighs) tend to be much weaker than the opposing adductor muscles.

How this exercise helps: Weakness in the abductors can allow the pelvis to drop on one side, which can cause groin muscles to tighten and become painful.

How to do it: Lie on the side that's not painful (or less painful) on a mat or a carpeted floor. Your painful side will be on top. Place your arm under your head, and bend your other leg's knee for better support and balance.

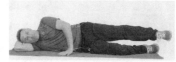

Slowly raise your affected leg, keeping it in line with your torso. Keep the knee straight, and don't roll forward or backward. Raise your leg only to hip height (a few inches). Then slowly lower your leg back to the starting position. After performing a set, roll over and repeat the exercise with the other leg, only after pain has eased in the affected leg. Otherwise, focus only on strengthening the painful side.

•**Hip flexor stretch.** This exercise is vital. Most of us spend a lot of time sitting, causing these muscles to shorten and tighten.

How this exercise helps: It stretches tight hip flexors, which can stress the low back.

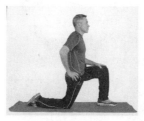

How to do it: Kneel on your right knee on a mat or a carpeted area. (If you need more padding, you can put a folded towel under the knee.) Place your left foot flat on the floor in front of you, with the knee bent. Rest your left hand on your left thigh and your right hand on your right hip. Keeping your back straight and abdominal muscles tight, lean forward so that more of your weight is on the front leg. You'll feel a stretch in your right upper thigh. Hold for 20 to 30 seconds. Switch sides.

•**Quad stretch.** Overly tight quad muscles can pull the pelvis downward—a common cause of low-back and hip pain.

How this exercise helps: Stretching the quads helps distribute weight evenly through the pelvis.

How to do it: Stand near a wall for support. Rest your right hand on the wall, then reach back with your left hand to grip your left foot/ankle. Pull your heel upward toward your buttocks—and eventually behind the hip. Keep pulling, gently, until you feel a stretch in the front of your thigh. Tighten your abdominal muscles. Hold for about 20 to 30 seconds. Repeat on the other side.

If your pain doesn't improve after a month of performing these exercises, consult your doctor.

It's Your Butt!

Chris Kolba, PhD, PT, a sports medicine physical therapist and clinical instructor at The Ohio State University Wexner Medical Center in Columbus. He developed The Ohio State Tactical Rehab and Conditioning Program to meet the needs of firefighters, police officers and other tactical operators.

Want to get to the bottom of your persistent back, knee or hip pain? Look behind you, and you'll find the likely cause.

Dormant butt syndrome is the name that I've coined for a serious problem that affects millions of Americans, especially those who spend most of the day sitting. Did you pull a hamstring while playing with your grandkids? Suffer from an aching back after a few hours of TV watching? Weak gluteal (butt) muscles are often the common link. A lack of strength in this area forces other muscles to compensate and do jobs that they're not designed to do alone, resulting in pain in unexpected parts of the body.

THE NEGLECTED CORE

The big muscles in the buttocks do more than give it shape. They absorb shocks and control movements necessary for walking and other activities. When the gluteal muscles are weak, other muscles and joints definitely take the hit.

Dormant butt syndrome strikes people who are generally sedentary—whether they're sitting behind a desk, driving a car or watching their favorite sitcoms. When you're positioned on your derriere for hours on end, the glutes aren't "firing" and there's more tightness in the hip flexor muscles, which can lead to hamstring injuries or back, hip

or knee pain. Runners and other athletes who do repetitive motion can also get tight hip flexors.

When I evaluate clients who have lower-body pain, I always check for adequate glute strength. To do this, I ask the patient to lie on his/her stomach and do a leg lift against resistance from my hand to determine how strong his glutes are.

I also put my fingertips lightly on the hamstring and gluteal muscles of the lifted leg to evaluate the "firing pattern" of muscles. Normally, the gluteal muscles will fire (or activate) first, followed by the hamstrings. If the pattern is reversed, I'll know that the gluteal muscles are weaker than they should be.

MORE BANG FOR YOUR BUTT

I advise clients to spend the majority of their waking hours standing, if possible. Since this isn't always practical, at least make an effort to increase your amount of upright time—staying on your feet when watching TV, for example, or standing (and pacing) when talking on the telephone. *Six other movements that help—do each one twice a week (except for the hip flexor stretch, which should be done daily)…**

•**Glute Bridge.** It is among the best exercises for targeting the glutes. It gives the abdominal core muscles a bit of a workout, too.

What to do: Lie on your back with your knees bent and your feet flat on the floor. Contract your abdominal muscles slightly. Next, raise your hips up about six inches and hold for a few seconds… then slowly lower yourself back down. Repeat this movement 10 to 12 times.

•**Lunges.** They strengthen the gluteal muscles, along with muscles in the hips and thighs.

What to do: Stand with your feet together and your hands on your hips. Take a step forward with your left leg, while simultaneously bending that leg until the thigh is parallel to the floor. Keep your front foot flat on the floor as you bend your knee (most of the weight should go onto your heel), and don't let the front knee extend farther forward than the toes. Return to the starting posi-

*Consult your doctor before beginning this regimen—or any other new exercise program, especially if you've had knee, hip or back surgery.

tion, then repeat with the other leg. Work up to 12 to 15 reps on each leg.

Note: If a deep knee bend is painful, don't go down as far.

•**Wall squats.** Squats are popular because they increase both gluteal and thigh strength. This exercise is easier than traditional squats because it requires only body weight and a wall for support.

What to do: Lean back against a wall with your feet shoulder-width apart and out a foot or two. Keep your back and hips against the wall.

Slide down until your thighs are parallel to the floor. Hold the position until your thighs start to say "enough," then rise back up. In the beginning, your thighs might start shaking after just a few seconds. Over time, try to work up to holding the position for 30 to 60 seconds.

If you're out of shape or have weak knees, you can lower yourself about halfway to the parallel position. Don't let your knees collapse inward, and stop if you feel any pain. Work your way toward the full bend as you build strength.

•**Side planks.** For those with dormant butt syndrome, it's important to stretch/strengthen surrounding muscles as well as the glutes themselves. This exercise activates muscles in the midsection, including the hips.

What to do: Lie on your right side, with your legs extended and "stacked" on top of each other. Prop up your upper body by supporting your weight on your forearm, keeping your shoulder aligned with your elbow. Contract the ab muscles and lift your hips and knees off the floor. Hold the position for 10 to 30 seconds, then lower back down. Repeat on the other side. Start with two to three sets, holding the position for 10 seconds, and gradually work up to one minute per set.

•**Single leg balance.** Most people lose some strength, balance and *rotational motion* (the ability of their joints to rotate) as they get older. This exercise is a good way to improve hip and core stability while challenging balance.

What to do: Stand on one leg, with your arms held slightly away from your body for balance.

Important: For safety, stand next to a counter to catch yourself if you start to topple over. Try to hold the position (without swaying) for 30 to 60 seconds. Then try it on the other leg. It's challenging at first! Once it gets too easy, lift the leg a bit higher and/or try to do it with your eyes closed. This is harder because vision helps the body orient itself.

•**Hip flexor stretch.** Tight hip flexors cause dormant butt syndrome. When these muscles are tight, there's *compensatory movement* throughout the lower back, which can lead to pain as well as disk damage in the lower back.

What to do: Kneel on your left knee, with your left hand on your hip and your right foot flat on the floor in front of you—the right knee should be bent and the right thigh should be roughly parallel to the floor. Move your left hip forward until it extends beyond the left knee. Don't bend forward during the movement. Hold the position for 20 to 30 seconds, then repeat for three or four reps. Change position and repeat on the other side.

Protect Your Knees with the Ultimate Knee Workout

Steven P. Weiniger, DC, a postgraduate instructor at Logan University in Chesterfield, Missouri, and a managing partner of BodyZone.com, a national online health information resource and referral directory for posture-exercise professionals. He is the author of *Stand Taller, Live Longer: An Anti-Aging Strategy.* StandTallerLiveLonger.com

Each year, more than 700,000 Americans undergo knee replacement to help relieve the pain associated with knee osteoarthritis, rheumatoid arthritis or other forms of degenerative joint disease—and the numbers just keep rising. This trend is due largely to an aging population and obesity, a leading cause of joint damage.

But is surgery really the right solution for all these people? Not necessarily.

Here's the catch: Many people who receive knee replacements could have avoided surgery—along with the risk for infection and the painful weeks of postsurgical rehabilitation—with simple exercises that strengthen the knee and help prevent deterioration of the tendons, ligaments and bones.

A HEALTHY-KNEE PROGRAM

In addition to exercise, normal body weight is critical for long-term knee health. If you're overweight or obese, your knees are subjected to unnecessary force. Research has shown that losing as little as 11 pounds can cut the risk of developing knee arthritis by 50%.

But if you're overweight, losing any amount of weight can help. One study, published in the journal *Arthritis & Rheumatism*, found that every pound of lost weight translates into a four-pound reduction in knee stress—with each and every step.

Why exercise helps: Patients who stretch and strengthen the muscles around the knees have better joint support. There is also an increase in synovial fluid, a gel-like substance that keeps the joints moving smoothly.

What's more, exercise increases bone density in these patients and results in better range of motion.

4 MUST-DO EXERCISES

Everyone can benefit from knee exercises. Even if you don't suffer from knee pain now, the following exercises may help prevent problems from developing. People who have received surgery to replace or repair a knee also can benefit by strengthening their muscles to help guard against future knee injuries.

The goal of knee exercises is to work the muscles around the joint. These include the quadriceps (on the front of the thigh)...the hamstrings (back of the thigh)...and the muscles in the calves. Strength and flexibility in these areas support the knees and help keep them aligned. Alignment is critical because asymmetry increases pressure and joint damage.

Perform the following regimen daily—it can be completed in about 15 to 30 minutes. If you have an advanced knee problem due to a condition such as rheumatoid arthritis, your doctor may also prescribe additional exercises that are targeted to address your specific issues.

Important: All of the exercises described in this article should be performed within a range of motion that does not cause pain. If a slight strain oc-

curs with the first repetition, that is acceptable, as long as the pain diminishes with subsequent repetitions. If the pain worsens with subsequent repetitions, stop the exercise.

Four must-do knee exercises...

1. Knee-to-Chest Stretch. This exercise improves flexibility in the lower back, hips and hamstrings. People who do this stretch will notice an

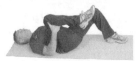

opening of their hips, allowing them to stand taller. This improvement in posture is important for reducing knee stress.

Bonus: You can use this movement to diagnose knee problems. If the knee you're bending doesn't come straight toward your shoulder and stay in line with your foot, you'll know that you have an alignment problem that needs to be corrected.

This knee exercise can be performed in bed if that is more comfortable than doing it on a carpeted floor or on a padded surface.

What to do...

• **Lie on your back with your knees bent and your feet flat on the floor (or bed).**

• **Using both hands, slowly pull one knee toward your chest.** (To avoid straining the knee, grip behind it, not on the front.) Go as far as you can without discomfort—you should feel a stretch in your lower back, but no pain.

Hold the position for 15 to 30 seconds, then slowly lower the leg. Perform the movement eight to 12 times. Repeat with the other leg.

2. Knee-to-Chest Stretch with Resistance. This is similar to the exercise described above, except that you use a latex exercise band (such as TheraBand) to increase resistance and strengthen muscles.

• **Lie on your back with your legs straight.** Loop the latex band around the bottom of one foot. Grip the loose ends of the band with both hands.

• **Use the band to pull your knee toward your chest.**

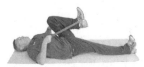

Hold the position for 15 to 30 seconds, then straighten the leg while pushing against the band

—hold the band taut to increase resistance. Do this eight to 12 times, then repeat with the other leg.

3. Standing One-Leg Balance. This move is more challenging than it looks because you're us-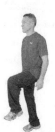ing the weight of your body to strengthen your legs as well as the "core" muscles in the abdomen. These muscles, which connect the torso and pelvis, help control motions in your whole body. Core weakness is a common cause of asymmetric motion, which often leads to knee problems.

•**Stand next to a wall, with your right shoulder just touching the wall.**

•**Lift your left knee until the foot is off the floor.** If you can, keep raising it until the thigh is about parallel to the floor. Make sure that your posture is upright at all times.

Hold the position for about 15 seconds, then lower your foot. Repeat eight to 12 times, then turn around and do the same thing with the other leg.

Important: If you can't balance for 15 seconds—or if you find yourself using the wall for support or moving your arms or dancing around to balance on one foot—your legs are weaker than they should be. This means you should definitely also do the next exercise.

Note: Even if you can easily perform the one-leg balance above, it's a good idea to do the one below to maintain your strength.

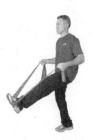**4. Standing One-Leg Balance with Resistance.** This is similar to the exercise that's described above, except that you use a latex band to strengthen muscles in the thighs and hamstrings. Stand with your right shoulder barely touching a wall. Loop a latex band under your left foot. Hold the loose ends of the band in each hand.

•**With your hands at waist level, raise your left foot until your thigh is about parallel to the floor.** Shorten the band by wrapping it around your hands to keep some tension on the band.

•**While holding the band taut and your knee elevated, slowly press your foot forward, as though you're taking a big step.** Keep the band taut to increase resistance. Maintain your balance!

•**Now, pull on the band to return to the bent-knee position.** Repeat eight to 12 times, then turn around and repeat with the other leg.

Sore Feet? Four Feel-Better Yoga Poses

Roger Cole, PhD, internationally recognized, certified Iyengar yoga teacher. Based in Del Mar, California, Dr. Cole has trained thousands of yoga teachers and taught yoga as a healing art to physicians, physical therapists, medical students and patients. RogerColeYoga.com

---

Our poor feet pay the price—in the form of pain, inflammation and misalignments—for our habit of wearing high-heeled, pointy-toed, stylish-but-not-sensible shoes. Along with all the other great things yoga postures can do for your body, this ancient practice can also help feet feel and function better.

The greatest thing yoga can do for foot health is to help restore normal "foot posture." That means equal weight on the inner and outer foot...arches lifted...toes spread apart evenly...and usually feet pointing straight ahead. The four poses below can help you achieve this correct foot posture.

WHY "FOOT YOGA" WORKS

The following three standing poses challenge your ability to keep weight equally distributed on the "four corners" of the foot—the ball of the big toe, ball of the little toe, inner heel and outer heel. Each pose makes the weight distribution uneven in one way or another, so the act of bringing the feet back to neutral strengthens certain muscles and stretches others, while also training your nervous system to "find center" with your feet. The fourth pose is a kneeling posture. It stretches the top of the foot while temporarily taking tension off the inflammation-prone *plantar fascia* (a band of tissue that runs the length of the sole).

Check with your doctor before beginning, as not all yoga poses are appropriate for all people. Start by holding the standing poses for five to 15 seconds per side, working your way up to 30 seconds per side...start by holding the kneeling pose for 10 to 30 seconds, gradually increasing to one minute. For best results, practice daily.

The basic instructions below will get you started. For more detailed instructions and photos of each pose, go to YogaJournal.com/poses. *Poses to try...*

•**Vrksasana (Tree pose).** Stand on right foot, right knee straight. Bend left knee and place sole of left foot on inner right thigh, so toes point down and left knee points out to side. Raise arms straight overhead and hold pose. Repeat on other side.

Foot focus: Concentrate on keeping weight evenly distributed among all four corners of the supporting foot. This strengthens the calf and shin muscles that balance the foot and stretches the plantar fascia.

•**Utthita Parsvakonasana (Extended side angle pose).** Stand with feet spread about three-and-a-half feet apart, right toes turned a little to the left and left toes facing sideways at a 90-degree angle. Bend left knee until knee is directly above ankle. Lean to left side by bending at left hip, placing left forearm on thigh or placing left hand on floor. Extend right arm diagonally overhead. Keeping torso facing forward (not turned toward floor), hold pose. Repeat on other side.

Foot focus: Press outer edge of back foot down into floor before you start going into the pose... keep it there throughout. Also, as you bend front leg, do not allow weight to shift to inner edge of that foot—keep knee aligned over ankle.

•**Virabhadrasana 1 (Warrior 1 pose).** Stand with left foot about three-and-a-half feet in front of right foot, toes facing forward. Now turn right foot outward so toes are on a 30-degree angle. Bend left knee, bit by bit, directly toward left foot. Keep hips facing forward. Raise arms straight overhead and hold pose. Repeat on other side.

Foot focus: Before bending front knee, press outer corner of back heel firmly into floor. Keeping that part of heel down, slowly begin to bend front knee. When outer corner of back heel begins to lift, press it firmly back into floor and don't bend front knee any further—you have gone as far as you should. This pose strengthens key muscles that lift the arch of the foot, while also stretching some of the muscles whose tightness can flatten the arch.

•**Virasana (Hero pose).** Kneel with tops of feet on floor. Keep knees close to each other but not touching...spread feet apart slightly wider than hip width. Place a prop (such as a yoga block or thick book) on floor between ankles, then lower pelvis so hips are supported by the prop.

Foot focus: Keep thighs parallel and feet pointing backward in line with shins. If the stretch at the top of the ankles is too intense, support the ankles by draping them over a rolled blanket.

Rebuilding Powerhouse Muscles Helps Conquer Pain

Eric Goodman, DC, founder and creator of Foundation Training. He is author of *True to Form: How to Use Foundation Training for Sustained Pain Relief and Everyday Fitness* and coauthor of *Foundation: Redefine Your Core, Conquer Back Pain, and Move with Confidence.* FoundationTraining.com

Not surprisingly, all the hunching, slumping and slouching of modern-day life are taking a toll on our bodies. Reading and working on our computers and smartphones...spending large amounts of time in the car...watching TV on the couch. Life in the 21st century is filled with many pleasurable conveniences and one giant modern-day nuisance—chronic pain.

Specifically, the sitting and slumping compress the spine and overtax the joints. Over time, poor posture weakens the muscles along the back of the body known as the posterior chain. These powerhouse muscles—the back, glutes and hamstrings—are intended to do the heavy lifting, working to protect the joints and skeleton.

Excess sitting and inactivity cause the posterior chain to weaken, while the chest and quadriceps overdevelop to compensate. This causes joint degeneration and all of its debilitating symptoms, such as headache, neck, back and hip pain, carpal tunnel syndrome, plantar fasciitis and more. Compression squeezes the internal organs, too, impacting your breathing, your digestion and your immune function.

I created Foundation Training, a series of corrective body-weight exercises that allows you to use gravity to counterbalance the physical changes caused by inactivity. It healed my own chronic back pain, and I've watched as thousands of patients—from former professional basketball players in their 40s to decorated Air Force veterans in their 70s—have experienced great success and eventual pain relief with this system.

When you reactivate and strengthen the chain, your body rediscovers how to move properly, the pain dissipates and, eventually, stops.

CORE MOVEMENTS

Here are four good starter exercises that will help engage your posterior chain and reactivate neglected muscles—without going to the gym or investing in any special equipment.

●**Decompression breathing.** The first of these exercises, called decompression breathing, is present in every future Foundation Training pose. It is the standard way to enter and exit the positions for all of the exercises.

A curled or hunched stance hinders the lungs' ability to expand and contract, leading to shallow breathing, which in turn shortchanges every other organ and process in the body. Decompression breathing works to actively lift and widen the 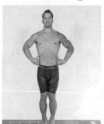 rib cage while simultaneously strengthening all of the muscles that are required to keep the rib cage there.

Stand tall, toes touching, an inch or so between the heels. Place your thumbs on the bottoms of your rib cage, pinkie fingers on the tops of your pelvic bones. Inhale deeply, broadening and elevating the rib cage as much as possible, and trying to increase the distance between your thumbs and pinkies. As your chest lifts up and expands, you begin to experience a widening of the rib cage in all directions. Remember to keep the back of your neck long and shoulders down.

As you exhale, imagine your rib cage remaining in its expanded state. The goal is to maintain that upper-torso expansion when you exhale. Inhale again, filling out even further, using slow and controlled breaths. Breathe in for three to five seconds, and breathe out for five to seven seconds with every decompression breath. Do this for 10 breaths, and you should instantly feel taller and more energized.

●**Supine decompression.** As with the previous move, this is about strengthening and expanding your lungs and lifting your chest so that your internal organs are no longer squished. Begin by lying down on a yoga mat, face up, with your hands resting on your chest and your legs and feet touching each other. Your neck should be long—imagine lots of space between the bottom of your head and the base of your neck. Move your hands to the ground, slightly away from your sides with your palms up.

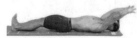 Start to squeeze your knees together, engaging the leg muscles. At the same time, flex your feet so that your toes point toward the ceiling (heels remain on the floor), and press your hands into the ground (try to get every fingernail touching the floor).

Keeping your knees squeezed and feet together and flexed, lift both knees a few inches off the ground—your knees will bend, and your heels will naturally move a few inches closer to your rear end as you do this. Extend your arms above your chest with your fingertips touching, forming a ball. Continue to lift your extended arms overhead with your fingertips still in the ball position, lifting your chest higher with each breath. You should feel tension in your pelvis, shins, arms and neck. Repeat the move 10 times, with the same breath count as you used for the standing decompression breathing.

REAWAKEN YOUR POSTERIOR CHAIN

Even active people can have weak posterior chains—back muscles, glutes and hamstrings—if they spend the majority of their time sitting or have chronic poor posture. Every time they exercise or go for a stroll, they're exercising the wrong muscles. The muscles in the front of the body end up doing the heavy lifting, so to speak, fighting gravity every step of the way. At the same time, the powerful muscles along the back of the legs and hips learn to live in a short, tight, underutilized position.

To shift the burden of supporting your body back to the strong posterior chain, you need to challenge those long-neglected glutes, hams and back muscles with these two very effective exercises…

•**The Founder.** Stand with your feet wide, about three feet apart. Your weight should be in your heels, arms down at your sides, chest up, shoulders down. Your chest should be fully expanded and held high (higher than what might feel natural or comfortable). Face forward and take a deep decompression breath, expanding the rib cage.

Next, begin to hinge at the hips, knees very slightly bent, extending your hips back behind you, as if you were starting to sit down in a chair. At the same time, reach your arms in front of you, as if you

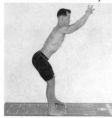

were pretending to touch the top of an imaginary doorway. (You'll be in a pose similar to a chair pose in yoga.) Look straight ahead, keeping your head in line with your spine. Hold for 10 seconds, breathing deeply while keeping your chest elevated. Let your back muscles burn—they're getting stronger! Lift your arms up a few more inches, pointing toward the seam where the wall meets the ceiling. Your gaze remains straight ahead. Hold for 10 more seconds. A few Founders a day will strengthen your muscles. When done well, it's a powerful pose.

•**The 8-point plank.** Begin by lying on a yoga mat, stomach down, head and upper body propped up as if you are in a sphinx pose. You'll

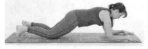

be propped up on your forearms, hands flat on the floor, elbows a few inches in front of your shoulders. Your forearms will point straight ahead, and your palms should be flat on the floor. Flex your feet so that your toes press into the ground. Your knees should continue touching the ground.

Note: You now have eight points of contact with the floor—two hands, two elbows, two knees, two feet.

Start decompression breathing. With each inhale, feel your ribs expand—you'll feel a lifting sensation in your upper body, almost as if your back is floating up toward the ceiling. Continue pressing your palms, forearms, knees and toes into the ground as your upper back lifts. Eventually, your pelvis will follow, lifting a few inches off the ground.

Note: The eight points all stay on the ground. Keep your neck long and your chin back, and gaze at your hands. Continue decompression breathing for five to 10 breaths, then gently lower yourself back down.

Perform several of these planks a day for three to six months to elicit a major shift in your posture, pain and overall health. The exercises will activate muscle connections. Each time you practice, you are improving upon a neurological pattern. You won't just get stronger, you'll get better.

You can find free tutorials for each of the exercises shown in this article by searching "Foundation Training" at YouTube.com.

Roll Away Your Pain

Joel Harper, a New York City–based personal trainer whose clients include several Olympic medalists. The creator of the PBS DVD *Joel Harper's Firming After 50,* he designed all of the personal workout chapters for Dr. Mehmet C. Oz and Dr. Michael F. Roizen's YOU series of books and accompanying workout DVDs. He is author of *Mind Your Body: 4 Weeks to a Leaner, Healthier Life* and the Bottom Line blog "Your Personal Mind-Body Coach." JoelHarperFitness.com.

Foam rollers are great for easing muscle tightness and relieving soreness by releasing knots in fascia, which surround the muscles, and increasing blood flow to enhance recovery.

Roll away muscle stiffness and pain in three common tight spots...

TIGHT-MUSCLE MOVES

Roll back and forth from the top to the bottom of each target muscle 25 times. Do one set per muscle. Repeat all exercises on both sides of your body. Never roll over joints.

•**IT Band Roll**—for the iliotibial band that runs along the outside of your thighs and helps keep your hips and knees stable. Lie on your right side with the roller under the middle of your thigh. Support your upper body with your right forearm on the ground and your left hand on the floor in front of your stomach. 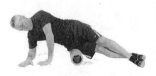 Keep your chin up and right elbow pressed back so that you stay on your side and avoid tilting forward with your upper body. Legs are together, ankles crossed. If this is too difficult, cross the top leg over the bottom one and anchor your left foot on the floor for balance. Use your hands and your core to shift your weight and help you roll along the full length of your quad.

•**Lat Roll**—releases tension in the muscles on the upper sides of your back. Lie on your right side, legs together and bent at right angles. Place the roller just below your armpit, perpendicular to your body. 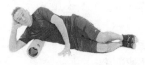 Your right elbow is bent in the air, and your right hand is holding your head. Using your left hand as a prop, use your hips and legs to roll two inches up and down along the muscles wherever you feel it is most needed. You also can tilt your body forward and back to get a cross-muscle massage as well.

•**Calf Roll.** Sit on the floor with legs straight, and place the roller under your calves (or under only your right calf with your left leg to the side if that is easier), just 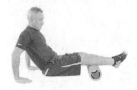 above the ankle. Lean your upper body back slightly, and place your hands flat on the floor for support, arms slightly bent. Use your hands and hips to help you roll up and down the length of your calves, tilting your legs slightly from side to side as you roll to find the area that needs it most. To add pressure, cross one leg over the other, bending the upper leg so that your foot is on the top of your calf...or for even more pressure, slide your foot down your calf to rest on your ankle. Switch legs and repeat.

Walking: A Drug-Free Rx for Arthritis

Susan Besser, MD, primary care physician, Mercy Personal Physicians in Baltimore, Maryland.

Study titled "Effectiveness of a Scaled-Up Arthritis Self-Management Program in Oregon: Walk With Ease," led by researchers at Oregon State University, published in *American Journal of Public Health.*

Painful, stiff joints make it hard to get moving, but moving is exactly what you need for pain relief when you have arthritis. What many people don't realize is that the world's simplest exercise—walking—is an amazingly powerful arthritis pain-buster. But the trick is, you need to know exactly how and when to walk, and what to do before and after, to get the full benefit. Taking these steps will also help you get over the fear that any movement will be painful, which keeps many people glued to a comfy chair.

Getting on a smart walking program can help with inflammatory conditions such as rheumatoid arthritis and psoriatic arthritis and "wear and tear" osteoarthritis.

Walking is so beneficial that it's considered a natural medication for arthritis. It makes your muscles stronger, which takes pressure off your joints...and boosts the health of your cartilage, your joints' shock absorbers, by increasing circulation and bringing nutrients and oxygen to the area. And while walking specifically targets the joints in your lower body, the feel-good endorphins released during exercise should make you feel better from head to toe.

As a calorie-burning exercise, walking can also help with weight loss—and every pound of overweight puts added pressure on your joints. Weigh less, and you have less pain.

Here's what to do...

How long to walk: Your goal is to walk for 30 to 60 minutes at a time, but if you can handle only five minutes to start, that's OK—start there and go a little longer every day.

How often to walk: Remember, walking is medicine for arthritis—so aim to take this medicine every day! If you're new to walking, begin with two or three days a week and build up from there.

How fast to walk: Walk fast enough to increase your heart rate while still being able to have a conversation. The key is to push yourself but not to the point that you're tiring too quickly or adding to your joint pain.

Of course, if you have any additional mobility issues or other chronic conditions, ask your doctor whether you should refine these guidelines.

You can follow a plan on your own, no gym membership needed. But you might find needed motivation through a walking group with friends or with a formal program such as Walk with Ease from the Arthritis Foundation. This six-week course, held in cities across the country, shows you how to manage arthritis as well as begin a walking routine. Researchers at Oregon State University surveyed 598 sedentary people with arthritis who participated in the program and found that those who completed it reported significantly less pain and fatigue. Not near a group? You can purchase a self-guided book ($12) with all the information and start reaping the benefits. Go to Arthritis.org and search "Walk with Ease."

To make your walks more comfortable, warm up for a few minutes with easy walking in place, then stretch. Stretch again after walking—you should be able to increase your range of motion as these muscles will be quite warm.

Whenever your joints feel sore, use a shorter stride. This puts less pressure on them.

Maintain good posture, with your core engaged and your upper body relaxed.

Don't let pride or even forgetfulness keep you from wearing a brace if your doctor has recommended one. The support it offers will help stabilize the joint, make walking easier, and potentially prevent a fall.

Note: If starting out walking on land is simply too painful for you, get in a pool. Walking in water is gentler on your joints yet adds some resistance, giving you an even better workout.

---

8 Stretches That Ease Your Aches and Pains

Karl Knopf, EdD, director of fitness therapy and senior fitness for the International Sports Sciences Association and retired director of adaptive fitness at Foothill College in Los Altos Hills, California. He is author of *Stretching for 50+* and *Foam Roller Workbook.*

Many older adults I meet don't see the importance of flexibility work until they are hunched over and in constant pain, looking and feeling older than their years.

Some of these individuals don't think that stretching is beneficial—and find it outright boring—and believe that they'll get more benefit by spending their time doing cardio and resistance exercises. The truth is that daily stretching is as important as regular aerobic exercise (five days a week) and weight training (two to three times a week).

STRETCHING TIPS

It's easy to sneak stretching into your life. Simply incorporate stretches into your normal routine or while working at your desk...watching TV...or between sips of tea while you read. *But stay safe...*

• **Warm up your muscles before you stretch by walking around for a few minutes first.**

• **Don't bounce through stretches.** Instead, hold steady, extending slightly on the outbreath, but push only as far as comfortable.

• **Hold stretches for at least 30 seconds or as tolerated,** not to one minute unless otherwise noted for individual stretches below.

You're unlikely to notice immediate changes in your flexibility and range of motion, but if you keep up with daily stretching, you'll notice subtle changes. It will be easier to bend over and tie your shoelaces…you'll feel less stiff when you get out of bed in the morning…and you'll have an easier time getting in and out of the car.

The following are effective but simple exercises that can improve posture, prevent injuries and target the most common sites of aches and pains…

NECK: THE TURTLE

This exercise reverses aches associated with sitting in front of a computer for hours a day and pushing your head forward. You can do it standing or sitting. Just be sure to keep your neck and back in alignment. The focus of the exercise is to pull the head back, which stretches the neck muscles.

1. Pretend you're holding an apple under your chin, or keep your chin parallel to the floor. Inhale deeply.

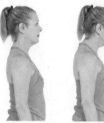

2. Exhale through your lips while pushing your chin forward.

3. Inhale through your nose, and slowly return your head to the neutral position you started with. Repeat as many times as you like to loosen up your neck.

SHOULDERS: THE ZIPPER

This exercise loosens the shoulder muscles. You can do it standing or sitting. As you become more flexible, you can eliminate the strap and try to grab your fingertips instead.

1. Hold a strap in your right hand, and raise your arm above your head. Bring your right hand down behind your head. Grab the end of the strap with your left hand.

2. Raise your right hand up as high as is comfortable, lifting the left hand along with it. Hold. Perform two times on each side.

3. Pull your left hand down to also bring your right hand down. Hold. Perform two times on each side.

4. Switch sides and repeat.

LOWER BACK: SEATED KNEE TO CHEST

This exercise stretches the lower back and gluteus maximus muscles and has been shown to improve blood flow and relieve muscle tension.

Sit with proper posture in a stable chair, and

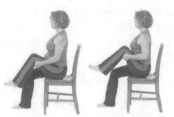

place your feet on the floor…or lie on the floor. Clasp both hands beneath your left leg.

Bring your left knee toward your chest. Hold, feeling the stretch in the gluteal region, Release the knee, switch sides, and repeat.

STRETCHING

Sitting for much of the day, as a lot of us do, can lead to tight hip flexors—the muscles that support the hip joints. To loosen them up, stand

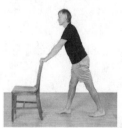

behind a sturdy chair with your hands on the back of it. Slide your left leg back a comfortable distance. Gently tuck your tailbone under and press your hips forward while keeping your rear heel down. When you can feel the stretch in your upper leg/hip region, hold.

Do two more times. Then do three repetitions on the other side.

LEGS: SEATED HAMSTRING MASSAGE

The hamstrings—the areas on the back side of the thighs that connect to both the hips and the knees—are prone to tightening up and are common areas of injury and pain. This exercise mas-

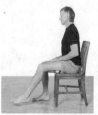

sages the area to boost blood flow and calm muscle tension.

Sit in a sturdy chair, and place a foam roller under one thigh… or, if you prefer, lie on the floor. Slowly and gently roll and press your leg along the roller. Hold

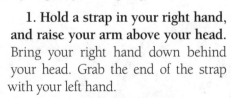

the roller there for five to 30 seconds. If you notice a particularly tense area, return to it. Repeat with the other leg.

WRISTS: SEATED WRIST STRETCH

With all of the computer work and driving we do, our hands and wrists are prone to tightening up and cramping. This exercise targets both the wrists and the forearms.

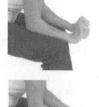

1. Sit in a chair, and rest your forearms on your thighs with your wrists dangling just beyond your knees. Make loose fists with your hands, and slowly lift your knuckles toward the ceiling. Hold.

2. Lower your knuckles slowly toward the floor. Hold.

Repeat this exercise as many times as feels comfortable.

FEET: ARCH ROCKS

Many people have trouble with foot cramping, stiffness and tightness as they age. This exercise helps to loosen the arches to relieve that discomfort.

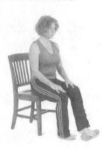

1. Sit in a chair with both feet on a foam roller.

2. Slowly roll your feet forward and then back to massage the bottom of your feet. If you feel particular areas of tension, apply additional pressure and concentrate on those areas.

HANDS: V-W STRETCH

This exercise targets the hands and fingers and can be helpful for wrist strain. While the instructions are for sitting, it also can be done standing.

1. Sit with proper posture in a stable chair. Rest your hands on your thighs, palms facing down. Squeeze all your fingers together.

2. Separate one finger at a time, starting with the little finger, then the ring finger, until you've separated all your fingers. Squeeze your fingers together, and repeat.

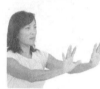

To increase the challenge: Hold your arms straight out in front of you. Instead of just separating your fingers, try to make a V and W with them.

To make a V: Spread your little finger and ring finger away from your index finger and middle finger.

To make a W: Put your ring finger and middle finger together and separate the little finger and index finger from the group.

Bathtub Stretch for Pain-Free Joints

Harris H. McIlwain, MD, a rheumatologist and pain specialist, McIlwain Medical Group, in Tampa. He is coauthor, with Debra Fulghum Bruce, PhD, of *Diet for a Pain-Free Life* and *Pain-Free Arthritis.*

Moist heat eases movement by increasing flow of blood, oxygen and nutrients to joints. During a warm bath or while seated on a shower stool, "circle" wrists by rotating hands, envisioning fingertips tracing the face of a clock. Next, circle ankles by rotating feet. Do these moves daily, working up to 15 repetitions of each.

13

Exercises for Special Conditions

Best Exercises If You Have Cardiovascular Disease, Diabetes, Lung Disease or Cancer

John P. Porcari, PhD, program director of the Clinical Exercise Physiology (CEP) program at the University of Wisconsin–La Crosse. A past president of the American Association of Cardiovascular and Pulmonary Rehabilitation, he has authored or coauthored more than 350 abstracts and 150 papers on exercise physiology.

Everyone agrees that exercise is good for you. The goal for most people should be at least 150 minutes of moderate aerobic activity a week, plus strength training two days a week, according to the Centers for Disease Control and Prevention.

But what if you have a chronic condition, such as heart disease, arthritis, lung disease or cancer, that makes exercise difficult—or raises your concern about injury?

While exercise is helpful for most chronic health problems, some activities are likely to be easier, more beneficial and less risky than others.* *Best workouts if you have…*

*Always talk to your doctor before starting a new exercise program. If you have a chronic illness, it may be useful to consult a physical therapist for advice on exercise dos and don'ts for your particular situation.

CARDIOVASCULAR DISEASE

A key benefit of exercise is reduced heart attack risk. But if you have already had a heart attack or undergone bypass surgery…or have symptoms, such as chest pain (angina), that signal established heart disease, you may worry that physical exertion is too risky.

For the vast majority of people with heart disease, it's not—if it's supervised. This usually involves initial and periodic testing to establish safe levels of exercise and monitoring of heart rate and blood pressure for some sessions. Once you're cleared, you can do most sessions on your own.

When performed at the proper intensity, standard aerobic activities are usually suitable. This means you can most likely walk, jog, use a stationary bike or treadmill (or even participate in aerobic dance) as long as you do it at a moderate level that doesn't raise your heart rate too high. Talk to your doctor about the heart rate you should strive for.

Once you have that number, you may want to wear a heart rate monitor—several models are widely available for under $100.

Another option: Use the "Talk Test." If you can talk while exercising, this will indicate with 95% accuracy that your heart rate is in a safe range.

If you have hypertension: Higher-intensity exercise may trigger potentially dangerous spikes in your blood pressure—talk to your doctor about appropriate heart rate goals, and remember to breathe (do not hold your breath) and stay away from heavier weights when doing strength training.

Important: Be sure to ask your doctor to reevaluate your target heart rate if you change blood pressure medication—some drugs, such as betablockers, will affect your heart rate.

DIABETES

Exercise can lower blood sugar almost as well as medication. Recent guidelines for people with diabetes recommend 150 minutes of moderate to strenuous aerobic exercise weekly, in addition to three strength-training sessions that work all the major muscle groups—increasing muscle mass is believed to be a particularly effective way of controlling blood sugar.

All aerobic exercises are beneficial, but those that use both your upper- and lower-body muscles are best because they help deliver blood glucose to muscle cells throughout your body—try an elliptical machine, the Schwinn Airdyne (a stationary bike that adds arm movements) or NuStep (a recumbent stepper that incorporates arm movements). If you walk, use poles to involve your arms. Try to do some type of exercise every day—this helps ensure its blood sugar–lowering benefits.

If you use insulin on a regular schedule: Exercise at the same time each day, if possible, to help maintain even, predictable blood sugar levels. Insulin should typically be used 60 to 90 minutes after your workout—check with your doctor or diabetes educator.

To prevent excessive drops in blood sugar: Eat something before or just after exercise and adjust your insulin dose on the days you work out. Talk to your doctor for specific advice.

JOINT AND BONE DISEASE

If you have arthritis, certain exercises may be painful. That's why swimming and/or aerobic exercise such as "water walking" in a warm-water pool are good options. If you don't have access to a pool, choose non–weight-bearing exercise, such as a stationary bike, to minimize stress on your joints.

With arthritis, it's especially helpful to consult your doctor or physical therapist before starting a new exercise program—so your workout can be tailored to your specific type of arthritis.

Good rule of thumb: If an exercise hurts, don't do it.

If you have bone disease, including osteoporosis or decreased bone density due to osteopenia: Weight-bearing exercise strengthens bone by exerting force against it. For this reason, walking is better than biking, for example, and swimming is usually the least likely to help.

Warning: Avoid exercises involving quick changes in direction, such as aerobic dance, which may increase fracture risk.

LUNG DISEASE

Asthma, one of the most common lung diseases in the US, generally does not interfere with exercise unless you are performing an activity that's especially strenuous such as running, which can trigger an attack ("exercise-induced asthma").

With exercise-induced asthma, the triggers vary from person to person. For example, working out in the cold is generally to be avoided (but a face mask or scarf may warm air sufficiently). Very vigorous exercise, such as squash or mountain biking, can cause difficulties for some people with asthma, who may do better alternating brief periods of intense and slower-paced activity (as used in interval training). Know your own triggers.

Swimming is also a good choice —the high humidity helps prevent drying of the airways, which can trigger an asthma attack.

If you use an inhaler such as albuterol to treat an asthma attack: Ask your doctor about taking a dose immediately before you exercise to help prevent an attack, and always carry your inhaler with you throughout the activity.

If you have chronic obstructive pulmonary disease (COPD): Exercise doesn't improve lung function, but it does build muscle endurance and improve one's tolerance for the shortness of breath that often accompanies COPD (a condition that typically includes chronic bronchitis and/or emphysema).

Aerobic exercises that work the lower body (like walking or stationary cycling) are good, but the Schwinn Airdyne or NuStep provides a lower- and upper-body workout with the option of stopping the upper-body workout if breathing becomes more difficult.

CANCER

Exercise may help fight the nausea and muscle wasting that sometimes occur with cancer and its treatment. In fact, a recent meta-analysis of 56 studies found that aerobic exercise, including walking and cycling—both during and after treatment—reduced fatigue in cancer patients.

Interestingly, strength training was *not* found to reduce fatigue. But because strength training helps maintain muscle mass, some use of weights or resistance machines should be included for 15 to 20 minutes twice a week, if possible.

Because cancer patients sometimes have trouble maintaining their body weight, it's especially important for those who are exercising to increase their calorie intake to compensate for what gets burned during their workouts.

Rx: Exercise and Call Me in the Morning

Jordan D. Metzl, MD, a sports medicine physician at the Hospital for Special Surgery in New York City. The author of *The Exercise Cure: A Doctor's All-Natural, No-Pill Prescription for Better Health & Longer Life.* Dr. Metzl maintains practices in New York City and Greenwich, Connecticut, and is a medical columnist for *Triathlete Magazine.* He has run in 31 marathons and finished 11 Ironman competitions.

A recent study made international headlines when it found that exercise was just as effective as—or sometimes even outperformed—drugs when treating such conditions as heart disease and stroke.

The details: After examining about 300 medical trials involving more than 330,000 patients, Harvard researchers found that frequent exercise and powerful drugs, such as beta-blockers and blood thinners, provided very similar results. And in the case of stroke recovery, regular workouts were actually more effective than taking anticoagulant medications.

A troubling fact: Only one-third of clinicians "prescribe" exercise, which could not only boost the health of Americans significantly but also save the average patient thousands of dollars a year in medical costs.

My recommendations for condition-specific routines that contribute to a healthy, disease-free future…*

HEART ATTACK AND STROKE

Drugs such as beta-blockers help treat heart disease, but side effects can include fatigue, dizziness, upset stomach and cold hands. Meanwhile, a single 40-minute session of aerobic exercise has been shown to lower blood pressure for 24 hours in hypertensive patients, and regular workouts can reduce both systolic (top number) and diastolic (bottom number) blood pressure by five to 10 points. Consistent exercise also can improve cholesterol levels.

Why exercise works: The heart is a muscle, and cardiovascular exercise forces it to pump longer and eventually makes it stronger, preventing the buildup of plaques that can rupture and lead to a heart attack or stroke. Many heart attack and stroke survivors are afraid to exercise, but it's crucial that they move past this fear. Those who exercise require less medication…need fewer major surgeries such as bypasses…and are 25% less likely to die from a second heart attack than their couch potato counterparts.

What to do: Five times a week, do 30 to 40 minutes of cardiovascular exercise at a level of exertion where conversation is just manageable. (You might breathe heavy, but not gasp for air.) You have lots of choices for this exercise. Options include very fast walking, jogging, swimming, using an ellipti-

*Be sure to check with your doctor before starting any fitness program. If your condition is severe, he/she may initially want you to use exercise as an adjunct to medication, not as a replacement. Never stop taking a prescribed drug without talking to your doctor. *Caution:* With any of these workouts, seek immediate medical attention if you experience chest pain, shortness of breath, nausea, blurred vision or significant bone or muscle pain while exercising.

cal machine or recumbent bike, or taking an aerobics class. Pick an activity you enjoy to help you stay committed. After just six weeks, you'll likely have lower blood pressure, and by three months, your cholesterol levels should be improved.

Note: People with heart failure, a condition in which the heart cannot pump enough blood to the rest of the body, should avoid resistance exercises, such as push-ups and heavy weight lifting, that force muscles to work against an immovable or very heavy object. Such activities can put an excessive burden on the heart and cause further injury to it.

DEPRESSION

Exercise really is nature's antidepressant. Several studies have shown that working out is just as effective, if not more so, than medication when it comes to treating mild-to-moderate depression. Exercise also can help reduce the amount of medication needed to treat severe cases of depression…and even prevent depression in some people.

What to do: The key is to boost your heart rate high enough to trigger the release of endorphins, feel-good chemicals that elicit a state of relaxed calm. Spend 30 to 45 minutes at a level of exertion where conversation is quite difficult, three to five days a week, to benefit.

You also may want to try exercising outdoors. A study published in *Environmental Science & Technology* found that outdoor exercise produces stronger feelings of revitalization, a bigger boost of energy and a greater reduction in depression and anger than exercising indoors.

Strength training also is effective in treating depression—lifting weights releases endorphins and builds a sense of empowerment. For a strength-training program, ask your doctor to recommend a physical therapist or personal trainer.

If it's difficult to motivate yourself to exercise when you're depressed, relying on a personal trainer—or a "workout buddy"—can help.

BACK PAIN

Back pain strikes roughly half of Americans. Pain medications are available, but many are addictive and merely mask the symptoms rather than address the underlying problem. Muscle relaxants cause drowsiness…overuse of nonsteroidal anti-inflammatory drugs (NSAIDs), such as *ibuprofen*, can lead to ulcers…and steroid injections, which can be given only a few times per year, can cause infection or nerve damage and long-term side effects such as osteoporosis or high blood pressure.

What to do: There's a very powerful low-tech solution—a foam roller. Widely available at sporting goods stores, these cylindrical rollers have a record of preventing and relieving back pain. With the cylinder on the floor, move various muscles (your hamstrings, quadriceps and lower back) back and forth over the foam roller slowly. Roll each area for one to two minutes. If you hit an especially tender spot, pause and roll slowly or hover in place until you feel a release. The entire routine should take about 10 minutes.

Note: Rolling muscles can feel uncomfortable and even painful at first. But the more painful it is, the more that muscle needs to be rolled. Frequency eases discomfort.

In addition to rolling your muscles, start a back- and core-strengthening program. Avoid using heavy weights, especially within an hour of waking—that's when your muscles are tighter and you're more likely to strain a muscle.

Exercise: The Secret Weapon for Fighting Parkinson's Disease

Alessandro Di Rocco, MD, professor of neurology at Donald and Barbara Zucker School of Medicine, Hofstra/Northwell in Hempstead, New York. He is the director of the Parkinson's and Movement Disorders Center at Northwell Health. He has published many articles in professional journals, including *The Journal of Neuroscience* and *Movement Disorders.*

Medical treatment has made an enormous difference in the lives of people with Parkinson's disease (PD). But in recent years, it has become clear that the way to deal with this disease is not just to take medicine—no matter how good that medicine may be. Living with PD now also means living actively.

This may be more easily said than done for PD patients. The very nature of PD makes it hard for people to move properly. The disease causes tremor (shaking of the hands, arms, legs, jaw or tongue) and rigid muscles. It generally slows down movement and disrupts balance and coordination. No matter how helpful PD medications are, the disease worsens as time passes.

And then there's the reaction to exercise that many PD patients may have. It can be difficult and frustrating for them to simply move, let alone exercise. Feelings of fatigue, discomfort and self-consciousness can lead to inactivity and cause withdrawal.

But PD patients at any stage of the disease are urged to get up and get active—because the benefits of exercise for them far outweigh any of the drawbacks. People with PD who keep their bodies fit are better able to meet the many challenges of the disease. They reduce the impact of symptoms at every stage of the disease, stay healthier for longer and may even slow down the progression of the disease.

In addition, PD patients who exercise also reduce their risk for other types of diseases, such as cardiovascular disease and osteoporosis, and boost mood and cognitive ability.

Find out why exercise is so crucial for PD patients…

COUNTERACT THE DOWNWARD SPIRAL

PD is a condition in which some brain cells function poorly and gradually die. Particularly affected are neurons that produce the messenger chemical dopamine in the area of the brain, the substantia nigra, that is part of the finely tuned brain circuitry that controls movement.

This is why as PD progresses it becomes much harder to move properly. Tremors and rigidity or stiffness of muscles slow patients down and disrupt their balance and coordination.

Exercise can counteract this downward spiral. Research shows that exercising activates "muscle memory circuits" in the brain   that govern how muscles work together—and even in PD patients,

exercise keeps these brain circuits strong and functioning well.

In addition, exercise has been shown to augment the production of proteins, such as *brain-derived neurotrophic factor* (BDNF) and *glial cell line-derived neurotrophic factor* (GDNF), that promote the growth and health of neurons and strengthen connections among them.

In fact, evidence from animal studies suggests that physical activity counteracts the loss of brain cells in PD that otherwise leads to decline.

WHAT EXERCISE IS BEST?

Research shows that many different types of exercise benefit PD patients. Activities that emphasize agility, coordination and rhythm, such as tai chi, yoga and dance, are especially beneficial since they help to maintain the ability to perform complex movement combinations that may otherwise be undermined by PD's stiffness and slowness.

Tai chi for PD patients made headlines when researchers at the Oregon Research Institute published a study in *The New England Journal of Medicine* reporting that tai chi improved balance and functional ability in people who have mild-to-moderate PD. It also was found to reduce falls.

Tai chi, which involves slow movement and shifting weight from one foot to another, was previously found to help older people gain balance and strength.

In general, PD patients also benefit from an exercise program that includes stretching, aerobic activity and strength training.

Aerobic exercise—activities such as swimming or walking that raise the heart rate—has also been studied for PD patients.

In one review of eight trials published in *The Cochrane Database of Systematic Reviews*, German researchers found that treadmill walking improved walking speed and normalized gait in PD patients.

Strength training also has been found to be beneficial. A small study by researchers at the University of Illinois at Chicago found that lifting weights and doing other muscle-building exercises helped reduce the severity of symptoms in PD patients.

ADD MUSIC

The areas of the brain that respond to music are closely linked to those that control body movement. Music makes you want to move, and rhythm organizes and normalizes how you move.

Many people with PD are troubled less by tremor and can walk faster and with a smoother gait when listening to music, according to a 2012 study in *Parkinsonism & Related Disorders.*

PD patients can either listen to their own music while exercising, or find out more about music therapy by searching for the topic at Parkinson.org.

GETTING STARTED

•**How much exercise.** The more you are able to do, the better. In addition, the more intense you can make the exercise, the better—as long as the intensity is compatible with your general health and level of physical fitness.

PD patients should check with their doctors before starting an exercise program—and work with a doctor or physical therapist to tailor the program to their particular needs. This is especially important if a patient's ability to move is impaired or if the patient has other medical problems, such as joint pain or low blood pressure.

It is also crucial to work with a health-care professional as the disease progresses—to ensure that the exercise program matches and augments the individual's specific capabilities.

•**Where and how.** Exercise programs designed specifically for people with PD are becoming increasingly common in hospitals, Ys, community centers, churches and synagogues. Your doctor or physical therapist may be able to help you find one.

Or reach out on your own—even if they don't have organized classes for PD, many community centers with gym facilities are very welcoming to people with all sorts of physical challenges.

Parkinson's support or online discussion groups often are a good source of information about exercise and exercise programs. You can find more resources for PD patients in your area by calling the Parkinson's Foundation at 800-327-4545.

If you have PD: Make exercise a priority, and take it as seriously as the medications you take.

It is not very easy for most people to stay motivated when it comes to exercise. For the PD patient, fatigue, difficulty moving and feeling self-conscious about his/her condition can lead to a sedentary lifestyle. But like anyone who exercises, you will feel better and move with more ease if exercise is a regular part of your life.

Movement for Better Brain Power

Teresa Liu-Ambrose, PhD, PT, professor of physical therapy, Canada Research Chair in Physical Activity, Mobility, and Cognitive Neuroscience, and director, Aging, Mobility, and Cognitive Neuroscience Laboratory, University of British Columbia, and co-director, Centre for Hip Health and Mobility, all in Vancouver, Canada. Her study was published in *Archives of Internal Medicine.*

You've probably seen elderly family members and friends slowly lose their memories, and you're determined to do everything that you can to stay sharp.

But if you think that keeping your brain healthy is something that's really difficult or time-consuming, then here's some very exciting news...

There's a trick, and it's not hard...nor is it very time-consuming.

The secret lies in strength training, according to Canadian researchers.

A SMARTER WORKOUT

They found that after six months of twice-weekly, hour-long workouts, people who performed strength training had better memory and brain function, compared with those who did moderate to brisk walking and those who did balance, stretching and relaxation movements (the control).

Over the course of the study, the control group showed no improvement on any of the following measures, but check out how much the strength-training group outperformed the aerobic group...

•**The strength-training group showed a 17% improvement in the brain's executive function,** which controls planning, organizing, strategizing and managing time and space, whereas the aerobic group improved just 2%!

•**In terms of associative memory function (the type of memory that links information together,** as in matching an acquaintance's name with his or her face), the aerobic group improved 47%. But that paled in comparison to the improvement made by those in the strength-training group—92%!

•**Brain imaging of the strength-training group members** showed that three regions of their brains associated with cognitive behavior had become more active. Members in the aerobic exercise group, however, did not see any improvements in this area.

We can only speculate as to why strength training came out on top. One reason may be physiological. For example, strength training may reduce systemic inflammation, increase growth factors that promote neuronal growth and maintain insulin sensitivity (conditions such as diabetes increase your risk for dementia). It may also be that during strength training, the exerciser must constantly monitor his or her actions, including breathing properly, counting the number of reps and sets and using correct form.

BUILD MUSCLE—AND BRAIN POWER

To boost your memory and cognitive function, incorporate strength training into your workout schedule. Now, strength training shouldn't replace aerobic exercises or balance/stretching/relaxation exercises—those types of workouts are critical for other reasons, such as improving heart function and flexibility and reducing stress. Instead, strength training should be added to your routine if you don't already do it.

While study subjects performed strength training twice a week, an hour at a time, if that's too much of a time commitment (or if that's too much for you to handle, physically, right now), even adding smaller amounts of strength training to your routine is likely to help your brain a little. *Here's how to get started…*

1. Warm up. To prevent injury or strain, warm up for at least 10 minutes with light aerobic activity that will elevate your heart rate, such as brisk walking, jogging, biking or doing jumping jacks.

2. Build strength. To improve strength in all the major muscle groups, study subjects used dumbbells (starting with two to five pounds) weight lifting machines or body weight resistance (such as push-ups, lunges or squats, for example).

How many exercises you can handle during one workout depends on your level of fitness, so ask a trainer—it's best to start with only a few exercises and then gradually add more as you get stronger. Try performing two sets of each exercise, doing six to eight reps in each set, and resting for one minute in between sets. A trainer can advise you on correct form and provide guidance about when it's time to progress to heavier weights.

3. Cool down. As with the warm-up, slow down your heart rate with at least 10 minutes of light aerobic activity. Then, to prevent stiffness, gently stretch the muscles that you exercised.

And enjoy your brain power!

Want to Boost Learning and Memory? Time Your Exercise

Study titled "Physical Exercise Performed Four Hours After Learning Improves Memory Retention and Increases Hippocampal Pattern Similarity During Retrieval," by researchers at the Radboud University Medical Center in the Netherlands, published in *Current Biology*.

Cynthia Green, PhD, one of America's foremost experts on brain health, and founding director of the Memory Enhancement Program at the Icahn School of Medicine at Mount Sinai, New York City. Her company Total Brain Health, develops evidence-based brain wellness classes and programs.

You already know that exercise is great for your mind as well as your body. Now brain researchers are uncovering exactly how exercise helps our brains learn and, more importantly, how best to retain what we've learned.

Exercise is key. But it's all in the timing.

To evaluate the new research, we spoke with cognitive health expert Cynthia Green, PhD, president and CEO of Total Brain Health.

LEARNING + TIME + EXERCISE = KNOWLEDGE

Researchers in the Netherlands asked 72 volunteers to learn 90 picture-location associations in a 40-minute exercise. The researchers did noninvasive brain scans to see how the different parts of the brains lit up.

Then the researchers asked about one-third of the volunteers to exercise immediately afterward… another third to exercise four hours later…and a third group to not exercise at all. The exercise was a garden-variety aerobic workout—35 minutes of interval training on an exercise bike, at an intensity of up to 80% of maximum recommended heart rate for each individual.

Then, two days later, all the volunteers were asked to repeat the task to see how well they retained what they had learned. They repeated the brain scans, too.

Results: Exercising immediately after didn't help—those folks didn't retain knowledge any better than those who didn't exercise at all. But the ones who exercised four hours later did significantly better than everyone else at retaining what they'd learned.

What happened inside their brains was even more interesting. For those who delayed exercise for four hours, the hippocampus—a part of the brain crucial to long-term memory—looked remarkably similar during the initial learning task and the one repeated two days later when they got correct answers. It lit up in the same pattern. For the other volunteers, not so much—when confronted with the same task again, they had to, in essence, relearn much of what they had learned earlier.

While this experiment didn't examine physiology directly, the researchers note that other studies have found that exercise boosts brain chemicals known as *catecholamines*, including dopamine and norepinephrine, which are key to memory and learning. Still, they're not sure why waiting four hours made a big difference. That's where future research will go. The study also didn't look at what happens if you exercise, say, two or three hours after learning something—or five. For now, all they know is that getting some aerobic exercise about four hours later helps you remember.

EXERCISE AND YOUR BRAIN

The next time you need to make sure new information sticks—when you've just immersed yourself in a big new work project—try heading to the gym or lace on your running shoes and go out for a jog four hours later.

We also need to see the big picture when it comes to exercise and our brains. We know exercise overall is one of the best things we can do for our brains, and studies have repeatedly demonstrated that aerobic activity benefits cognition. Regular aerobic exercise—a rough total target of 150 minutes a week—is also key to maintaining cognitive health as you age, and it helps prevent dementia. But there's also growing evidence that strength training is also important for maintaining cognitive performance.

In other words, even if you don't care how buff you look, if you value your brain, when it comes to exercise—just do it.

Better Time to Walk

Andrew Reynolds, PhD, researcher, department of human nutrition, University of Otago, Dunedin, New Zealand.

Walking for 10 minutes after breakfast, lunch and dinner lowered post-meal blood sugar in people with diabetes about 12% more than taking a half-hour walk at any other time of day.

Especially helpful: A 10-minute walk after dinner, which tends to be the meal with the most carbs, had the biggest impact on blood sugar.

Theory: Blood sugar is needed to fuel muscles during exercise, so walking has the most impact when done after meals, when blood sugar levels are highest.

Got Diabetes? Don't Let Exercise Mess with Your Blood Sugar

Richard Cotton, MA, ACSM-CEP, exercise physiologist and national director of certification, American College of Sports Medicine, Indianapolis.

If you've been diagnosed with type 2 diabetes, you know that exercise is key for long-term blood sugar control. But it also can affect your blood sugar levels in the short term—and not always in good ways. Exercise too enthusiastically, and you could find your blood sugar level dropping too low—or even spiking.

Here's how people with type 2 diabetes can handle (and even better, avoid) the two most common exercise/blood sugar problems…

PROBLEM #1:
BLOOD SUGAR DROPS DURING EXERCISE

When you exercise, your body gets energy first by using blood sugar (glucose) and then by depleting *glycogen*, the storage form of glucose, from your muscles and liver. (You may also start burning fat for energy.)

The short-term effect is that blood sugar levels fall—and can stay reduced for as long as 24 hours. That's the benefit. But if levels fall too low (hypoglycemia)—below 70 mg/dL if your meter measures whole blood, or below 80 mg/dL if it measures plasma glucose—you may feel symptoms, including shakiness, clammy skin, blurred vision and confusion. A severe drop can be scary or even dangerous.

The good news is that it's rare—and easily prevented. Exercise-induced hypoglycemia is most common in people who take insulin—that is, everyone with type 1 diabetes and some people with type 2. It can also happen if you are taking certain medications that promote insulin secretion, including sulfonylureas and glinides. If low blood sugar during or after exercise happens to you regularly, talk to your doctor about possible solutions such as eating a small snack before (and maybe during) exercise, adjusting your medication dose—or both.

Exercise If You Take Insulin? This Online Calculator Makes It Easy

If you have diabetes, you know that regular exercise should be a key part of your life—it even might allow you to reduce your medication. But if you're taking insulin—like all people with type 1 diabetes and about 30% to 40% of people with type 2—exercise can be tricky. If you don't time your snacks and insulin right with the intensity and duration of your exercise routine, you might have an episode of low blood sugar (hypoglycemia), which is no fun—and can be dangerous.

There's an easy way to calculate what you need to do. It's called Excarbs. (The name comes from the need to figure out how many extra carbs you need when you exercise.) It's an easy-to-use calculator developed by the nonprofit Sansum Diabetes Research Institute in Santa Barbara, California. Go to Excarbs.sansum.org/exercise-intensity-calculator.

The online calculator helps you adjust your carb intake and insulin doses according to the kind of exercise you plan to do and when you're going to do it. To use it, type in your weight, how long and how vigorously you plan to exercise and some details about your medical management of your diabetes such as how much insulin you take, and then hit the button to get a personalized plan for your next workout. If you're eating a meal within two hours before working out, for example, you'll get a sample plan with advice to either reduce your insulin dose by a certain amount or increase your carb grams by a certain amount to account for the effect of exercise on blood sugar levels.

If you haven't been exercising regularly, talk to your doctor before using the Excarbs calculator. The goal of the Sansum Diabetes Center is to support people with insulin-dependent diabetes in exercising safely, and you'll want your doctor's input at first to make sure that's what happens.

—Richard Cotton

Fortunately, exercise-induced hypoglycemia is quite rare in people who manage their diabetes with lifestyle alone or with a medication such as *metformin*, which instead of promoting insulin secretion makes your body more sensitive to the insulin it already makes. Still, it's possible for a mild drop in blood sugar to happen, especially if you train really hard or for more than an hour. Even a mild blood sugar drop might make you feel tired afterward.

The best advice for everyone with diabetes, especially at the beginning of a new exercise program, is to test your blood sugar three times—before, during and after your workout. Once you get a sense of how your exercise routine is affecting your blood sugar, you can cut back on the testing. Just make sure that you have access to a quick energy source such as an energy bar or fruit juice in case your blood sugar drops.

Tip: To reduce your risk for hypoglycemia, do resistance exercise *before* aerobic exercise.

PROBLEM #2:
BLOOD SUGAR IS TOO HIGH BEFORE OR DURING EXERCISE

Sometimes, blood sugar levels get too high—250 mg/dL or 300 mg/dL or even higher—which can cause you to feel symptoms such as thirst, headache, blurred vision and fatigue. It's called hyperglycemia. It's an indication that you need to adjust your eating pattern, your medications or both so that you can bring blood sugar to more acceptable levels, such as the mid-100s.

Is it safe to exercise if your blood sugar is already somewhat elevated? The answer is yes as long as you're feeling good. Exercise can bring high blood sugar levels down quickly. Indeed, with exercise your muscles can burn up glucose at almost 20 times their normal rate. That's a key reason that regular exercise is so effective in controlling diabetes. Exercising, even a nice brisk walk, is one good way to bring levels down. Make sure you're staying well-hydrated, too, since high blood sugar can lead to frequent urination and thus dehydration.

Exception: Sometimes, if you start exercising when your blood sugar is already running high, rising adrenalin or other exercise-stimulated hormones can stimulate your body to release even more sugar into the blood—temporarily overwhelming the sugar-burning effect of exercise. If that happens, don't sweat it. Just cool down as you would any time you exercise aerobically and then sit quietly to allow your body to rest. After 30 minutes, when you test your blood sugar again, you should find that your blood sugar has gone down to more normal levels. In some cases, it might take an hour.

TAILORING YOUR EXERCISE PROGRAM TO YOUR BLOOD SUGAR PATTERN

The good news is that for most people with diabetes, exercise won't cause any short-term blood sugar problems—and it's one of the best things you can do to control your diabetes.

Check with your doctor before starting a new routine to see if you have any exercise limitations. If you're planning exercise more intense than walking and you have certain risk factors or conditions (such as high blood pressure, high cholesterol, heart disease, kidney problems), your doctor may also recommend that you undergo exercise stress testing, which involves walking fast on a treadmill while your heart is monitored. But most people with diabetes don't need this test.

If you have health issues such as foot problems, eyesight issues, arthritis or other limitations, your doctor can help you tailor an exercise plan that works for you or can refer you to a diabetes educator or an exercise physiologist who can help. It's a good thing that exercise is so safe, because it's so beneficial for people with diabetes.

The Heart-Health Workout

Barry A. Franklin, PhD, director of preventive cardiology/cardiac rehabilitation at Beaumont Health in Royal Oak, Michigan. He is a past president of the American Association of Cardiovascular and Pulmonary Rehabilitation and the American College of Sports Medicine.

What if there were a piece of exercise equipment that could cut your risk of dying from heart disease by nearly half?

This is actually possible by simply using a treadmill—in a strategic way. The approach is not complicated or even that difficult, but few people take advantage of it.

THE "MET" SECRET

We all know that walking is an excellent form of exercise. What makes a treadmill so efficient is that you can control your pace and/or incline so that you maintain your desired intensity and get the maximum benefit from your exercise routine.

The treadmill's winning secret is that it gives you the ability to monitor energy expenditure, also called a MET, which stands for metabolic equivalent. Every one MET increase in your fitness level cuts your risk for death from heart disease by 15%, so increasing METs by three, for example, will cut risk by 45%. Many treadmills display METs readings. You can also estimate METs with an app for your smartphone or tablet. The Exercise Calculator for the iPhone or iPad displays METs when you enter your weight, type of activity and length of time exercising.

Simply put, METs allow you to track the intensity of your workout by estimating the amount of oxygen your muscles are burning to fuel you through various activities. For example, sitting requires one MET…and normal walking requires two to three METs—that is, two to three times as much oxygen and calories as you'd burn while relaxing in a chair. Light jogging requires eight METs…and running at a 6 mph pace, 10 METs.

With immediate feedback from your METs reading, you can effectively gauge how hard you're working out…and receive the motivation to push yourself at the safest and most effective intensity levels.

Important: If you've been sedentary, start your treadmill walking at 2 mph to 3 mph with no incline. Gradually increase your speed over the next eight to 10 weeks, then progress to graded treadmill walking or slow jogging. If symptoms such as shortness of breath, dizziness and/or chest pain develop, stop and tell your doctor.

Here's how to most effectively use a treadmill for specific exercise goals…

• **Quick but effective workout.**

What to use: Incline and speed. When it comes to getting the most out of exercise, intensity and duration are inversely related. By combining higher treadmill inclines with increased speeds, you'll bolster your MET level and reach your target heart rate sooner. Working at your target heart rate helps improve fitness. With fast, graded treadmill walking, you can get a great workout in just 20 to 30 minutes.

Example: Increase speed slightly (0.1 mph to 0.2 mph) every minute for five minutes. Then increase the incline setting, which is measured as a percentage, by 0.5% (for example, going from 1% to 1.5% incline) and walk for five minutes. Alternate this sequence once or twice (increasing speed and incline each time) until you feel you're working hard, but can still carry on a conversation.

• **Weight loss.**

What to use: Incline. With incline walking, more muscle mass—especially in the quadriceps and glutes—is activated with each stride. And the more treadmill incline you use, the more calories you'll burn.

A mere increase of just 1% on the incline setting (for example, going from 1% to 2%) at a comfortable walking speed (such as 1.5 mph to 2.5 mph) will boost your energy expenditure by about 10%, and I'll bet you won't even feel a difference. If you walk faster, you'll burn even more calories because you'll be working at a higher MET level.

Research shows that regular brisk walks of at least 30 minutes five or more days a week is the best approach to weight loss. Walking on level ground at 2 mph or 3 mph equates to about two or three METs. To help protect your knees, slow your pace as you gradually work up to higher levels of inclines.

Good news: At high inclines, walking may burn as many calories as jogging or running.

DON'T FORGET STRENGTH TRAINING

To get the most from your treadmill walking—or any cardio activity—be sure to add some resistance or strength training to further build your muscle strength. Strength training complements aerobic exercise, reducing your risk for heart disease. You'll also improve your insulin sensitivity (to help fight diabetes) and boost your bone mass (to guard against osteoporosis).

Best: Target various upper and lower body muscle groups, including the chest, back, shoulders, abdomen, quadriceps and hamstrings, using hand weights and/or weight machines. Some yoga poses can also increase muscle strength and endurance.

Aim for eight to 10 exercises…and do at least one set of 10 to 15 reps per set, at least twice a week.

BONUS TOOLS

You've probably seen people at the gym wearing ankle weights while walking on the treadmill. I'm not a fan. They can strain the lower extremities, increasing your risk for orthopedic or musculoskeletal problems.

Better approach: Try walking with a backpack carrying a comfortable amount of weight. You'll burn more calories than you would if you were walking without one. A snug fit will keep the weight close to your spine and hips—which may help you avoid balance problems and improve your bone density.

And don't forget your headphones. Music (whatever genre you like) can reduce perceived exertion and may make your workout seem easier. It can be more motivating than watching TV.

TREADMILL SAFETY

Treadmills are generally a safe way to exercise, but accidental falls can happen. *To stay safe…*

•**Always straddle the treadmill** before turning it on, and don't assume it will always start at a slow, comfortable speed.

•**Lightly hold the handrail** for support while walking.

•**Always warm up and cool down** before and after the aerobic phase of your workout. Never suddenly stop the treadmill.

Yoga for High Blood Pressure

Beryl Bender Birch, founder of the Hard & the Soft Yoga Institute and the nonprofit Give Back Yoga Foundation, Give BackYoga.org, both based in East Hampton, New York. She is the author of *Power Yoga, Beyond Power Yoga* and *Boomer Yoga.*

A single 10-minute session of "slow breathing" can result in a temporary lowering of both systolic (top number) and diastolic (bottom number) blood pressure. How much depends on such factors as diet, stress level and genetics.

My recommendation: Do Face Up Dog Posture and Face Down Dog Posture followed by Child's Pose.

What to do: For Face Up Dog, start by lying facedown on the floor with your feet (tops flat on floor) in line with your hips. Place your arms at the sides of your chest and hands directly under your shoulders. While keeping your knees on the floor, push into your arms straightening them, roll your shoulders back, arch your back slightly and keep your neck aligned with your spine. Hold for five breaths. Then exhale into Face Down Dog (by turning your feet so that your heels are flat on the ground, and pushing up and back into an upside-down V). For Child's Pose, kneel with your feet folded under flat and extend your arms straight in front of your head, palms flat on your mat. Touch your forehead to the ground if possible.

Which Workout for What Heart Problem?

Aaron Baggish, MD, director, cardiovascular performance program, Massachusetts General Hospital Heart Center, Boston.

It doesn't take a scientist to figure out that the hearts of athletes are stronger than those of people who don't exercise. But scientists have been studying it nonetheless, and have learned that there are substantial differences in the size and thickness of the heart chambers of athletes, attributes that support the value of regular exercise for a healthy

Exercises for Special Conditions

heart. Further research is revealing that there are specific relationships between the kind of exercise you do and how it affects the heart, which may one day lead to prescription of exercise routines to address individual cardiovascular needs.

HOW AND WHY EXERCISE HELPS THE HEART

Up until now, the studies have just looked at a single snapshot of the heart function of athletes. So researchers at Massachusetts General Hospital studied the effect of different forms of exercise on heart function and structure.

The researchers selected student athletes from Harvard teams at the start of their fall semester. From the crew team, they enrolled 20 male and 20 female rowers in a trial testing the effects of endurance training, and from the football roster, they recruited 35 male players to test the effects of strength training. The researchers looked specifically for athletes who were not at an elite level of performance and fitness, so change could be measured over time. The athletes' training routines weren't altered for this study—they simply followed the regimen and practice schedules that had been developed by their coaches for their individual sports. Researchers took daily data on how long the young men and women trained and what type of training (endurance versus strength) they did, over a 90-day period.

For the endurance athletes, training consisted of long-duration open water sessions and indoor rowing machine workouts at 70% to 80% of maximum heart rate. Strength athletes did tackling drills, sprint training, weight lifting and plyometric (power jumping) exercises. All participants trained five or more days a week. They were questioned in private about previous steroid use, and those who had a history of using the drugs were excluded from the study.

IT'S ALL GOOD

At the start and end of the study, participants were given an echocardiogram to measure changes in heart structure and function against baseline measures, which led to the finding that both groups exhibited change. What was especially interesting was that there were considerable differences be-tween the cardiac changes in each group. The endurance athletes experienced significant increases in the size of their left and right ventricle chambers (the large pumping chambers in the heart), while the strength athletes showed thickening of their left ventricle wall.

Implication: Observations that the heart responds to exercise in a sport-specific fashion points to how exercise can be used for the treatment of different types of heart disease. Future work will reveal more about the optimal combination of endurance and strength training for heart conditions such as congestive heart failure, hypertension and coronary heart disease.

For now, however, this much is clear: Exercise that includes both aerobic and strength training is beneficial for health.

The Ultimate Exercise Rx for Peripheral Artery Disease

Neel P. Chokshi, MD, MBA, associate professor of clinical medicine, Perelman School of Medicine, medical director, Sports Cardiology and Fitness Program, University of Pennsylvania, Philadelphia.

If your calves cramp while walking or climbing stairs—especially if the pain eases when you stop—it's a red flag that you may have *peripheral artery disease* (PAD). With PAD, your arteries are narrowed due to plaque buildup, which prevents the muscles in your extremities (usually your legs) from getting enough blood flow to keep up with the increased oxygen demand when you are active.

It's no small matter—if PAD goes untreated, the condition can lead to infection, loss of the function of the limb and, in severe cases of blockage, amputation.

Here's the irony of treating PAD: People who have this circulatory problem, with its telltale pain while walking, are often prescribed (you guessed it!) walking to relieve their pain. Even though it hurts, walking—when done according to certain guidelines (see next page)—does actually improve the symptoms of PAD and slow its progression. In fact, exercise works as well as any medication or surgery, according to research published in *Circulation*.

WALK THIS WAY

What's so great about walking? When you repeatedly put one foot in front of the other, it brings more oxygen to your muscles, which improves your circulation and eases the pain of PAD. The exact reasons why walking helps aren't known, but it's well-established that the more you walk, the farther you'll be able to walk…and with less pain.

Important: If you suspect that you have PAD but haven't been diagnosed, it's important to see your doctor for an evaluation. This will include an ankle-brachial exam, which compares the blood pressure in your arms to that in your feet, to show how well your blood is flowing, and possibly other tests such as an ultrasound. You may also have other related factors, such as high blood pressure, that need to be addressed.

To get the best results from your walking program…

•**Stretch.** Before getting started, your calf muscles need a good stretch to increase blood flow to the area.

What works best: Stand in front of a low step (a curb works fine, too). Place the toes of one foot on the step and drop your heel just enough to feel a stretch in your calf. Don't overdo it…stop at the point of tightness. Hold it for 10 to 15 seconds, then switch feet.

To warm up your thigh muscles, stand on one leg and raise the other foot behind you by bending the knee. Do not pull up on your foot…just rest that ankle in your hand and hold that position long enough to feel a slight stretch in your thigh (usually 10 to 15 seconds). Switch legs and repeat. (If you can't reach your ankle, try standing with a wall behind you and place that foot against the wall to hold it up.)

•**Walk.** Find a flat, safe surface for your walks (neighborhood streets, a local track, a shopping mall or a treadmill).

What works best: Start by walking for five minutes at a pace that causes some pain. On a pain scale from one to five, where one is mild pain and five is severe pain, aim to walk at a three or four.

•**Rest.** After walking for five minutes with moderate pain, stop and rest until the pain goes away.

Helpful: If you like to walk in an area where there aren't any benches for your rest period, treat yourself to a cane with a folding seat attachment. It's not too heavy to carry and gives you a place to sit during your rest stops.

•**Repeat.** Once the pain has dissipated, try to walk for another five minutes. If you find that it's impossible to do the additional five minutes without severe pain, try slowing down your pace to achieve a few extra minutes.

•**Stay focused on your goal.** Try to walk at least three—ideally, five—times a week. During the first two months, build up slowly to a total of 35 minutes of walking during each session, not counting the rest breaks. After you can manage that, keep adding a few minutes each week until you're at the ultimate goal of walking 50 minutes per session.

•**Cool down.** You should always finish by walking slowly for five minutes. Then stretch your calf and thigh muscles again to help minimize muscle soreness after walking.

SMART STRATEGIES

To give yourself the best possible odds of succeeding at your walking program, you should also…

•**Track your progress.** To stay motivated, jot down the total time and distance of your walks. Or wear a fitness tracker, such as Fitbit, or use a phone app, like MapMyWalk, to help track your time, effort and distance.

•**Avoid boredom! If you walk outside, vary your route.** If you prefer a treadmill, listen to music or a podcast…or watch a 30-minute TV show.

Also helpful: Find a walking buddy—the social aspect can help keep you on target.

FOR AN EXTRA BOOST

Working with a physical therapist to start a walking program is smart, since supervised programs seem to be more effective by helping to ensure that you keep up with your walking program and hit the required pain thresholds. You're also likely to get help paying for your sessions with a physical therapist.

Recent development: Medicare Part B now covers comprehensive cardiac rehabilitation programs that include exercise, education and counseling for patients with PAD. The specific amount you'll owe may depend on several things, such as the Medigap insurance (if any) you have and the type of facility you choose. Check with your insurer.

AN ALTERNATIVE TO WALKING

If any amount of walking is too painful or too dangerous for you, don't give up. New research shows that you can get comparable results with arm exercises.

Important recent finding: In a study that was conducted at University of Minnesota School of Nursing in Minneapolis, researchers randomly divided 28 people with PAD (average age 65.6) into three different groups—no exercise…treadmill walking…or arm exercise. Participants assigned to arm exercises used an arm ergometer (a device with bicycle-like pedals that are operated by the arms). After three months of training for three hours a week, people in both exercise groups could walk farther without pain.

Other possibilities: It's likely that bike riding, dancing, swimming or pool walking, which haven't yet been tested in people with PAD, may also help relieve symptoms. If you enjoy those activities, talk to your doctor about giving them a try!

Stronger Body = Stronger Heart

Stefanos Tyrovolas, PhD, principal investigator, Frailty, Sarcopenia and Nutrition Group, Parc Sanitari Sant Joan de Déu, Barcelona, Spain.

Men and women with the highest muscle volume were 81% less likely to suffer heart at-tack or stroke compared with those who have the lowest, according to a 10-year study of 2,020 adults, ages 45 and older.

Theory: Muscle mass helps maintain normal inflammatory, endocrine and metabolic function, which can stave off cardiovascular disease.

Takeaway: Include resistance training in your exercise routine.

Pain-Relieving Stretch for Peripheral Artery Disease

Neel P. Chokshi, MD, MBA, associate professor of clinical medicine, Perelman School of Medicine, medical director, Sports Cardiology and Fitness Program, University of Pennsylvania, Philadelphia. Study presented at the American Heart Association's Arteriosclerosis, Thrombosis and Vascular Biology/Peripheral Vascular Disease Scientific Sessions.

For people with *peripheral artery disease* (PAD), a buildup of fatty deposits in arteries that prevents sufficient blood and oxygen from reaching muscles, exercise is not just good for cardiovascular health—it can mean the difference between keeping their legs and needing amputation. That's because exercise increases vital circulation to the limbs. There's a catch-22, however. Having PAD can make activities such as walking, climbing stairs and just moving around so painful that many of the 8.5 million American adults who have the disease avoid exercise as much as possible.

In a small study from Florida State University College of Medicine in Tallahassee, patients with PAD who stretched their calf muscles for 30 minutes a day, five days a week for a month improved both blood flow to their calves and their walking ability. They were able to walk farther during a timed period (six minutes)…and they were able to walk for a longer distance without needing to stop and rest because of discomfort.

While it's premature to recommend any specific stretching protocol based on just this small study, it does suggest that if you have PAD, calf stretching can help you better manage the condition. For the study, participants stretched using a special splint that flexed their ankles about 15%, pulling their toes up toward their legs. But you don't need splints to stretch your calf muscles. A physical therapist can show you how to do it—and recommend for how long and how often you should do it.

You Can Use Exercise to Fight Cancer

Study titled "Voluntary Running Suppresses Tumor Growth through Epinephrine- and IL-6-Dependent NK Cell Mobilization and Redistribution" by researchers at University of Copenhagen, Copenhagen University Hospital, Chalmers University of Technology, Göteborg, Sweden, Oak Ridge National Laboratory, Oak Ridge, Tennessee, University Hospital Essen, Germany, published in *Cell Metabolism.*

The big news in cancer treatment these days is a new kind of high-tech immunotherapy that unleashes the body's own ability to target and kill tumor cells.

But research has found that there may be something very similar that goes on in your body—any day you exercise a certain way—that unleashes the body's tumor-fighting response in a way that may both prevent and treat cancer. The research involved mice, but those results often transfer to humans. *Here's what was discovered…*

HOW EXERCISE PROTECTS

In a series of experiments, researchers trained one set of mice to run on treadmills while another group was more sedentary. They then injected the mice with tumor-producing carcinogens.

The exercising mice fought the tumors better. They had fewer tumors, and the tumors that they did develop were smaller and lighter, with fewer growth factors and less metastasis. Compared with couch-potato mice, their tumor burden was reduced by more than 60%.

The how was even more illuminating. Certain kinds of exercise stimulated a specific immunological response that sent the body's natural killer immune cells directly into tumors to destroy them—a kind of "immunological spark" that ignites other cells in the immune system to fight cancer, according to the study's authors.

The key was adrenalin, a "stress" hormone also known as epinephrine. When you exercise vigorously enough to get your heart really pumping, your body sends out more adrenalin—and it's that adrenalin surge, the researchers report, that stimulates natural killer cells to scour and destroy tumors.

Human studies will be needed to pinpoint exactly how intense exercise needs to be to optimize this immune response. But we already know that exercise that raises your heart rate significantly and makes you break a sweat causes the release of much more adrenalin than milder exercise. You don't have to be an Olympic athlete to reach those levels.

WORK AT YOUR OWN PACE

Of course, if you're not fit, you'll want to start slowly and safely. But becoming fit has its own separate reward—people who exercise regularly and are more fit tend to produce more adrenalin for the same level of exercise intensity compared to less fit people. In short, training boosts the adrenalin response.

If you're being treated for cancer, it's understandable if you don't have much energy for vigorous exercise. Do what you can, and talk with your doctor about ways to get more exercise. Even moderate exercise like walking has wonderful benefits for people undergoing cancer treatment, from reducing nausea to improving muscle tone to enhancing mood. But if you can work out hard, that adrenalin rush may be adding an immunological boost to your cancer fight, too. And once you've beaten the cancer, regular heart-pumping exercise may help prevent it from ever coming back.

Exercises Protect Head and Neck Cancer Patients' Ability to Swallow

Victor M. Duarte, MD, board-certified otolaryngologist in Modesto, California. His study was published in *Otolaryngology—Head and Neck Surgery.*

You take a bite and you chew, but you just can't swallow. The food stays in your mouth, turning to mush…or it gets stuck in your throat and makes you choke…or it finally goes down, but it hurts. This happens again and again, with every bite, until you're afraid to eat or drink at all.

That scenario is all too real for patients with head and neck cancers (cancer of the throat, larynx, oral cavity, salivary gland or paranasal sinuses). Radiation is often a part of the typical treatment for head and neck cancers—and the majority of such patients who receive radiation develop *dysphagia* (swallowing difficulties). Often they end up on a diet of puréed foods or even just liquids…in extreme cases, they need feeding tubes.

You can imagine the terrible impact that this has on patients' quality of life, not to mention their nutritional status. And sadly, the swallowing problems often remain for the rest of their lives.

Very good news: Specially designed mouth and throat exercises (including gargling!) help decrease these terrible problems, an exciting study shows—but only if the exercises are started in time.

GET WITH THE PROGRAM…

Patients with head and neck cancers often are sent for "swallowing rehab" after radiation treatment, once dysphagia has developed. But for this study, researchers wanted to see whether swallowing problems could be prevented or minimized if patients performed targeted exercises before and during their cancer treatment.

The study included 85 patients with head and neck cancer who were about to be treated with either radiation alone or chemotherapy plus radiation. Two weeks before beginning their cancer treatment, the participants were instructed in the swallow preservation protocol. Taught by a speech-language pathologist, the protocol consisted of a series of exercises designed to maintain range of motion of the mouth and neck muscles involved in swallowing and to counter the effects of the fibrosis (scar tissue formation and stiffening) that often occurs after radiation.

Exercises included gargling…sticking out the tongue…effortful swallowing ("swallowing hard")…"chug-a-lugging" several ounces of liquid all at once…and more. Participants were advised to repeat each exercise 10 times per session (except the chug-a-lug) and to complete three sessions per day, starting two weeks prior to treatment and continuing for two months after treatment ended. During treatment, participants also were encouraged to continue eating and drinking as they normally would—even if it hurt to swallow or if they experienced a distorted, unpleasant taste (a common side effect of chemotherapy).

…AND STICK WITH THE PROGRAM

Participants kept records to track how frequently they performed the exercises. Of the 85 participants, 57 were considered compliant with the program because they completed at least one full set of exercises each day. The remaining 28 patients, who did not do at least one complete set of exercises daily, were deemed noncompliant. *One month after treatment ended, here's where things stood…*

• **A regular chewable diet** (not purée or liquid) was being managed by 54% of compliant patients… but just 21% of noncompliant patients could chew regular food.

• **A feeding tube was required for only 23% of compliant patients**…compared with 54% of noncompliant patients.

• **Abnormal esophageal narrowing (stenosis)** occurred in just 7% of the compliant group…as opposed to 32% of the noncompliant group.

• **All in all, the benefits for the people who really followed the advice were tremendous!**

Now, you might think that the people who were noncompliant (and who had worse outcomes) tended to be noncompliant because their conditions were worse to begin with and/or because they suffered greater side effects from treatment—either or both of which could make the exercises more difficult. However, that wasn't the case, the researchers said. There were no significant differences between the compliant and noncompliant groups in terms of tumor stage, treatment type, radiation dose or the diet they could tolerate pretreatment...nor were there any significant differences in the two groups' pain levels after treatment.

Bottom line: Should you or a loved one ever need radiation for head or neck cancer, ask your doctor about starting swallow therapy before your treatment and continuing right through your post-treatment period whether or not you are having swallowing difficulties. Your doctor can refer you to a speech-language pathologist with expertise in swallow therapy...or you can find such a therapist through the American Speech-Language-Hearing Association, ASHA.org.

To Ease Chemo Pain, Walk This Way

Abstract titled "A URCC NCORP nationwide randomized controlled trial investigating the effect of exercise on chemotherapy-induced peripheral neuropathy in 314 cancer patients," by **Ian Kleckner, PhD,** research assistant professor, University of Rochester Medical Center, New York, and colleagues, presented at the American Society of Clinical Oncology meeting.

A whopping 38% of people being treated with multiple drugs for cancer develop nerve pain—resulting in tingling, shooting pains, movement problems and/or numbness. It's called *chemotherapy-induced peripheral neuropathy* (CIPN), and it's so painful that some people drop out of lifesaving chemo, and the pain can last for years. There are no FDA-approved drugs to prevent it—or treat it.

But there is something incredibly simple that you can do yourself that makes a real difference. It's a gentle exercise program that's easy to do at home.

A WAY TO EXERCISE WHILE YOU ARE IN CHEMO

The program is called Exercise for Cancer Patients (EXCAP), and it's the brainchild of Karen M. Mustian, PhD, MPH, at the University of Rochester Medical Center. She has conducted trials on the effect of exercise on cancer patients since 2007.

EXCAP is deceptively simple, especially for something that can transform cancer patients' lives. It's daily walking plus a set of exercises using stretchy elastic resistance bands to build muscle strength. That's all—but it's tailored to each individual's fitness needs...it's based at home...and it includes coaching by a trained instructor who can help each patient progress (and overcome any obstacles encountered). The goal is to slowly build endurance and strength with daily exercise—by increasing the number of steps walked and with progressively challenging resistance band exercises. It lasts six weeks, although it's easy to continue on your own after the official program ends.

FIGHTING NEUROPATHY WITH YOUR OWN TWO FEET (AND ARMS)

In this study, researchers identified 314 patients in the ongoing clinical trials on EXCAP who were getting chemo drugs known to contribute to nerve pain, including platinum, *vinca alkaloid* and *taxane*. (If you are being treated with one of these drugs, the chance that you'll get CIPN is 60%.) These drugs often are used to treat breast cancer, and indeed three-quarters of the patients were being treated for breast cancer. Everyone got chemo, but about half of the patients were also enrolled in EXCAP.

Results: Exercisers had significantly less chemo-induced nerve pain—especially older ones.

How does exercise help? The exact mechanisms aren't known, but other EXCAP studies have shown that the program reduces chronic inflammation. It has other benefits, too, such as reducing cognitive impairment—aka, "chemo brain"—in people being treated with drugs for cancer. Plus, regular exercise reduces the risk for cancer recurrence and it even may make cancer treatments more effective.

How much exercise is enough to minimize cancer treatment side effects such as nerve pain? There aren't any official guidelines yet, so your best bet is to discuss an exercise plan with your doctor, who may be able to recommend a physical therapist or exercise trainer you can work with. Use common sense—start slowly and build up very gradually. Don't overdo it. Chemo is taxing and exhausting, but the good news is that this very mild exercise program, tailored to your energy level, may help you get through the process with less pain now—and in the future—and will also improve your circulation so that toxic compounds that result from chemotherapy move out of your body faster. (And if you haven't started cancer treatment yet, make sure that exercise is part of your cancer prehab program.)

A Boost for Cancer Treatment

Study led by researchers at Kansas State University, Manhattan, published in *Journal of the National Cancer Institute*.

Moderate exercise may boost cancer treatment. Regular activities that use 30% to 60% of a patient's aerobic capacity—not less and not more—can make radiation treatment for cancer more effective by enhancing oxygen delivery and blood flow to the tumors. Examples of this type of exercise are a brisk walk or a slow jog. Too much exercise may have a negative impact by shutting down blood flow to the tumor region or harming the immune system. Each patient should talk to his/her doctor for specific recommendations.

Exercise—at Any Age—Cuts Risk for Breast Cancer

In a study of more than 3,000 women (both premenopausal and postmenopausal), those who did 10 hours of moderate exercise a week—including walking and gardening—had a 30% lower risk for breast cancer than those who were sedentary.

Theory: Besides reducing body fat, exercise may increase antioxidant capacity and enhance cell repair.

Lauren McCullough, PhD, epidemiologist, The University of North Carolina at Chapel Hill.

Prostate Cancer Recovery Tip

Siobhan M. Phillips, PhD, assistant professor of preventive medicine, Northwestern University Feinberg School of Medicine, Chicago.

Just a little exercise goes a long way in healing after prostate cancer. A review of more than 51,500 prostate cancer survivors found that those who walked at an easy pace for three hours per week had less fatigue, depression and weight problems (common post-treatment issues) than those who didn't walk as much. Picking up the pace was also beneficial—men who walked briskly for only 90 minutes a week showed similar improvements. About half the men had surgery, and 40% received radiation as their primary treatment.

Is the Way You Walk Giving You a Warning?

Mary Harward, MD, a geriatrician in private practice in Orange, California. She specializes in the diagnosis and treatment of gait disorders and other diseases affecting older adults.

When you go to the doctor, odds are that you are taken to an exam room and asked to "have a seat" until the doctor arrives. The problem is, you'll probably stay seated during the entire visit, and your doctor may miss a symptom—a dangerous gait—that's just as important as abnormal X-rays or blood tests.

TAKE IT SERIOUSLY

It's never normal to shuffle, be off-balance or have an unusual posture. A gait disorder always means that something—or, in most cases, a combination of factors—is awry.

Problems with gait affect about 15% of adults age 60 and older and more than 80% of those age 85 and older. Gait disorders, which interfere with stability and balance, are not only among the most common causes of falls and subsequent hospitalizations, but also can be one of the first health problems that eventually leads to nursing home care.

My advice: Doctors should ask every patient if he/she has fallen in the last year. In addition, if you're age 65 or older, you should ask your doctor to check your gait at least once a year.

WHAT'S BEHIND IT?

Patients often assume that problems with one's gait are due to neurological disorders, such as Parkinson's disease or multiple sclerosis (MS). With Parkinson's disease, patients also experience a resting tremor or shaking of one hand, muscle rigidity and slow movements, while MS typically is accompanied by vision problems, dizziness and trouble speaking. *But there are other possible causes of gait problems…*

•**Arthritis.** Gait problems are common in patients with arthritis, particularly osteoarthritis of the knee or hip. If you have knee or hip pain, you may favor that side and use other muscles to compensate. This throws off your posture and body mechanics, which may cause you to limp or take tentative steps.

Helpful: Ask your doctor if it's appropriate to see a physical therapist for advice on exercises to strengthen the muscles around the arthritic joint—this will help you walk normally and with less pain.

Pain control is also very important. Apart from making you more comfortable, it will help you do the exercises that you need for a better gait. If you don't get adequate relief from over-the-counter pain relievers, talk to your doctor about stronger forms of pain control. Stretching, massage, heating pads, cold packs and/or acupuncture are helpful to some people.

•**Back problems.** A gait problem often is due to a painful back. Patients with lumbar stenosis, for example, will frequently experience nerve pressure from damaged vertebrae in the spine, affecting their ability to walk. Patients with sciatica (nerve pain that often accompanies lower-back problems) will have difficulty walking or standing. Suspect nerve problems if you have back or leg pain that gets worse when you walk or stand for more than a few minutes and gets better when you're off your feet. See your doctor for treatment advice.

•**Balance disorders.** If you sometimes feel as though you're about to fall (even when you're not), see a doctor right away. Problems with balance—often accompanied by dizziness, spinning sensations, etc.—are a major cause of falls. Potential causes include ear infections, inner-ear disorders, neuropathy (nerve damage) and circulatory problems.

Also: Ask your doctor to test your vitamin B-12 level. Older adults often have low levels of intrinsic factor, a protein that's needed for B-12 absorption. It's also common for vegetarians to be deficient in this vitamin because meat is a major source of B-12. Low B-12 can make you feel light-headed, cause numbness and/or tingling in the feet and make it difficult to walk.

Similar foot and leg symptoms are caused by diabetic neuropathy, nerve damage that may occur in patients with poorly managed (or undiagnosed) diabetes. Bunions and other foot conditions also can contribute to gait disorders.

•**Drug side effects.** It's not surprising that sedating medications such as *diazepam* (Valium) can increase fall risk. What many people don't realize is that nonsedating medications also can be an issue.

Example: Medications that lower blood pressure, such as diuretics, can cause orthostatic hypotension, a sudden drop in blood pressure that can make you dizzy or light-headed. Some blood pressure drugs also decrease magnesium, which can cause leg weakness or cramps. Your doctor might advise changing medications. Alcohol or drugs that lower blood sugar or affect mood or sleep also can change one's gait.

Important: Be especially careful after eating. Studies have shown that dizziness and gait problems tend to get worse about 30 minutes after meals—blood travels to the digestive tract after meals, sometimes lowering blood pressure.

•**Reduced brain circulation.** Gait disorders are often the first sign of infarcts, areas of brain damage caused by impaired circulation. Infarcts occur in patients who have had a stroke or other problems that affect blood vessels in the brain, such as hypertension or high cholesterol.

A patient who has multiple infarcts might walk very slowly…take short steps…stand with his feet wider apart than usual…and/or hesitate when starting to walk or have trouble slowing momentum when stopping.

HOW'S YOUR GAIT?

If you've noticed changes in the ways in which you move, see your doctor for an evaluation. *He/she will give you tests that may include…*

•**The timed get-up-and-go test. This measures the time it takes you to get up from a chair (without using your hands to push off from the armrests),** walk 10 feet, turn around and walk back to the chair. You should be able to complete the sequence safely in 14 seconds or less. If it takes longer than 20 seconds, your gait is seriously impaired.

The Ultimate Exercise Plan for Restless Legs—You May Not Need Drugs After All…

Roger A. Herr, PT, a New York City–based physical therapist and a the Secretary of the Board of Directors of the American Physical Therapy Association. He has worked in a variety of acute and post-acute care settings in New York, Washington and California. To find a physical therapist near you, go to MoveForwardPT.com.

If you have ever had throbbing, pins-and-needles, creepy-crawling or other uncomfortable sensations in your legs while sitting or lying down—especially if they are accompanied by a strong urge to move your legs—then chances are good that you have *restless legs syndrome* (RLS).

It's an annoying condition that many people try to cope with on their own in its early stages. But most people with RLS suffer so much that they need more help and often turn to medications, such as *ropinirole* (Requip) and *pramipexole* (Mirapex). While these drugs may provide short-term relief, they can actually worsen symptoms in many people who use them long term.

So what's the solution if you'd rather avoid medication?

Getting regular exercise has been shown to reduce the severity of symptoms by approximately 50%. But it's crucial that you get the *correct* type of exercise—and in the correct amounts. For that reason, it's wise to follow the simple exercise plan in this article, which is specially designed for people with RLS.

THE EXERCISE SOLUTION

With RLS, also known as Willis-Ekborn disease after the doctors who discovered it, the key is to not do too much of any one activity (sitting, standing, walking or even lying in one position) for too long.

Your fitness level will determine your tolerance for physical activity. Recognize your limits and avoid overexertion, which can trigger RLS. Also, don't sit for more than two hours at a time—get up and walk even if you're at a movie, in a meeting or traveling.

Research shows that the foundation of an effective RLS exercise plan is a combination of gentle lower-body resistance training (such as gentle lunges and knee bends) as well as moderate aerobic activity (such as walking, cycling or water aerobics).

Aim for 30 minutes at least three days a week—ideally, you should work up to 60 minutes each session. But to truly have the best odds of reducing your RLS symptoms, you also need to do the following exercises, which don't take long to perform and are carefully selected for the condition.

Important: In some people, exercise can interfere with sleep, so be sure that your workout is at least two hours before bedtime. And stay away from high-impact activities, such as jogging, kickboxing and jumping jacks—these exercises can overtax the leg muscles.

WHAT WORKS FOR RLS

Leg stretches are particularly useful because people with RLS tend to have tight leg muscles, often due to long hours of sitting or standing. These tight muscles (even in the upper legs) limit mobility, increasing risk for RLS discomfort in the lower legs. *In addition to walking and resistance training, do the following stretches two or three times a day…*

•**Calf Stretch.**

What to do: Stand a little less than arm's length from a wall. Put your palms against the wall, and step your right leg forward with your left leg behind you. Slowly bend your right knee, and press down with your left heel to stretch your left calf. Hold for 30 to 60 seconds. Repeat with the other leg.

●**Hamstring Stretch.**

What to do: Lie on the floor on your back, and position yourself near a doorframe. Put your left leg through the doorway, and raise your right leg as high as you comfortably can with your right heel resting against the doorframe. Gently straighten your right leg until you feel a stretch along the back of your right thigh. Hold for about 30 to 60 seconds. Switch legs and repeat.

●**Quadriceps Stretch.**

What to do: While standing near a wall in case you need support, raise your right leg and grasp your right ankle behind you. Gently pull your right heel up until you feel a stretch in the front of your right thigh. Hold for 30 to 60 seconds. Repeat with left leg.

FOR IMMEDIATE RELIEF

Exercises that can offer instant relief from an RLS attack…

●**Ankle Pumps.** When your legs bother you, ankle pumps get the blood flowing. These exercises can be done while sitting or while lying on your back in bed or on a couch.

What to do: Extend your legs straight in front of your body. Flex your ankles so that your toes point toward your upper body, then point your toes and feet away from your body. Do this 10 or 20 times, every other hour if necessary. If RLS wakes you up at night, do ankle pumps, and you may be able to get back to sleep quickly.

●**Walking.** If ankle pumps don't provide enough relief within a minute or two, get up and walk at a comfortable pace around the room. This gets your blood flowing even more than ankle pumps. Walking is also rhythmic, which is relaxing and may help you get back to sleep.

The New Anti-Snoring Workout

Murray Grossan, MD, ear, nose and throat specialist, Cedars-Sinai Medical Center in Los Angeles. GrossanInstitute. com

S noring can be a nightmare—both for the sufferer and his/her bed partner. But until recently, the treatments have been limited. A snorer might be told to lose weight, for example, wear a mouth guard or a mask (part of a continuous positive airway pressure, or CPAP, system) that delivers a steady stream of air at night…change his sleeping position…or, in severe cases, get surgery.

Recent development: In a 2015 study of 39 men who snored or had mild *obstructive sleep apnea* (OSA), a common cause of snoring, scientists found that performing mouth and tongue exercises reduced the frequency and intensity of snoring by up to 59%—a reduction on par with other therapies, including mouth guards or surgery.

And while snoring may seem like more of an annoyance than a health problem, that is simply not true. Snoring has been linked to medical conditions, including heart attack, stroke and glaucoma. *How mouth and tongue exercises can help…*

SIT-UPS FOR YOUR THROAT

If your bed partner has complained of your snoring or you have unexplained daytime sleepiness, consider trying the following exercises.

About half of my patients improve enough after doing these exercises (think of them as "throat sit-ups") for five minutes three times a day for six weeks to avoid surgery or other inconvenient therapies such as wearing a mouth guard or using CPAP. They also awaken feeling more refreshed and reduce their odds of developing OSA.

Here are the main exercises included in the recent study mentioned above (led by Geraldo Lorenzi-Filho, MD, PhD)—along with some slight variations that I have found to be effective for my patients. The tongue positions for these exercises strengthen your tongue muscle and the sides of your throat. However, my variations give these muscles a more rigorous strength-training workout.

● **Tongue Push.**

What to do: Push the tip of your tongue forcefully behind your upper front teeth and move it all the way back along the roof of your mouth (palate) 20 times.

My variation: Say the vowel sounds "A, E, I, O, U" while doing the exercise.

● **Flat Tongue Press.**

What to do: Suck your tongue up against the roof of your mouth, pressing the entire tongue against your palate 20 times.

My variation: Repeat "A, E, I, O, U" while doing the exercise.

● **Say "Ahhh."**

What to do: Focus on raising the back of the roof of the mouth and *uvula* (the fleshy appendage in the throat that's responsible for the rattling sound made by snorers) 20 times.

My variation: Say the vowel "A" (or "Ahhh") while doing the exercise.

THESE THERAPIES HELP, TOO

Colds, allergies and sinus infections can cause nasal congestion and/or postnasal drip—two common conditions that can make your throat swell, increasing your risk for snoring. *What helps…*

● **Nasal lavage** (using a saline solution to irrigate and cleanse the nasal cavity) helps clear nasal congestion and postnasal drip. Subjects in the study mentioned above performed nasal lavage three times a day. Based on my clinical experience, once a day does the job.

A product that I created called The Hydro Pulse Sinus System ($69.99, HydroMedOnline.com) works well. It includes a special throat attachment that directs pulsating irrigation to the tonsils and throat to ease swelling. But you could also use a neti pot (*typical cost*: $10)—just be sure to keep it clean and sanitized between uses and use distilled or sterile water to prevent a sinus infection. Or you can buy sterile squeeze bottles filled with nasal saline.

Yoga and Tai Chi for Asthma

Yoga Pose for Asthma

In a recent study of 20 people with asthma, those who took two one-hour yoga classes plus a half-hour home class weekly for 10 weeks reported reduced symptoms.

Specific pose: Do the Extended Side Angle Posture. It increases lung capacity by stretching and activating the intercostal muscles between each rib, which expand when you inhale and contract when you exhale.

What to do: From a standing position at the top of your mat, inhale and step back with the right foot, taking your feet wide apart, about four to five feet. Turn your left foot out and your right foot in about 45°, and raise your arms parallel to the floor. Exhale while bending your left knee directly over your ankle as you rest your left forearm on your left thigh. Reach your right hand out over your head and ear. Keep your head in alignment with the spine and your abdomen pulled in. Look up and take five breaths. Inhale, come up out of the posture. Reverse your feet and arms and exhale down to the other side, repeating the stretch.

Beryl Bender Birch, founder of the Hard & the Soft Yoga Institue and the nonprofit Give Back Yoga Foundation, GiveBackYoga.org, both based in East Hampton, New York. She is the author of *Power Yoga, Beyond Power Yoga* and *Boomer Yoga.*

Tai Chi Helps Control Asthma

When 17 asthma patients took classes in tai chi (an ancient Chinese practice that coordinates breathing and slow body movements) once weekly for six weeks and performed daily exercises for 30 minutes using audiovisual aids at home, patients showed significant improvements in asthma control and reduced their use of short-acting asthma relief medication.

Theory: Tai chi strengthens respiratory muscles.

If you have asthma: Check for tai chi classes at your local community center or health club.

Sumalee Kiatboonsri, MD, professor of medicine, division of pulmonary and critical care medicine, Ramathibodi Hospital, Bangkok, Thailand.

•**Nose taping.** With age, the tip of one's nose naturally begins to droop some. This can obstruct the nasal valve, which impedes breathing and contributes to snoring.

Try this simple test: Use your finger to press the tip of your nose up. If breathing feels easier when you do this, try taping your nose up before bedtime.

What to do: Cut a three-inch strip of one-half-inch medical grade tape. Place it under the nose at the center, without blocking the airway. Gently lift the nose as you run the tape up the midline of the nose to the area between the eyes. The taping should be comfortable and is for use during sleep.

Important: Commercial nasal strips, such as Breathe Right, spread the sides of the nose apart. Taping up the nose, as described above, also does this, with the additional advantage of opening the nasal valve.

Take Care Where You Exercise

Neil Schachter, MD, medical director of the respiratory care department at Mount Sinai Hospital and the Maurice Hexter Professor of Pulmonary Medicine at the Icahn School of Medicine at Mount Sinai, both in New York City. He is the author of *The Good Doctor's Guide to Colds and Flu* and serves on the American Lung Association's Northeast Board of Directors.

Air pollution still ranks high on the list of health threats—especially for people with asthma and other chronic lung conditions.

Exercise away from major roads. Levels of PM2.5 particles tend to be much higher in areas with heavy traffic. If you like to walk, jog or bike, do it as close to nature as possible—and away from busy streets. Pollution is usually highest within 50 feet of roads.

Best Exercise for COPD Patients

Renae McNamara, PhD, BAppSc (Phty), clinical specialist physiotherapist in pulmonary rehabilitation, Prince of Wales Hospital, New South Wales, Australia.

Water workouts are great for a variety of ailments. There's something about being in a pool with an instructor and other folks soothed by the surrounding heated water. Water activity tends to be more fun than working out on land—splashing around can make us feel like kids again.

Now you can add chronic obstructive pulmonary disease to the list of conditions a water workout can benefit. A recent study out of Australia shows that aquatic exercise builds more endurance and decreases fatigue and shortness of breath more substantially for people with COPD than land exercise—and this finding may apply to people with other sorts of respiratory problems and chronic conditions, too.

WATER WORKOUTS: LESS PAIN, MORE GAIN

The research focused specifically on people who had both COPD, an all-too-common respiratory problem that is a leading cause of death in the US, and an additional chronic condition that makes exercise difficult—such as obesity, joint problems or back pain. But there's every reason to think that the study's results will apply to people with other sorts of medical issues, especially those with respiratory conditions. Future studies will need to examine that.

Researchers were interested in finding out which type of workout would help people find the most relief—land-based exercise (a mixture of walking, cycling, aerobics and dumbbell lifts) or water-based exercise (aquatic calisthenics done in chest-to-neck high water in a pool heated to 93°F).

The patients were split into three groups. One group did one-hour water exercises three times a week for eight weeks with a trained physiotherapist. Another group did land exercises for the same amount of time with the same trained physiotherapist. And a third group performed no exercise (the control).

At the end of the study, when each group was asked to perform a walking test to measure endurance, members of the water group could walk 118% farther than they could at the start of the study, on average...the land group's distance improved, too, but by only 53%...and the control group actually got weaker—their distance was 13% shorter.

Also, the people who had been exercising in a pool saw a 9% decrease in shortness of breath and a 13% decrease in fatigue by the end of the study... while the people who had been exercising on land saw only a 4% decrease in shortness of breath and a 3% decrease in fatigue.

CONTRA-CONVENTIONAL WISDOM

So why did water workouts come out on top? Water may have helped more for a few reasons. First of all, you have the effect of buoyancy, which supports your weight and reduces impact on your joints. Warm water also helps with pain control and increases blood flow to muscles. Plus, water offers resistance to all your movements, so your muscles work harder, and that strengthens them.

What's ironic is that it wasn't all that long ago that people with COPD were warned not to do water-based exercise. Doctors worried that the water would compress the chest and that the exertion would stress the heart. But studies that have analyzed COPD and water exercise under controlled conditions (as in, when patients were under the watchful eye of a health professional) have shown that these fears are unfounded.

GET YOUR GOGGLES ON!

Now that we have these study results, if you suffer from COPD as well as obesity, joint problems or back pain, you owe it to yourself to talk to your doctor or physical therapist about trying pool-based therapy with a trained health professional. (If you have COPD but none of those other conditions... or if you have one of the other conditions but not COPD...or if you suffer from a different type of respiratory problem...you may still find pool-based therapy to be more beneficial than land exercises, so it's worth a try.)

Group classes are usually easier to find than individual classes (plus, they tend to be cheaper and more fun). But either type of class is useful. To find one, call your local YMCA (ymca.net) or a community recreation center that has a pool or a hospital with an aquatic rehab center.

You May Have a Broken Back and Not Know It...

David Borenstein, MD, clinical professor of medicine at George Washington University Medical Center in Washington, DC. He maintains a private practice at Arthritis and Rheumatism Associates in Maryland and Washington, DC and is author of *Back in Control!*

Don't assume that an aching back means just a pulled muscle. It's among the most common symptoms of vertebral fractures, small cracks in the vertebrae of the spine.

About 25% of postmenopausal women in the US eventually will develop a vertebral fracture. Men over age 60 are prone to them, too. Up to two-thirds of these fractures never are diagnosed because the pain is so minor that patients don't bother to tell their doctors—or, as is often the case, because there's no pain at all.

The risk: Hairline cracks in the vertebrae eventually can cause the bone to crumble and collapse, a condition known as a vertebral compression fracture. When you see someone with a hunched-over posture, the so-called dowager's hump, you'll know that he/she has a compression fracture. These fractures also can cause patients to lose inches in height over the years.

Studies have shown that patients with compression fractures face a 23% higher risk for death than those with stronger bones. Difficulty breathing and pneumonia also can occur in severe cases because the stooped-over posture often interferes with normal lung function.

BONE LOSS

Unless you've had a severe injury (from a car accident, for example), vertebral factures usually are due to osteoporosis, the leading cause of bone loss. They also can be caused by osteopenia, less severe bone weakening that can start decades before the development of full-fledged osteoporosis. People who have one fracture are at greater risk of developing another.

For women, the main cause of bone loss is the postmenopausal decline of estrogen. In the first five years after menopause, women can lose up to 25% of their bone density.

Men have thicker bones to begin with, and they lose bone more slowly, but they're not immune to fractures. About 25% of men develop osteoporosis by age 70. By the time they reach 75 to 80, they're just as likely as women to have severe bone weakening.

The only way to know that you have osteoporosis is to get a bone-density test. The most accurate test is a *dual-energy X-ray absorptiometry* (DXA). The test is painless, takes about 10 minutes and exposes patients to less radiation than a chest X-ray.

Cost: $150 to $200. The test usually is covered by insurance. Newer DXA machines also are able to scan the spine to detect spinal fractures. This test is referred to as a *vertebral fracture assessment* (VFA).

You might see kiosks at pharmacies and malls that offer a heel sonogram. It's a fast, inexpensive test that measures bone density in the heel. It can indicate which patients might have low bone density. However, the test is not as accurate as DXA. I don't recommend it.

Every woman should get a DXA test around the time of menopause. Men should have the test if they have a family history of osteoporosis…if they're taking steroids (which can cause bone loss) for another condition…or if they have low testosterone, which also leads to bone weakness.

PREVENTING FRACTURES

Early diagnosis of osteoporosis and then adopting bone-building strategies can protect the spine. Patients with low bone density who don't improve with lifestyle measures may need to take bisphosphonates (such as Fosamax) or other medications. Drug therapy can improve bone density by at least 4% a year and reduce the risk for future fractures by 30% to 40%. The general recommendation for bisphosphonates is to take them for five years because long-term bisphosphonate therapy has been linked to a rare type of thigh fracture.

Here, important lifestyle steps…

•**Get more calcium.** It improves the body's ability to develop new bone. Women need 1,200 milligrams (mg) daily until menopause and 1,500 mg afterward. Men should get 1,000 mg until age 65 and 1,500 mg thereafter.

Dairy foods and fortified juices and cereals are the best dietary sources of calcium. (One cup of milk or fortified juice has about 300 mg of calcium.)

Supplements can help if you don't eat a lot of high-calcium foods. Both forms of supplements —calcium citrate and calcium carbonate—are effective.

Helpful: Take calcium supplements with meals. The stomach's acidic environment during digestion improves calcium absorption.

•**Supplement with vitamin D.** A majority of Americans are low in this nutrient, which is needed for calcium absorption. The recommended daily amount is 600 international units (IU) for those ages 51 to 70 and 800 IU after that. However, higher amounts—usually between 1,000 IU and 2,000 IU daily—often are recommended, particularly for those who have dark skin and/or those who don't get a lot of sun exposure.

•**Eat leafy green vegetables, such as spinach and kale.** These are high in vitamin K, which helps calcium in the blood enter the bones. The Harvard Nurses' Health Study found that women who ate at least one daily serving of leafy green vegetables were 50% less likely to suffer a hip fracture than those who ate less. It's not known whether these foods protect the vertebrae, but increasing vitamin K intake as part of a healthy diet is probably helpful.

•**Walk for 30 minutes four times a week.** Walking and other types of weight-bearing exercise (in which the muscles and joints work against gravity) significantly increase bone density. People who exercise regularly throughout their lives put more bone "in the bank" to protect against future fractures.

Riding a bicycle (including a stationary bike) has similar effects. The spine benefits from any exercise that requires you to be upright. This includes jogging, aerobics, yoga and jumping.

•**Swim for pain relief.** Swimming isn't a weight-bearing exercise, so it won't increase spinal strength—but it's very useful for strengthening the muscles that surround the spine and helping to prevent pain and stiffness.

•**Strengthen abdominal muscles.** Strengthening the muscles that surround the spine and abdomen (the so-called "core muscles") can help reduce back pain if you have a fracture. Also by improving muscular support around the spine, strong core muscles may help protect the back from future injuries.

Try this: Lie on your back with your knees bent and your feet flat on the floor. Tighten the abdominal muscles while gently pressing your lower back toward the floor. Hold the tension for five to 10 seconds, relax, then repeat the movement 10 times. Do this daily.

You also can do crunches to strengthen the core muscles in the abdomen and lower back. Crunches are safe for most patients, but they do put pressure on the spine—talk to your doctor before doing them if you have significant bone loss and/or fractures.

To do them: Lie on your back with your knees slightly bent…cross your arms over your chest… and gently raise your shoulders a few inches off the floor. Hold the stretch for a second, then relax. Repeat 10 times. Do this daily.

•**Use heat and/or cold for pain.** To relieve pain initially, apply an ice pack to your lower back. Keep it there for about 10 minutes. Do this several times during the first 48 hours.

After that, heat reduces muscle spasms and can minimize back pain. It also increases circulation, which flushes out pain-causing chemicals from the injured area. Apply a hot water bottle or heating pad to your lower back for 10 to 20 minutes several times daily.

This Yoga Pose Improves Scoliosis

Study of people with scoliosis by researchers at College of Physicians and Surgeons, Columbia University, New York City, published in *Global Advances in Health and Medicine.*

Yoga position that improves scoliosis: Side plank. People with scoliosis who held the side plank pose for one to two minutes a day for several days a week reduced the curvature of their spines by an average of 32%. Those who did the pose at least four times a week had the most improvement.

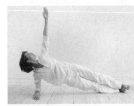

Caution: Do not attempt the pose on your own—talk to your doctor, and get professional yoga instruction.

Photo: iStock

Even if You Have Arthritis, High-Impact Exercise Can Help Your Knees

Derek H. Ochiai, MD, a surgeon and specialist in sports medicine at Nirschl Orthopaedic Center, Arlington, Virginia.

Study titled "Effect of Exercise on Patellar Cartilage in Women with Mild Knee Osteoarthritis" by researchers at Central Finland Central Hospital, Oulu University Hospital, University of Oulu, University of Helsinki and Helsinki University Hospital, Finland, published in *Medicine & Science in Sports & Exercise.*

When your knees hurt climbing the stairs, you don't exactly feel like jumping for joy. But that may be exactly what you need to do to strengthen the cartilage in your knees and slow the progression of osteoarthritis. While you shouldn't run outside and starting playing hopscotch right away, a carefully structured jumping program may benefit your knees without hurting them.

STEP JUMPING BUILDS CARTILAGE

Until now, high-impact exercise has been thought to be harmful to people with knee arthritis. The surprising finding that it may not only be safe but actually beneficial comes from a new Finnish study. It helps build knee cartilage, which no- or low-impact aerobic exercise has not been shown to do.

The researchers looked at the effect of a high-impact exercise program on knee cartilage, osteo-arthritis symptoms and physical function in 76 women, ages 50 to 65, who had knee pain on most days. The women had *patellofemoral joint osteoar-thritis*, a common form of the disease that causes pain under the kneecap (aka the patella) and often makes climbing stairs painful. Sound familiar? Men often get this kind of knee arthritis, too, so let's all pay attention.

The women were randomly assigned to either an exercise group or a control group. The control group went about their normal daily routines. The exercise group went to supervised classes of about an hour three times a week.

Their jumping exercises started out very gentle and gradually increased in intensity. The women did aerobics while jumping over foam blocks that were two inches from the ground and jumped up and down steps that were four inches high. Every three months, the heights were raised until eventually they were about eight inches for both the aerobics and the steps. There were no deep squats. (Squats can be very tough on knees.) On average, each exerciser did 44 high-impact jumps per exercise session, which is less pounding than you'd get from, say, running for the same amount of time. A few women (six, to be exact) had some joint problems at one time or another, but they just took a week or more off and then returned to the classes.

The results were modest but significant. At the end of the 12-month period, the investigators found that when measured via magnetic resonance imaging (MRI), the thickness of the kneecap cartilage among women assigned to the jumping group had a 7% increase. For the control-group there was no improvement. They also found the knee extension force of those in the jumping group increased by 11% compared with controls. Self-reported pain was about the same in the jumping and the control group. The women got a little fitter, too.

Added bonus: Although this study did not look at bone strength, high-impact exercise is exactly what's been shown to help strengthen bones against osteoporosis.

SHOULD YOU JUMP TO IT?

The current study suggests that adding a little jumping—carefully—to your routine might be reasonable. But don't neglect low-impact exercises such as cycling or aquatic classes either. In the end, any exercise that doesn't hurt you is good for your knees. You might call it the arthritis paradox—it may hurt to be active, but being active reduces the hurt. When it comes to the knees in particular, there is growing evidence that exercise reduces pain and improves function.

Being more active may also help you lose weight and, it's amazing how little weight loss it takes to reduce the pressure on your knees.

For gym rats, try the elliptical machine, the recumbent bike and, of course, swimming. It is a great aerobic exercise and it puts very little pressure on your knees. The stair climber is a little too much stress on the knees, though. Whatever you do, start off slowly and build up intensity gradually, just as the women in this study did.

Sprain-Proof Your Ankles: This Injury Can Lead to Arthritis and Other Problems

Luke T. Donovan, PhD, ATC, an assistant professor in the department of kinesiology at the University of North Carolina at Charlotte, and past program director of the Post-Professional Athletic Training Program at The University of Toledo. His research interests include chronic ankle instability.

I f you haven't sprained an ankle yet, it may be just a matter of time. About 25,000 Americans suffer from these painful injuries every day—that's a total of 9 million such injuries each year.

But an ankle sprain is not that serious, right? We've all seen athletes limping off the field, only to return to the game soon after. You've probably done the same thing yourself. You take a wrong step… your foot turns…you hobble for a while…and you forget about it.

What you may not realize: An ankle sprain can cause a lifetime of problems, including persistent ankle weakness, difficulty walking and even arthritis of the ankle. *What you need to know to protect yourself…*

LINGERING DAMAGE

An ankle sprain occurs when a ligament (the band of tissue that connects bone to bone) stretches beyond its normal limits. The more a ligament stretches—or even tears—the more severe the sprain.

Most people who sprain an ankle never see a doctor. They assume that a little rest—along with an over-the-counter pain reliever and perhaps some ice packs—will take care of things. It's true that the immediate symptoms usually clear up quickly… within a matter of days or weeks. But what happens after that?

Studies have shown that more than 30% of people who sprain an ankle go on to develop chronic ankle instability. The joint feels as though it might "give" at any time. As a result, their health may suffer—they tend to exercise less…gain weight…and have more limitations in their daily movements. People who have sprained an ankle are also twice as likely to reinjure it.

To be clear, an ankle sprain does not cause high blood pressure or diabetes, for example, but it often does interfere with the types of activities that help prevent these and other serious chronic conditions. Ankle sprains have also been linked to a 13% to 16% increased risk for arthritic ankles.

SPRAIN-PROOF YOUR ANKLES

The ankles are uniquely prone to injuries due to the mobility and wide range of motion of the ankle joint…and the fact that the ankles support the weight of your entire body.

For these reasons, it's wise for all adults—and especially those who have suffered previous ankle injuries (even if they were years ago)—to do a simple daily regimen of stretching, strengthening and balancing exercises.

Try to do all of the exercises below a few times a day—together, they take only about 10 minutes…

•**Stand on one foot.** This balancing exercise helps prevent ankle sprains by improving ankle muscle reflexes and *proprioception*, the body's ability to orient itself in space. I tell people to do the exercise when they're standing in line…talking on the phone…or even brushing their teeth.

What to do: Simply stand on one foot near a chair or any other stationary object that you can grab on to if you lose your balance. Stand on one foot for about 30 seconds, then switch sides. Work up to a minute or two on each side.

When it starts to feel easy: Close your eyes while you balance. Taking away the visual feedback forces the muscles and nerves to work harder.

•**Soft-surface stands.** To further improve ankle muscle function and your sense of balance, do one-legged stands (as described above) on a pillow, a foam pad or a balance disc (they're also called balance trainer balls and are available at sporting-goods stores and online).

The unstable surface forces your body to adapt to changes in balance and weight distribution. It makes your muscles more reactive, which can help you adjust to sudden changes in walking surfaces, posture, foot movements, etc.

•**Calf stretches.** The calf muscles connect to the Achilles tendon in the ankle. Stretching and strengthening the calves improves stability and range of motion.

What to do: While facing a wall, stand back about one foot with your palms on the wall for support. Take one step back with your right foot and slightly bend your left leg. You'll feel the stretch in your right calf/ankle. Hold the position for about 10 seconds, then repeat on the other side. Perform the stretch three times on each side and work up to holding it for 30 seconds.

•**Ankle/calf raises.** As mentioned above, stronger calves and Achilles tendons improve ankle stability. This exercise strengthens both.

261

What to do: While still facing a wall, with your palms on the wall for support, rise up on your toes as far as you can. Hold the stretch for a few seconds, then lower your heels to the floor. Repeat eight to 10 times. It's harder than it sounds! As your muscles get stronger, you can increase the difficulty by taking one foot off the floor when rising/lowering with the other foot.

●**Resistance exercises.** With an elastic resistance band, you can strengthen the ankle by moving it in its complete range of motion.

What to do: While sitting in a chair, wrap an elastic resistance band under the ball of your foot. While holding the band tightly, move the foot/ankle up, down, left and right. Repeat a few times in each direction. Then perform on the other foot.

WHEN TO GET HELP

What if you think that you've actually sprained an ankle? First, see a doctor. You'll need an X-ray to determine whether you have a bone fracture, which typically requires the foot/ankle to be immobilized by a hard cast or boot.

If you have a sprain, don't try to simply "walk it off." The best thing you can do is keep weight off the ankle as much as possible until the pain and swelling are completely gone. An elastic bandage (such as ACE) can help minimize swelling.

During this time, you may also want to immobilize the joint with a brace (such as Aircast) for four to six weeks. Such braces are available online and at most drugstores for about $20 and up.

Also helpful: To reduce pain and swelling, apply a cold pack (or ice wrapped in a towel) to the ankle for 20 minutes, once every hour for up to eight hours a day. Continue with this frequency for at least the first day after the sprain. After that, let pain be your guide—apply cold as long as the pain is severe and cut back as it eases.

To help prevent long-term problems: I advise getting some form of rehabilitation—from a physical therapist or an athletic trainer—after the injury heals.

Best Treatments for Ankle Arthritis

Judith F. Baumhauer, MD, MPH, professor and associate chair of the department of orthopedics at University of Rochester School of Medicine, New York. She was the recipient of the American Orthopaedic Foot & Ankle Society's Roger A. Mann Award for outstanding clinical study.

Remember that sprained ankle you suffered years ago? Or maybe it was an ankle fracture that left you hobbling around for weeks. Whatever the specific problem, be forewarned that ankle injuries can come back to haunt you—years or even decades later. *Here's how…*

SELF-CARE FOR ARTHRITIS

The ankle is vulnerable to the same types of arthritis that affect other joints. Post-traumatic arthritis is the most common form in the ankle, followed by age-related osteoarthritis and rheumatoid arthritis. For these forms of ankle arthritis, you might be able to manage discomfort with simple remedies.

But self-care is tricky. You can't "go easy" on the ankles in the same way that you would with certain other joints. People use their ankles all day, every day. *My advice for people with ankle arthritis…*

●**Choose activities that minimize ankle wear and tear.** To stay active and keep the muscles supporting the ankle strong, try biking, swimming, walking, rowing, elliptical workouts or other low-impact, weight-bearing exercises that don't cause relentless pounding.

●**Keep your weight down.** People with ankle arthritis tend to gain weight because they find it too painful to walk or exercise much…and the extra pounds accelerate joint damage by increasing the weight load on the ankles.

Helpful: Losing even five pounds can reduce the ankle load by 20 pounds, which may be enough to minimize symptoms.

●**Exercise the ankles.** Ankle-specific exercises will build up the muscles surrounding the joint, keep the joint from getting stiff and reduce the bone-on-bone friction that occurs with arthritis.

Example: Several times a day, flex your foot upward (*dorsiflexion*) as far as it will go…hold for a few seconds…then flex it downward (*plantar flexion*). You can find dozens of ankle exercises on the Internet (or see next page for an ankle-strengthening exercise).

•**Wear shock-absorbing shoes.** Also known as "stability sneakers," they have a densely cushioned heel/sole that absorbs shocks when you walk, exercise, etc.

NOT READY FOR SURGERY

In addition to the steps above, some simple therapies can help slow the progression of arthritis. For example, it may help to wear an over-the-counter ankle brace that gives support and stability…apply cold packs when the ankle is hurting…and/or take as-needed doses of a nonsteroidal anti-inflammatory drug (NSAID), such as *ibuprofen* (Motrin) or *naproxen* (Aleve).* If you're lucky, these and other self-care therapies—including physical therapy—may be the only treatments you'll ever need.

Very helpful: A cortisone injection. Cortisone (sometimes combined with lidocaine) is a strong anti-inflammatory that can reduce or eliminate pain within a day. The shot is good for patients who are having moderate daily pain—and might be helpful for an upcoming vacation, for example, or when the pain is unusually severe. This shot won't stop the arthritis but can get you through a rough patch. In some cases, hyaluronic acid injections may be used but may not be covered by insurance.

WHEN SURGERY IS NEEDED

Even with the approaches described earlier, many people will eventually develop "end-stage" arthritis that does not improve and interferes with their daily activities.

Until about 10 years ago, most patients with end-stage ankle arthritis were advised to have a procedure called *ankle arthrodesis*, commonly known as ankle fusion because affected bones are fused together to reduce pain and inflammation. Now, patients (based on their age and other factors) have a second option—a total ankle replacement.

*Discuss the use of NSAIDs with your physician—they can cause side effects such as stomach upset, ulcers and high blood pressure.

Because long-term comprehensive studies haven't yet been done, there's still debate about which approach is better. Both procedures are effective…and both have downsides that patients need to know about. *Specifically…*

•**With ankle fusion, the affected bones are locked together (with screws alone or plates and screws) and eventually fuse into a solid mass of bone.** This eliminates the rubbing/friction that causes the pain and disability of ankle arthritis. Most patients will walk in a shoe (without a cast) in eight to 12 weeks. And unlike ankle replacement (discussed below), the procedure is permanent. You're unlikely to require an additional procedure unless it doesn't fuse.

Downside: Bone fusion eliminates ankle mobility. You might walk haltingly when you go up hills or down a flight of stairs. And because the ankle is locked in place, other structures in the foot assume more of the burden of daily movements—and could become more susceptible to arthritis.

•**With a total ankle replacement, the arthritic surfaces are replaced**—as also occurs with a knee or hip replacement—with an artificial joint. Surgeons advise patients that the implants might last for eight to 12 years. A recent study found that 73% were still working after 15 years.

The advantage of total ankle replacement is that the ankle will flex. Patients retain a greater degree of motion and experience less stress on surrounding joints.

Downside: The risk for additional procedures to repair/replace a damaged implant.

My take: I might recommend joint replacement for someone who's over age 60 and in good health but has other arthritis in the foot…or a person who is active with sports, such as tennis, that involve jumping and cutting. However, the choice between fusion and replacement is highly individualized.

Important: See a surgeon who's experienced in both procedures to get an unbiased opinion about the pros and cons of each. To find such a surgeon near you, consult the American Orthopaedic Foot & Ankle Society, AOFAS.org.

Insurance typically covers these procedures, but be sure to ask.

Feels Like Your Ankle Is About to Give Out? Here's an Easy Exercise to Strengthen

Luke Donovan, PhD, ATC, assistant professor of kinesiology, University of North Carolina at Charlotte.

Years or even decades after an ankle sprain, some of the symptoms of the original injury can linger, and a person may feel like his/her ankle will give out at times and have cyclic swelling and pain. In fact, about 40% of people who suffer an ankle sprain develop this chronic ankle instability (CAI), which can affect a person of any age.

But aging also can be a primary cause of ankle instability. As we age, there's a natural decline in muscle and tendon function as well as neuromuscular control.

SIMPLE EXERCISES HELP

The exercises below are best done barefoot and on both sides of the body. Perform them daily, doing strength exercises and balance exercises on alternating days.

To strengthen ankle-supporting muscles, stand on one foot and roll from heel to toes, then reverse and roll from your toes to heel. Repeat three sets of 10 to 15 reps three to four times a week. Next, walk a few feet just on your heels…then the insides of your feet…the outsides of your feet…and finally on your toes. When muscles start to tire, try to take a few more steps and then work a new muscle group. Balance exercises, such as standing on each leg for 30 to 60 seconds up to three times a day, have been shown to improve neuromuscular control. To make this more challenging, close your eyes.

Note: If you have a balance disorder, check with a doctor before doing these exercises. Also, if any exercise starts to become painful, stop and try another time. And always be sure to stand next to something sturdy that you can grab onto in case you lose your balance.

Helpful: A lace-up ankle brace for support.

If your ankle worsens, see a foot and ankle surgeon, who may advise physical therapy or surgery to repair ligaments.

Easy Exercises for Foot Health

Jonathan D. Rose, DPM, a podiatrist in private practice in Baltimore. He is coauthor of *The Foot Book: A Complete Guide to Healthy Feet.* PodiatryAssociates.org

The right exercises can help keep your toes and feet limber and strong.

EXERCISE #1: **Pick up marbles.** This will strengthen muscles in the bottom of your feet and may help prevent plantar fasciitis. Place marbles on the floor. Pick up one marble at a time with your toes, and drop it into a nearby bowl or cup. Repeat with your other foot.

EXERCISE #2: **Grasp a towel with your toes.** This exercise encourages you to do toe curls that will strengthen the tops of your feet. Sit in a straight-back chair with a small towel at your feet. Use the toes of one foot to scrunch the towel and pull it toward you. Repeat with the other foot.

EXERCISE #3: **Trace the alphabet.** This exercise helps ankle mobility. Sit down and extend your leg. Trace the alphabet in the air with your big toe. Repeat with the other foot.

EXERCISE #4: **Do toe raises.** This exercise helps to strengthen the Achilles tendon and the arch of the foot. Stand with your hands resting on the back of a sturdy chair, and slowly rise up on your toes and come back down. Toe raises can be done in three sets of 10. Repeat two to three times a week.

Note: Toe raises are not recommended for people suffering with plantar fasciitis. Instead, you want to stretch the calf by bringing the toes and feet upward toward the shin.

14

For Women Only

Safe Workouts for Women

Wayne Westcott, PhD, professor of exercise science and chair of the Exercise Science Program at Quincy College, Quincy, Massachusetts. He is author or coauthor of several books, including *Get Stronger, Feel Younger*.

Exercise machines can provide excellent workouts. But unfortunately, a woman may wind up with injuries if she uses a machine improperly—or if the machine is not suitable for a person her size.

Benefits: Cardiovascular exercise helps you control or lose weight…reduces blood pressure and cholesterol…and boosts energy and mood.*

Do a cardio workout for 30 minutes or more at least three times a week. Begin with a five-minute warm-up, working up to your target speed…and end with a five-minute cooldown, gradually slowing your pace. For the 20 minutes in between, work hard enough to give your heart a workout, but not so hard that you risk overtaxing it.

To gauge effort: If you can talk normally, work harder…if you barely have the breath to get a word out, ease up. Interval workouts—alternating every few minutes between bursts of intense activity and periods of lighter activity—burn more calories than a single sustained pace.

*Consult your doctor before beginning any exercise plan.

RECOMMENDED: TREADMILL

You walk or run on a flat or inclined surface as the treadmill records your time, mileage, heart rate and/or calories burned. A preset program can automatically generate varying speeds and inclines.

Especially beneficial for: Women with or at risk for osteoporosis (brittle bone disease). Walking is a weight-bearing exercise that increases bone density…and the treadmill's shock-absorbing platform is easier on joints than pavement.

To use: Start by setting the speed at two miles per hour, then slowly increase your pace. Move naturally, keeping your head up and staying in the center of the belt.

Safety alert: Holding the handrails while walking rapidly or running forces your body into an unnatural posture, increasing the risk for muscle strain—so once you have your balance, let go. Use a safety key with a cord that clips to your clothing and connects to the emergency "off" switch so that the treadmill belt will immediately stop moving if you fall.

RECOMMENDED: STATIONARY BICYCLE

An upright bike looks and feels like a regular road bike. With a recumbent bike, the rider sits on a wide saddle, leaning against a backrest, legs out in front. Both types give an equally good cardio workout.

Especially beneficial for: Women with balance problems, because there is no risk of falling...and overweight women, because it supports the body and allows adjustable levels of external resistance rather than working against the user's own body weight. A recumbent bike is most comfortable for people with back problems or limited mobility.

To use: Every few minutes, alternate "sprints" of fast, low-resistance pedaling..."climbs" of slow, high-resistance pedaling...and recovery intervals of moderately paced, medium-resistance pedaling. To work shin muscles, use pedal straps or toe clips so that you can pull up as well as push down while pedaling.

Safety alert: Improper seat height can lead to knee injuries. When one pedal is pushed all the way down, your knee should be slightly bent—never fully extended. If the seat adjusts forward and aft, position it so that knees align with your ankles rather than extending beyond your toes. If you have narrow hips and the distance between the pedals seems too wide, see if a different brand of bike feels more comfortable. To reduce back and shoulder strain on an upright bike, raise the handlebars.

USE WITH CAUTION: STAIR STEPPER

This machine provides a challenging workout because you work against your own body weight and your center of gravity moves up and down with every step.

Problem: Users may lean heavily on the handrails to keep their balance and to take weight off the legs. This increases the risk for injury to the wrists...and misaligns the spine, which can strain the back.

Solution: To avoid falls, keep only your fingertips on the rails, using a light touch...maintain a moderate pace that does not challenge your balance. Do not set the height of the rise too high (as if taking stairs two at a time)—the stepping motion should feel natural. For good posture, keep shoulders and hips aligned and imagine trying to touch the top of your head to the ceiling.

Note: The stair stepper may not be appropriate if you are overweight or new to exercise and feel discouraged by the difficulty of the workout...have problems with your joints...or have any trouble with balance.

USE WITH CAUTION: ELLIPTICAL TRAINER

This low-impact machine combines the leg motions of stair climbing with cross-country skiing to work the lower body. Some styles include movable arm poles, adding an upper-body component.

Problem: For short-legged women, the elliptical can force a longer-than-normal stride that may strain the knees, hips and/or lower back.

Solution: The goal is to move smoothly with good posture. If your movement feels awkward or jerky, decrease the stride setting (try 16 inches). If this does not help, avoid the elliptical trainer.

HOW TO SAFELY WORK WITH STRENGTH-TRAINING MACHINES

Next, add strength-training machines, which build muscle...fortify tendons and ligaments...increase bone density...improve posture...boost mood...and raise metabolic rate so that you burn more fat.

Best: Do a strength-training workout two to three times per week, leaving at least one day between workouts so that muscles can recover. Start with a gentle warm-up of three to five minutes, doing an activity that involves the whole body, such as jumping jacks. Then use the machines for a total of 20 to 30 minutes.

Machine styles and weight increments vary depending on the manufacturer. If the machines in your gym do not have the same increments as the starting weight guidelines below, ask a trainer if it is possible to modify the options. *On each machine...*

●**Perform one to three sets of eight to 12 repetitions, resting for one minute between sets.**

●**If you can't complete eight repetitions using the starting guidelines, reduce the weight.** When it becomes easy to complete one set of 12 reps, try two sets, then three. When it becomes easy to do three sets, increase the weight.

●**Control the motion at all times.** Count slowly to two as you raise the weight...count to four as you lower the weight.

•**Exhale as you raise the weight...inhale as you lower the weight.** This helps keep blood pressure down.

Finish workouts with a three-minute walk to cool down. Then do three minutes of gentle stretching to maintain flexibility, holding each stretch for 15 to 30 seconds.

New research: Stretching promotes additional gains in strength.

Address each major muscle group to keep muscles in balance—otherwise the weaker muscles could be prone to injury. *A complete workout typically includes...*

•**Lat pull-down.**

Muscles worked: The latissimus dorsi (upper back) and biceps—muscles used in daily life for lifting and carrying (for example, grocery bags).

To use: Sit tall, facing the machine, with thighs tucked beneath the pads to stabilize your lower body. Reach up, palms facing you and slightly farther than shoulder-width apart, and grasp the bar hanging overhead. Squeeze shoulder blades together as you pull the bar down a few inches in front of your face...stop at chin level...then raise the bar to starting position. Start with 35 pounds if you're in your 40s...32.5 pounds in your 50s...30 pounds in your 60s...27.5 pounds in your 70s...25 pounds in your 80s and beyond.

Safety alert: Never pull the bar behind your head. This can injure the neck and shoulders. It is safe to grasp the bar with palms facing away—but muscles get a better workout when palms face you.

•**Shoulder press.**

Muscles worked: Shoulders, triceps (back of the arms) and base of the neck—used when placing items on a high shelf.

To use: Sit erect, hips and shoulder blades pressed against the backrest. With hands at shoulder height, palms facing forward and arms bent, grasp the outer set of handles and push up until arms are nearly straight...then lower to starting position. Start with 30 pounds if you're in your 40s...27.5 pounds in your 50s...25 pounds in your 60s...22.5 pounds in your 70s...20 pounds in your 80s and beyond.

Safety alert: If you have shoulder problems, such as with your rotator cuff, use the inner handles, palms facing each other—this is easier.

•**Chest press.**

Muscles worked: Pectorals (front of the chest) and triceps—used for pushing a lawn mower or wheelchair.

To use: Sit erect with arms bent, hands at chest height, palms facing forward. Grasp handles and press forward, elbows pointing to the sides (not down), until arms are nearly straight...then bend elbows and return to starting position. Start with 35 pounds if you're in your 40s...32.5 pounds in your 50s...30 pounds in your 60s...27.5 pounds in your 70s...25 pounds in your 80s and beyond.

Safety alert: Do not lean forward—keep head up and entire back pressed against the backrest to avoid neck and low-back strain.

•**Biceps curl.**

Muscles worked: Biceps and forearms—needed for lifting and carrying.

To use: Sit with arms out in front, elbows resting on the padded platform. Palms facing you, grasp handles and bend elbows to bring hands toward your chest...then straighten arms to return to starting position. Start with 30 pounds if you're in your 40s...27.5 pounds in your 50s...25 pounds in your 60s...22.5 pounds in your 70s...20 pounds in your 80s and beyond.

Safety alert: Elbows are prone to hyperextension—so to prevent joint injury when lowering the bar, stop when elbows are still slightly bent. If your lower back arches, reduce the weight to prevent back strain.

•**Leg press.**

Muscles worked: Quadriceps and hamstrings (fronts and backs of thighs), inner thighs and buttocks—vital for walking and climbing stairs.

To use: Sit and recline against the backrest, legs raised in front of you, knees at a 90-degree angle, feet flat and hip-width apart on the movable platform. Slowly straighten legs until knees are almost straight, pressing with heels to push platform away...then bend knees to return to starting position. Start with 85 pounds if you're in your 40s...80 pounds in your 50s...75 pounds in your 60s...70 pounds in your 70s...65 pounds in your 80s and beyond.

Safety alert: To protect knees, do not straighten legs completely...keep thighs parallel to align knees.

• **Ab crunch machine.**

Muscles worked: Abdominals—which help maintain posture and combat belly bulge.

To use: Sit and place feet behind ankle pads to stabilize lower body...grip handles and place elbows on padded rests to stabilize upper body. Using abdominal muscles, curl upper body forward to bring your chest toward your knees... then uncurl as far as possible without letting weights return to the resting position. Start with 40 pounds if you're in your 40s...37.5 pounds in your 50s...35 pounds in your 60s...32.5 pounds in your 70s...30 pounds in your 80s and beyond.

Safety alert: Keep head and spine aligned to prevent neck injury.

Better Bone Health

Miriam Bredella, MD, assistant professor of radiology, Massachusetts General Hospital, Boston.

When researchers studied the bones of 50 overweight women, those with more deep fat around the belly had significantly lower bone mineral density, and therefore higher osteoporosis risk, than those with more fat around the buttocks and hips.

Theory: Visceral (belly) fat leads to lower levels of growth hormone and insulin-like growth factor, both of which promote bone health.

If you are a woman with a waist circumference greater than 34.6 inches: Eat a healthful diet, and exercise to bring your waist size.

Best Workouts for the Plus-Sized Woman

James Hagberg, PhD, professor of exercise physiology, department of kinesiology at the University of Maryland in College Park.

You begin with good intentions, determined to exercise away those excess pounds. But a workout that is too challenging for your full figure and fitness level may leave you discouraged—or possibly even injured. *Here's how heavier women can exercise safely, effectively and enjoyably...*

• **Have fun.** In school, did you dread gym because you felt self-conscious in shorts or because running laps was used as punishment? Find an activity that lets you feel good about yourself and brings you pleasure—aqua aerobics, square dancing, Zumba, kayaking (yes, kayaks are made for all sizes!).

• **Start slowly.** If you're daunted by the idea of a daily half-hour hike, begin with a five-minute walk three times a week. It doesn't matter if it takes six months to work your way up. Fitness is a lifetime commitment, not a "gotta do it now" goal.

• **Protect your joints.** For heavier women, jogging and aerobics put excess stress on knees and ankles, because body weight comes down hard with each footfall.

Better: Use an elliptical machine, which simulates fast walking, stepping or running yet involves little impact because feet remain grounded on the pedals...or swim, because the water supports your weight.

• **Maintain a stable center of gravity.** Sports such as tennis require quickly shifting your center of gravity up and down and side to side. The heavier you are, the more energy this takes—and the more quickly you may become exhausted and give up. Opt instead for an activity in which your center of gravity does not have to shift much, such as bicycling or rowing.

• **Forget about "winning."** Competitive team sports that pit you against fitter people might be discouraging. If it's your dream to play basketball, go for it—but find a league that focuses on fun.

Satisfying: Try yoga or tai chi, using personal progress as your measure of success.

Taking Off Just a Few Pounds Protects Your Breasts

Anne McTiernan, MD, PhD, professor of epidemiology, Fred Hutchinson Cancer Research Center and a research professor in the departments of epidemiology and geriatrics at the University of Washington, both in Seattle. She is the senior author of a study on weight loss and breast cancer risk published in *Journal of Clinical Oncology.*

Have you heard the news about the big payback for shedding just a little extra body baggage?

Here's the scoop: If you're postmenopausal and overweight, dropping just 5% of your body weight—that's a mere nine pounds if you currently weigh 180—can significantly reduce levels of hormones linked to breast cancer, a new study shows.

Background: Overweight and obese postmenopausal women are considered to be at elevated risk for breast cancer. That's because, after menopause, fat tissue becomes a major source of various estrogens and other sex hormones that are implicated in tumor growth. Overweight women produce more of these sex hormones than thin women because they have more fat tissue.

For the new study, participants included 439 sedentary, overweight women ages 50 to 75. One group did 45 minutes of aerobic exercise, such as brisk walking, five days a week…a second group was assigned a diet of 1,200 to 2,000 calories a day…a third group followed both the diet and exercise regimens…the control group did not change their usual diet or exercise routines. Blood tests were done at the start and end of the study to measure levels of hormones linked with breast cancer risk.

After one year: In the control group, there was no change in weight, and hormone levels actually worsened…in the exercise-only group, weight loss and hormone reductions were very modest (though of course exercise has other health benefits).

In contrast: Women in the diet-only group lost 11% of their body weight, on average, while those in the diet-plus-exercise group lost 12%. And in both groups, sex hormone blood levels dropped significantly—by 10% to as much as 26%, on average, depending on the hormone. Such changes, according to previous research, suggest about a 50% decrease in breast cancer risk. Generally, the greater the weight loss, the greater the improvement in hormone levels…yet even participants who lost just 5% of their body weight experienced hormone level changes suggestive of a 22% reduction in breast cancer risk.

Bottom line: If you are overweight, start today to make the lifestyle changes that will take off some of those pounds. Besides all the other well-known benefits, slimming down a bit may help you avoid breast cancer!

10,000 Step "Rule" Revisited

I-Min Lee, MD, ScD, professor of medicine, Harvard Medical School, Boston.

When about 17,000 women (average age 72) wore an activity tracker for seven days as they went about their day-to-day lives, those who took an average of 4,400 steps each day were 41% less likely to die during the four-year follow-up period than women who took fewer than 2,700 steps, regardless of how fast they walked. Longevity continued to improve with more steps taken… up to 7,500 steps per day. There was no further reduction in the risk for death when additional steps were taken.

Sleeping with Light Linked to Weight Gain

Yong-Moon "Mark" Park, MD, PhD, epidemiologist, National Institute of Environmental Health Sciences, Research Triangle Park, North Carolina.

Women who slept while exposed to light—either from a lamp or the TV—were 17% more likely to gain 11 pounds or more over an average of five-and-a-half years, according to a study of nearly 44,000 women ages 35 to 74.

Theory: Artificial light suppresses production of the sleep hormone melatonin and may affect metabolic processes that contribute to weight gain. A small night-light did not affect weight. Researchers believe the findings would be similar in men.

High Physical Fitness = Lower Dementia Risk

Helena Hörder, PhD, researcher, University of Gothenburg, Sweden, and leader of a study of 191 women, published in *Neurology.*

Women with the highest level of physical fitness in middle age were nearly 90% less likely to develop dementia in later life than women with a moderate fitness level. And when highly fit women did develop dementia, its onset was an average of 11 years later—at age 90 rather than 79.

The study used a bicycle exercise test to measure cardiovascular capacity of women at an average age of 50. It then followed the women for 44 years, testing for dementia six times. Among women judged highly fit, 5% developed dementia…compared with 25% of those judged moderately fit, 32% of those with low fitness and 45% of those who had to stop the test because of cardiovascular problems.

The study involved a relatively small number of women, all of them from Sweden, and their fitness levels were measured only once. Changes over time were not considered.

How Women Can Look Forward to Working Out

Ro Di Brezzo, PhD, is a professor of kinesiology and director of the Human Performance Laboratory at the University of Arkansas in Fayetteville. Over her 35-year career, she has coauthored more than 50 journal articles and received many awards, including the Research Award from the Southern Academy of Women in Physical Activity, Sport and Health.

Many men find physical activity fun… whereas many women tend to see a workout as work (because we're all about getting things done). What are the specifics behind the workout-enjoyment gender gap? Research recently published in the *Journal of Physical Education, Recreation and Dance* explains…

•**Men tend to feel more confident.** Fun depends a lot on how confident and capable you feel. Older women in particular—many of whom did not grow up playing sports or lifting weights—may worry about injury or find it hard to relax when exercising. Women who are out of shape also may lack self-assurance. Many gyms cater to people who are already fit, and this can be intimidating to women who are just beginning an exercise program.

•**Men are more competitive.** Guys love to best their buddies and earn bragging rights by lifting heftier weights or scoring more points. But this notion is foreign to many women.

•**Women fill their minds with harsh self-talk.** They chide themselves inwardly for being fat or weak or tell themselves that they'll never master a certain skill. Such negative thoughts sap motivation along with any possibility of enjoyment.

•**Women often set unrealistic goals.** Then when they fall short, they feel frustrated and stressed out, which diminishes their fun and makes them more likely to give up.

Suggestions for pumping up the pleasure…

•**Get a workout buddy.** Women tend to be sociable, so take advantage of this trait. Make plans to meet a friend at the gym or on the tennis court. Not only will you enjoy yourself more, you'll also be more likely to stick with it—because even if you would be tempted to renege on your own exercise plans, you wouldn't let down a friend.

•**Find a fitness facility that fits you.** Is your gym a singles scene for buff 20-year-olds? No woman who is 50 or 60 wants to walk into a gym and feel like she's on *The Dating Game.* You'll feel more comfortable surrounded by patrons who are similar to you in age, appearance and exercise ability.

•**Choose an activity that suits your personal sense of fun.** Do you love the outdoors? Try walking, hiking or golf. If you like to socialize, sign up for a bowling league or softball team. For a contemplative workout, consider yoga, tai chi or swimming laps. If you did ballet or another type of dance in your youth, now is the time to try Zumba or ballroom dancing. If you enjoy exploring new trends, look into pickleball. This racquet sport combines elements of badminton, tennis and Ping-Pong (see page 100 for more information).

•**Hire a trainer or instructor.** An expert can show you how to use unfamiliar equipment, teach you to perform exercises properly, help you improve your skills at your chosen activity and familiarize you with sport-specific lingo. Once you know what you're doing, you'll have more fun, make swifter progress and be safer. You don't need to work with the trainer or instructor forever—just learn the basics, then check in every now and again to advance your skills.

•**End each session on a high note.** Hate squats? Get them over with early in your workout…and save your favorite moves for last, so you take away a pleasurable memory.

•**Keep records on your progress over time— how many push-ups you can do, how much weight you can lift, how far you walk each day.** It will give you a satisfying sense of accomplishment to see how far you've come…and make you look forward to the workouts to come.

Maximum Heart Rates for Women Are Wrong! (Your Workout Just Got Easier)

Martha Gulati, MD, professor of medicine and chief of cardiology, University of Arizona, Phoenix and author of *Saving Women's Hearts.*

There are two fitness formulas that most people think are as accurate as 2+2=4.

Maximum heart rate is the highest heart rate you can safely achieve. The formula to calculate it: 220 minus age.

Target heart rate is the heart rate during exercise that works to keep you fit. The formula to calculate it: 65% to 85% of your maximum heart rate.

Example: A 60-year-old has a maximum heart rate of 160 (220 minus age) and a target heart rate of 104 (75% of maximum) to 136 (85% of maximum).

For women, there's just one problem with the maximum heart rate formula.

It's wrong.

Recent study: The unisex formula for maximum heart rate produces a number that is too high for women, perhaps leading women to unnecessarily tough workouts that discourage them from exercising.

NEW FORMULA FOR WOMEN'S HEARTS

Martha. Gulati, MD, cardiologist, professor of medicine and chief of cardiolgy at the University of Arizona, conducted a 16-year study on the heart health of 5,437 women, aged 35 to 93, which involved regular treadmill stress tests during which the women exercised as hard as they could.

Analyzing results from her study, she found that the correct formula to figure out an accurate maximum heart rate for women is slightly different than the existing formula.

The new formula: 206 minus 88% of a woman's age.

Example: A 60-year-old woman would have a maximum heart rate of 153 (not 160). Her target heart rate of 65 to 85% of maximum would be 100 to 130 (not 104 to 136).

"I'd seen enough women patients who couldn't achieve their target heart rate that I didn't believe the general formula could be correct for women—and it wasn't," Dr. Gulati said. The study results were published in the medical journal *Circulation.*

Unfortunately, the inaccurate formula is programmed into just about every heart monitor and exercise machine.

What to do: If you're already comfortably achieving your target heart rate with the old formula, don't worry.

Just keep doing what you're already doing.

But if you start an exercise program and can't achieve your target heart rate using the old formula, don't think you're a fitness failure—use the new formula.

What's most important, however, is not whether or not you meet your target heart rate during exercise—it's whether or not you exercise regularly.

Physical activity and physical fitness is essential for maintaining the health of your heart and your overall health.

In fact, an earlier study conducted by Dr. Gulati showed that fit women were three times less likely to die from any cause compared with women who weren't fit.

THE BEST FITNESS MEASUREMENT

The measurement Dr. Gulati used in that study to determine physical fitness wasn't maximum heart rate or target heart rate.

It was a measurement called *metabolic equivalents* (METs), or the amount of oxygen required for any physical activity.

If you're able to perform an exercise at a certain level of METs, you're physically fit for your age, she says.

Here are her calculations for "age-predicted fitness level" of METs, and examples of activity that are at or near that level…

- **30 years old, 11 METs (jumping rope)**
- **40, 9.5 (singles tennis)**
- **50, 8.2 (rowing)**
- **60, 7 (jogging at 5 miles per hour)**
- **70, 5.6 (walking briskly)**
- **80, 4.3 (leisurely biking, at less than 10 miles per hour)**

If your fitness level is less than 100% of your age-predicted fitness level—in other words, if you can't do the type of exercise for your age that indicates you're fit—your first goal should be to become active.

Your second goal should be to get as fit as possible and try to achieve your age-related fitness level for some duration of your workout. (She points out that most exercise machines in gyms display METs.)

Dr. Gulati sums up her guidelines for women's fitness with these five rules…

Rule #1: Just be active—doing something is better than doing nothing.

Rule #2: Make changes gradually, not abruptly, to avoid injury.

Rule #3: Before you start any exercise program, discuss with your doctor if it is safe to do so.

Rule #4: Do activities you enjoy…dancing, gardening or taking the dog for a walk. Have fun!

Rule #5: Remember that more is better. So move, move, move!

What You Really Need for Toned Arms

Edward Weiss, PhD, a nutrition and exercise specialist at St. Louis University with Rebecca Shannonhouse, editor-in-chief, health content, Bottom Line Inc.

Anthony Youn, MD, a plastic surgeon in Troy, Michigan, and author of *The Age Fix.* DrYoun.com

Have all those photos of the ultra-toned arms of hard-bodied celebrities gone to people's heads?

You might wonder if that's the case when considering this surprising statistic: In 2000, 300 patients (mostly women) underwent fat-removing liposuction and/or "arm-lift" surgery called *brachioplasty* to remove saggy skin from their arms. By 2019, that number had skyrocketed to more than 18,000 procedures!

Many of these procedures are occurring after weight-loss surgery, which can cause a surfeit of saggy skin on the upper arms. But brachioplasty is no walk in the park. It costs about $5,000 (typically not covered by insurance), involves weeks or even months of recovery time due to swelling and usually leaves a scar that runs from armpit to elbow.

While arm-lift surgery may be a reasonable option for some who have had extreme weight loss, it's not for everyone. If you have mild-to-moderate underarm sag, the best way to reduce excess fat throughout the body—including the upper arms—is through healthful eating and aerobic workouts (such as fast walking).

Eating lots of vegetables and fruit helps minimize oxidative stress and inflammation throughout the body, which could help connective tissue in skin "heal" after being stretched by excess fat, explains Edward Weiss, PhD, a nutrition and exercise specialist at St. Louis University.

Also, for relatively lean arms, here are two exercises to help tone triceps…

Exercise 1: While holding dumbbells (start with 5-pound weights), position your arms straight up, then slowly bend at the elbows and straighten.

Exercise 2: Stand with feet shoulder width or slightly wider apart and arms raised, holding the weights above your head. While bending your elbows, slowly lower the weights toward the back of your head…then lift them back up to the starting position, again making sure to keep your elbows slightly bent when your arms are extended.

Work up to 25 reps of each exercise with 10-pound weights three times a week.

The Cellulite Solution

Wayne Westcott, PhD, professor of exercise science and chair of the Exercise Science Program at Quincy College, Quincy, Massachusetts. He is author or coauthor of several books, including *Get Stronger, Feel Younger.*

When scientists say there's "no such thing" as cellulite, they mean that cellulite is not a distinct type of body tissue, but it is ordinary fat. Yet for nearly nine out of 10 women, that unwanted dimpling on the hips and thighs is undeniably real.

How it got there: Fibrous cords connect the skin to the underlying muscle. When the fat layer that lies between the skin and the muscle is too thick, the cords are pulled tight and fat cells bulge out between them, causing that "cottage cheese" look. *And cellulite gets worse with age…*

• **The typical woman loses muscle mass at an average rate of about five pounds per decade from ages 20 to 50…and perhaps more rapidly after menopause.**

• **As muscle mass decreases, metabolism slows, the body burns fewer calories and the ratio of fat to muscle rises.**

• **Supporting connective tissues (such as collagen) break down and lose elasticity, making cellulite more pronounced.**

What doesn't help: A swarm of creams, wraps, massage techniques and mechanical devices purport to eliminate cellulite, typically by "melting away fat." None addresses the underlying physiological causes. Even dieting can backfire if you overdo it, because your body may break down muscle as well as fat to get the energy that it needs, raising your fat-to-muscle ratio.

What does help: Strength training, which rebuilds muscle, burns calories and boosts metabolism.

Best: Three times a week, do the following exercises. The routine takes about 20 minutes.*

*Check with your doctor before beginning any exercise program.

You need only three simple kinds of equipment. Go to a gym or buy your own equipment at a sporting-goods store or online (try Spri.com). Within four to six weeks, you should see a noticeable reduction in cellulite.

MEDICINE BALL

A medicine ball is a weighted ball about six to eight inches in diameter. Holding one while doing the following two moves adds extra weight that makes your lower body work harder—and as a bonus, tones the upper body, too. To start, choose a ball with which you can do eight to 12 repetitions per side. Once you work your way up to 15 reps, switch to a ball about one to two pounds heavier. Typically, a woman starts with a two- to four-pound ball and works up to six, eight or 10 pounds.

Cost: About $20 to $40 per ball.

Target zones: Front and back of thighs...buttocks.

•**Lunge.** Stand with feet shoulder-width apart, holding ball between hands at waist level, about six to eight inches in front of you. Bend elbows to bring ball up to chest level...at the same time, with your

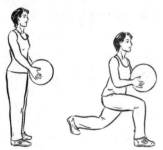

right foot, lunge forward about two to three feet, bending right knee to a 90-degree angle so that it is directly above foot. Step out far enough so that your knee does not move past your ankle (left leg will be slightly bent, heel up). Hold lunge position for three seconds, keeping back straight...then push off with your right foot and return to standing, bringing ball back down. Do 10 to 15 reps, then repeat on left. (Avoid lunges if you have knee problems.)

•**Knee lift.** Stand with feet shoulder-width apart, holding ball between hands at waist level.

Step right foot back about two to two-and-a-half feet, keeping your right leg straight and

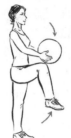

bending your left knee slightly. Elbows straight, raise ball in front of you to head height.

Bring right knee forward and up as high as you can...bend elbows and bring ball down to touch knee...then step back again with right foot as you straighten arms and raise ball to head height. Do 10 to 15 reps, then repeat on left.

RESISTANCE TUBES

Resistance tubes are elastic tubes about four feet long with handles on each end. They vary in thickness—start with a tube with which you can do eight to 12 reps per side. When you can do 15 reps, switch to a thicker tube.

Cost: About $5 to $15 per tube.

Target zones: Inner and outer thighs.

•**Hip adduction.** Attach one handle to a secure anchor (such as around a bed leg). Loop other

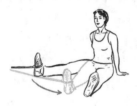

handle securely around your right foot (push past toes as far as possible so it doesn't fly off).

Sit on floor, with knees straight and legs spread, so tube is straight out to the right of your right foot. With hands on floor behind you, use inner thigh muscles to slide right leg in to meet left leg. Hold three seconds, then slowly slide right leg back out to spread-leg position. Do 10 to 15 reps, then repeat with left leg.

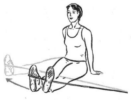

•**Hip abduction.** Attach one handle to a secure anchor, and loop other handle around right foot (as in the previous exercise).

Sit on floor, with knees straight and legs together, so tube is straight out to the left of your right foot, crossing over left ankle. With your hands on the floor behind you, use outer thigh muscles to slide right leg out to the right until legs are spread as much as possible. Hold three seconds, then slowly slide right leg back to meet left leg. Do 10 to 15 reps, then repeat with left leg.

DUMBBELLS

To start, use a pair of dumbbells (hand weights) with which you can do eight to 12 reps. When you are able to do 15 reps, switch to weights two to three pounds heavier. Typically a woman starts with five-pound weights, increasing to eight, then 10, then 12, then 15 pounds.

Cost: About $10 to $30 per pair.

Target zones: Front and back of thighs...buttocks.

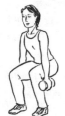

•**Squat.** Stand with feet shoulder-width apart, one weight in each hand, arms down at sides. Keeping torso erect and head in line with spine, bend knees (as if sitting on a chair) until thighs are nearly parallel to floor. Do not allow knees to move forward past toes. Hold for three seconds, then return to standing. Do 10 to 15 reps.

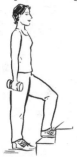

•**Step-Up.** Stand at bottom of a stairway, facing steps, one weight in each hand, arms down at sides. (If you have balance problems, hold a weight in one hand and hold onto banister with the other hand.)

Place entire left foot flat on first step, then rise until you are standing on the stair. Step back down, again moving left foot first. Do 10 to 15 reps, then repeat on the right side.

Exercise illustrations by Shawn Banner.

Three Simple Steps to Sleeker Thighs

Karen Burke, MD, PhD, a dermatologist in private practice in New York City and author of *Thin Thighs: Exercises and Recipes for Trim, Toned Thighs.*

Lumpy cellulite plagues women of all sizes. Though composed of ordinary fat, cellulite has a distinctive dimpled appearance.

Why women have it worse: Women have sacs of soft, spongy fat cells divided by connective tissues arranged in a series of arches that point outward, rippling the skin's surface, especially on hips and thighs. In men, fat sacs are smaller...connective tissues are more netlike...and skin is thicker—so the surface is smoother. *Helpful...*

•**Adopt an anti-cellulite diet.** Losing excess weight shrinks fat cells—but what you eat is as important as how much (even if you are slim).

Best: Eat less fat—dietary fat converts easily into body fat and triggers production of *galanin*, a hormone that increases cravings for yet more fatty food. Avoid sugar and alcohol—these raise insulin levels, inhibiting fat breakdown and facilitating fat storage. Get more fiber and protein—these digest slowly, so you feel fuller longer.

•**Do the right type of exercise.** Stretching and toning activities (yoga, tai chi, ballet) and isometrics (in which you hold contracted muscles in a static position) lengthen and smooth muscles, giving thighs a sleeker appearance.

Try this: Stand with feet shoulder-width apart. Contract abdominal muscles, and squeeze buttocks together...hold for 10 seconds...release...repeat 10 times.

•**Use daily self-massage.** Physically manipulating cellulite improves circulation, inhibiting blood vessel constriction that exacerbates lumpiness... and makes massaged areas swell slightly, so skin looks smoother for about a day. Some lab studies suggest that anti-cellulite creams with caffeine and vitamin E help break down stored fat and promote skin elasticity (though no human studies confirm this). Try these creams if you choose to...or apply any lotion or oil to your thighs so your hands glide smoothly. Massage for five to 15 minutes, applying firm pressure with the heels of your hands and stroking from the toes toward the tops of the legs, following the direction that blood flows as it returns to the heart.

Six Easy Exercises That Increase Your Pleasure in Bed

Hilda Hutcherson, MD, is professor of obstetrics and gynecology, Columbia University Medical Center, New York City, and author of three books, including *Pleasure: A Woman's Guide to Getting the Sex You Want, Need, and Deserve.*

Have you noticed that sex is not as enjoyable as it was before menopause? Maybe the "big O" has become a "mini O" because your orgasms are not as powerful as they were. Kegels—exercises that help with incontinence and also intensify climax—can help, but maybe not enough. Plus, loss of flexibility can make it hard to find a comfortable position for sex, further detracting from your pleasure. Time to give up on sex? Absolutely not! Try these special exercises recommended by a gynecologist—do them at least four times a week—and enjoy the results!

Vaginal Weight Training intensifies orgasms by improving strength and function of pelvic floor muscles. After each use, wash your weights with soap and water, then air-dry. *What to try…*

●**Vaginal barbell is a thin weight about seven inches long,** with rounded ends of two different sizes (try Natural Contours Energie, $35).

To use: Lubricate the larger end of the barbell with a water-based lubricant. Lie on your back with knees bent, and gently insert the lubricated end into your vagina until one-third of the barbell is inside and the rest is outside. Using your vaginal muscles to squeeze the hidden end of the weight, try to make the visible end move up and down. Gradually work your way up to 50 squeezes. When you master that, try inserting the smaller end of the barbell and moving the larger end.

●**Vaginal cones are small egg-shaped weights that typically come in sets of four or five.** Each has a line attached, like a tampon, for easy removal.

Online source: ShopInPrivate.com, about $50.

To use: After lubricating the lightest cone, gently insert it all the way into the vagina. Then walk around for five to 15 minutes, trying to keep the cone inside by squeezing your vaginal muscles. If it falls out, rinse the cone and insert it again. When you can easily manage 15 minutes, switch to a heavier cone.

Pelvic Flexibility and Strength Enhancers to increase the number of sexual positions you can comfortably get into, boosting stimulation of your pleasure spots. To practice, place an exercise mat or blanket on the floor. *The moves to do…*

●**Butterfly stretch improves hip flexibility and inner thigh strength.** Sit on the floor, knees bent, soles of your feet touching so that your knees fall open. Grasp your ankles, and gently pull your feet toward your groin. Rest your elbows on your knees and gently press your knees down. Hold for 10 seconds…rest…repeat 20 times.

●**Pelvic tilt increases your ability to arch your back and thrust your hips.** Lie on your back, knees bent, feet flat on floor and arms at your sides. Keeping your shoulder blades on the floor, lift your pelvis and your lower back as far as you comfortably can…also squeeze your vaginal muscles. Hold for 10 seconds…slowly lower to the floor and rest… repeat 20 times.

Back Stretches and Strengtheners help prevent sex-induced back pain. *Try these…*

●**Beach ball stretches and soothes low-back muscles.** Lie on your back, knees bent, feet flat on the floor. Grasp the backs of your knees and draw them to your chest. Hold for 10 seconds… slowly return to starting position…rest…repeat 20 times.

●**Cobra improves back strength and flexibility.** Lie on your stomach, elbows bent and hands by your ears. Push with your hands, slowly raising your upper body (not your pelvis) off the floor and arching your back. Hold for 10 seconds…slowly lower to the floor…rest…repeat 20 times.

Restore Your Pelvic Floor: Real Help for Incontinence, Pelvic Pain and More

Lesli Lo, DPT, women's health physical therapist, Northwestern Medical Group and instructor of obstetrics and gynecology at Northwestern University Feinberg School of Medicine, both in Chicago.

If you're a woman who pees when you laugh or cough or sometimes feels overcome with a sudden nearly uncontrollable urge to pee—that is, if you have urinary incontinence—you've undoubtedly heard of Kegel exercises, and maybe even tried them. The simple do-anywhere pelvic exercises often are recommended for this condition—and a wide variety of other pelvic problems including fecal (bowel) incontinence, chronic pain and pelvic organ prolapse, in which the bladder or uterus can bulge into the vagina.

But doing Kegels may be exactly the wrong thing for you. They actually could be making your problem worse. It's not that you're doing them wrong, although many people do. In fact, it's especially an issue if you do Kegels right.

If you suffer from incontinence and have performed hundreds of Kegels with no improvement or if you have chronic pelvic pain but think it can't be fixed, you are not alone—and there is help. Eventually, Kegels can be part of the solution, but there are steps you need to take first.

Read on to learn new ways to beat incontinence and other pelvic floor disorders.

A PELVIC FLOOR PRIMER—THE MENOPAUSE CONNECTION

The pelvic floor is a network of muscles, ligaments and tissue that acts like a sling to support a woman's pelvic organs—the uterus, vagina, bladder/urethra and rectum. You control your bowel and bladder by contracting and relaxing these muscles and tissues. Twenty-seven percent of women ages 40 to 59 will experience pelvic floor dysfunction (PFD) in their lifetime.

There's a strong menopause link: The estrogen drop that typically begins some time in your 40s during perimenopause and is typically complete when you enter menopause (usually by your early 50s) can cause the pelvic floor to thin out, making prolapse more likely. Plus age, obesity, repeated heavy lifting, traumatic injury—such as may happen during childbirth or from a hip or back injury—can cause pelvic muscles and connective tissues to become sensitive, strained and weak. Over time, the likelihood of a pelvic floor disorder increases.

WHAT MOST WOMEN GET WRONG ABOUT KEGELS

Women with PFD often think their internal muscles are too weak and do Kegels in an effort to strengthen them. While that often is true, it's not the biggest problem. For 99% of my patients, the real problem is muscles that are too tight.

These too-tight muscles often get stuck in a contracted position, unable to control the flow of urine or to fully relax and contract in a pleasurable way during intercourse. For these women, Kegels can worsen the situation by strengthening already too-tight muscles. What they really need is to relax them.

The first step: Bring up your symptoms with your internist, ob/gyn, urogynecologist or urologist. He/she can rule out any concerns that are not musculoskeletal, and if physical therapy is the next best course of treatment, he can refer you to a women's health physical therapist (WHPT). WHPTs partner with ob/gyns, urologists and other specialists to diagnose and treat not just the pelvic floor, but the body as a whole. Three to six months of weekly or biweekly manual therapy sessions, combined with homework, can typically ease symptoms of urinary incontinence, painful intercourse and/or pelvic pain.

A WHPT will perform an internal exam to assess your areas of strength and weakness and design a plan to retrain your muscles. You can find a WHPT with the locator on the website of the American Physical Therapy Association, APTAPelvicHealth.org. Insurance typically covers these services. (*Note:* Some chiropractors, occupational therapists and naturopaths may also perform similar treatments, but I am not familiar enough with their exact practices to recommend them. Midwives are typically not trained in these techniques.)

TONING THE PELVIC FLOOR—THE RIGHT WAY

A crucial component of treatment with a WHPT is manual therapy. It may take some getting used to, but it's the gold standard of practice. In manual therapy, a WHPT uses her hands to gently massage, stretch and release spasms and trigger points within the deep and soft tissues of the vagina. This helps reduce tightness and tension and can even break up scar tissue that's further restricting tissues, allowing the pelvic floor muscles to fully relax and contract. Though manual therapy can feel uncomfortable initially, any pain quickly recedes as the muscles and tissues relax.

Manual therapy is a prime opportunity to assess how you do Kegels. Many women do it so that it only strengthens, never relaxes. During such therapy, I will insert one finger into the vagina and then ask my patient to perform a Kegel by imagining she is stopping the flow of urine midstream. (Once a woman learns how to do this correctly, she can do it herself.) Two out of three women do this incorrectly, tightening their pelvic floor muscles but not releasing them all the way back down—or not tightening their pelvic floor at all, recruiting their abs or glutes instead. The goal is to teach them how to relax their muscles all the way down to starting position. *Some ways to teach this technique…*

●**Reverse Kegels.** In a conventional Kegel, you tighten your pelvic floor muscles, hold the contraction for 10 seconds, then fully relax back down, maintaining the relaxed position for 10 seconds. (Sometimes I tell patients to imagine they are controlling an elevator with their vagina and send it to the top floor, hold it there, then send it down to the basement.) In a reverse Kegel, you begin "in the basement," so to speak, relaxing the muscles as you do when you've just sat down on the toilet with a full bladder and are able to urinate. You should feel your anus relax as well. After relaxing for 10 seconds, send the elevator back up to the top and hold 10 seconds, then release again.

●**Biofeedback.** This pain-free, nonsurgical technique allows patients to see their pelvic muscles at rest and while contracted—and improves their ability to retrain the pelvic floor. A sensor or small weight is inserted into the vagina, while a nearby computer provides visual feedback. More than 75% of PFD patients who try biofeedback benefit from it.

●**New: Home biofeedback.** The apps Elvie Trainer ($199, Apple/Android) and PeriCoach ($299, Apple/Android) use intravaginal devices to assess the strength and endurance of vaginal contractions, and then send data to your smartphone via Bluetooth. I only recommend them for women who've had a professional pelvic floor assessment, because if you're not performing Kegels correctly, a product like this could contribute to further tightness/tension. But if you've learned to do Kegels so that you relax as well as strengthen, they can be helpful.

LIFESTYLE SOLUTIONS

Shallow chest breathing also can contribute to pelvic floor disorders.

Reason: The diaphragm, a sheet of muscle that separates the chest cavity from the abdomen, gets stuck in a contracted position—causing pelvic muscles to contract, too.

Solution: Learn diaphragmatic (belly) breathing. Lying down, pretend your belly is a balloon and fill it with air, keeping your chest still (you may need to start with shallow breaths). Now exhale, deflating the balloon. Try this once an hour for five breaths, and again for five minutes before bed. In two to three weeks, you should notice a change in the way you breathe.

In general, chronic stress can make urinary incontinence worse, so mind-body relaxation methods, such as meditation and yoga, also help.

One final tip: Sit-ups can put even asymptomatic women at risk of developing incontinence, prolapse or other PFD issues.

A better way to strengthen your abs: Plank.

15

Exercises for Better Vision

Why Sunlight Can Be Good for Your Eyes

Marc Grossman, OD, LAc, doctor of optometry and licensed acupuncturist in New Paltz and Somers, New York. He is coauthor of *Natural Eye Care: Your Guide to Healthy Vision.* A holistic eye doctor, his multidisciplinary approach uses nutrition, lifestyle changes and Traditional Chinese Medicine to tackle eye problems. NaturalEyeCare.com

You think you take good care of your eyes. You wear sunglasses outdoors and get regular eye exams. But did you know that exercise, stress and even mindfulness practices can impact eye health? Holistic optometrist Dr. Marc Grossman suggests several natural ways to show your eyes some love—and see your way to healthy vision for years to come.

•**Pay attention to your posture.** The eyes are extensions of the brain and part of our central nervous system. Signals and messages are sent from the eyes to the visual cortex in the brain, which processes and sends the information down the spinal cord to the rest of the body. Poor posture can disrupt these connections and lead to blurred vision, and conversely, visual strain can result in poor posture. To avoid this, when sitting, keep your chest up, shoulders back and weight over your seat so that both eyes are at task level and an equal dis-

tance from what is being seen. Always sit upright while reading or watching television instead of lying on your back, side or stomach.

•**Seek out sunlight.** Walking is one of the best things we can do for exercise, and depending where you walk, it has another benefit—natural sunlight. The eyes are light-sensing organs. It's important to get enough sunlight so that your eyes operate optimally. In fact, a recent study published in *JAMA Ophthalmology* found that increased exposure to sunlight reduces your risk for myopia (nearsightedness). Aim for at least 20 minutes of natural sunlight a day—just be sure to wear sunglasses that provide 100% UV protection and filter out both UVA and UVB rays.

•**Get moving.** Aerobic exercise not only benefits your heart, it also has been linked to improved retinal health and prevention of eye disease. Exercise raises oxygen levels in the cells and increases lymph and blood circulation. This increased circulation is a prerequisite for good vision. In addition, research published in *The Journal of Neuroscience* has found that moderate aerobic exercise may be able to delay the progression of *age-related macular degeneration* (AMD) by preserving the structure and function of the nerve cells in the retina. Get 20 minutes of aerobic exercise daily by walking, swimming or doing any other activity that you enjoy.

•**Don't forget about vision fitness.** Simple eye exercises will ease discomfort and support healthy vision. *Try figure eights to increase the flexibility of your eye muscles in a relaxed way…*

•Stand or sit with your feet shoulder-width apart, hands at your sides.

•Imagine a horizontal figure eight (as wide as is comfortable) about 10 feet away.

•Without moving your head, trace the figure eight with your eyes in one direction, then in the opposite direction. Remember to breathe normally and blink your eyes regularly as they move along the figure eight. Repeat several times. Do this for two minutes twice a day.

•**Change focus.** Don't keep your eyes locked on a computer or television or any other screen for a sustained period of time. Doing so causes tension on the visual system. We don't blink as much when we're staring at something, which dries out the cornea and exhausts the eye muscles. To change your focus when you're doing close-up work, look up and away often—such as out a window—to give your eyes a break.

Try the 20-20-20 rule: Every 20 minutes, look at something 20 feet away for 20 seconds.

•**Relax your eyes.** Relax the muscles around your eyes, and bring healing energy to your eyes through increased circulation and energy flow with a technique called palming. This is especially useful after long periods of computer use. *How to do it…*

•Remove your glasses or contact lenses, and sit leaning forward with your elbows resting on a table and your eyes closed.

•Place the palm of your left hand over your left eye, with your fingers on your forehead, the hollow of your palm directly over your eye (but not touching it), and the heel of your hand resting on your left cheekbone.

•Do the same thing with your right palm over the right eye and the right fingers crossing over the fingers of your left hand and the heel of your hand resting on your right cheekbone.

•Remain this way for three minutes, remembering to breathe normally.

•**Go the distance.** The eye muscles are most relaxed when using our distance vision because that's what they were designed for. Nowadays, to keep your eyes in top shape, make an effort to perform outdoor activities that require seeing at a distance, such as playing golf or tennis, riding a bike or just walking. When walking, keep your head up and scan the horizon. Indoors, do reading, writing or close-up work with an eye-to-activity distance of roughly 14 to 16 inches for adults. Watch TV from a distance of about eight to 10 feet for most large-screen TVs.

•**Be mindful.** It's no secret that mental stress affects the immune and respiratory systems and causes inflammation throughout the body. But did you know that stress-reduction techniques can have a specific impact on glaucoma? Your body can't deliver essential nutrients to your eyes if stress is impairing circulation and digestion. Destress by practicing proven mindfulness techniques such as meditation, deep breathing and yoga. Inversion poses in yoga, such as downward dog, also benefit vision because they increase blood flow to the head (consult your doctor first if you have glaucoma or high blood pressure).

An intriguing new study published in *Journal of Glaucoma* found that meditation in particular may be especially helpful for glaucoma patients. Hour-long, daily mindful-meditation sessions for just three weeks resulted in a significant reduction in eye pressure and in levels of the stress hormone *cortisol*, helping to minimize optic damage. Even five to 20 minutes a day can be very helpful.

Get Moving for Healthy Eyes

Marc Grossman, OD, LAc, doctor of optometry and licensed acupuncturist in New Paltz and Somers, New York. He is coauthor of *Natural Eye Care: Your Guide to Healthy Vision & Healing.* NaturalEyeCare.com

The more you get your heart pumping, the healthier your eyes will be. Researchers compared the physical activity levels and vision quality of 6,634 Brits. Being inactive was associated with being twice as likely to have only fair or poor vision. Although the study involved adults age 65 and older, you're never too young to establish a healthy, regular exercise habit if you haven't done so already. Getting in shape and staying there will also help you avoid high blood pressure and diabetes, both of which can lead to eye conditions that may cause vision loss.

Better Vision in 6 Weeks or Less: Without New Glasses or Surgery

Larry Jebrock, OD, a board-certified, licensed optometrist who emphasizes nonsurgical vision improvement and behavioral optometry. He is founder and director of Natural Vision Correction, Orthokeratology & Vision Therapy, in Novato, California. He is a former instructor for the California Optometric Association and a consultant for companies on the effects of prolonged computer use and video display terminals on the vision system. EyeExercises.com

If you're over 40, it's likely that you're not seeing as well as when you were younger—and if you're over 60, it's nearly certain that your eyesight has declined.

Breakthrough approach: Behavioral optometry—using eye exercises to improve vision—is an effective but usually overlooked method for stopping, slowing and even reversing the age-related decline of eyesight.

VISION PROBLEMS

If your eyesight has declined, you probably have *presbyopia*, a decrease in your ability to focus and see clearly at close distances, such as when you're reading or looking at the computer.

You also might have diminished *contrast sensitivity*—less light is reaching the retina, the lining at the back of the inner eye that transforms light into electrical impulses that are sent to the visual cortex in the brain. As a result, vision is "washed out" and the contrast between objects becomes less distinct. It may be difficult to see the difference between the

sidewalk curb and the street, for example. Lessened contrast sensitivity also worsens glare from headlights at night or sun reflecting off windshields during the day.

The danger: Poor contrast sensitivity increases the risk for falls and car accidents.

Aging also decreases overall visual acuity, or sharpness of vision. And visual reaction time is diminished. It takes longer for the brain to register what has been seen.

The typical solutions to declining vision are corrective lenses (eyeglasses or contacts) and Lasik laser surgery, in which the cornea is reshaped. But for many people, stronger corrective lenses are needed every six to 18 months, as vision continues to worsen…and Lasik surgery often is not covered by insurance, doesn't always restore perfect vision and can cause dry eyes, glare and hazy vision.

EXERCISES WORK

New scientific evidence: Researchers from University of California, Riverside and Brown University used eye exercises to improve the eyesight of 16 younger people (average age 22) and 16 older people (average age 71), and published their results in *Psychological Science.*

After just seven days, diminished contrast sensitivity was eliminated in the older group—in other words, their contrast sensitivity reversed, becoming the same as that of the younger group. And both younger and older adults had improved visual acuity in the problem areas common to their age—older people saw near objects more clearly, and younger people saw far objects more clearly.

Here are three vision-restoring exercises you can do at home. Results can be immediate or take up to six weeks. Once your eyes have improved, keep up the exercises, but you can do them less often. Your eyeglass/contact prescription may change, so see your eye-care professional.

•**Improve near vision and far vision.** Practice this simple eye exercise for three or four minutes a few days a week.

Instructions: Look at a calendar on a wall about 10 feet away. In your hand, have another object with numbers or letters, such as a small calendar or an open book. Cover the left eye with your hand. Look back and forth from the far object to the near object, focusing on and calling out a letter or number from each.

Example: The "J" in June from the far calendar and the "12" in June 12 from the near calendar. Do this five to 10 times, calling out a different letter or number each time. Cover the right eye, and repeat the exercise. (You also can use an eye patch to cover one eye and then the other.)

Bonus benefit: It's common after a car accident for the person who is at fault to say that he "never saw" the other vehicle. I call this inattentional blindness—your eyes are on the road, but your vision system is not fully activated, because you're thinking or moving or otherwise preoccupied. The near-far exercise also improves visual attention.

•**Improve peripheral vision**—the "other" visual system. Corrective lenses correct only central vision, when the eyes focus straight ahead, so that you can read, drive and see details sharply. But there are two key parts to the visual system—central and peripheral vision. And improving peripheral vision improves every aspect of seeing, from visual acuity to contrast sensitivity.

Everyday enemy of peripheral vision: Stress. Under stress, people see less, remember less and typically the visual field constricts. But there's a simple exercise called "palming" that relieves stress and eases eyestrain.

Instructions: Sit at a table with your elbows on the table. (Put a pillow under your elbows if that's more comfortable.) Breathe easily and deeply, relaxing your body. Close your eyes, and notice what you're seeing—it's likely there will be visual "chatter," such as spots and flashes of light. Now cup your palms over your closed eyes, and visualize (create mental imagery of) blackness.

Example: Visualize yourself out on the ocean on a moonless night on a black ship on a black sea. The goal of the exercise is to see complete blackness.

Relaxing, breathing deeply, blocking out light and "visual chatter"—and even the warmth of your palms—relaxes the visual system and helps to open up peripheral vision.

Do the exercise for as long as you like, from 30 seconds to 30 minutes.

•**Improve "binocularity"**—seeing out of both eyes. A common but little-recognized vision problem in older adults is a lack of binocularity—one eye is not processing visual detail, which decreases visual acuity and depth perception (crucial for stepping off a curb or walking up stairs without stumbling or falling). This exercise can help you see with both eyes.

For this exercise you'll need a Brock String, named after its inventor, the optometrist Frederick Brock. It's a simple device—a 10- or 12-foot string with several colored beads on it. (The Brock String is widely available online for around $10 or less.)

Instructions: Attach one end of the string securely to a wall with a nail, tack or tape. Sit 10 feet away from the wall, holding the string so that there is no slack. The closest bead should be about four feet from your eyes.

Hold the string to the side of your nose and look directly at the closest bead, using both eyes—you should see two strings going toward the bead and crossing either in front of or behind the bead. You're "seeing double" because the device is engineered to generate a double-image, similar to what you might see when your eyes are relaxed and unfocused. This experience helps you become aware that you're seeing out of both eyes. If you see only one string, you're not seeing fully out of both eyes. And if the strings cross in front of or behind the bead, your eyes aren't aimed right at the bead. *The goals of the exercise…*

•**Keep both strings "turned on"** (your eyes will get a "feel" for how to do this).

•**The strings should cross at the bead**—if the string crosses ahead of the bead, look a few inches beyond the bead…if the string crosses behind the bead, look in front of the bead.

Do the exercise for three or four minutes, two or three times a week.

Can We Say Good-Bye to Reading Glasses?

Marc Grossman, OD, LAc, director of optometry and licensed acupuncturist in New Paltz and Somers, New York. He is coauthor of *Natural Eyecare: Your Guide to Healthy Vision.* A holistic eye doctor, his multidisciplinary approach use nutrition, lifestyle changes and Traditional Chinese Medicine to tackle eye problems. NaturalEyeCare.com

When it comes to signs of aging, different people have different pet peeves. Some of us really don't like those gray hairs… others sigh over a lost silhouette…still others hate needing reading glasses to see what's on the menu.

Since exercise improves the strength, flexibility and function of our bodies, it makes sense that eye exercises could improve our ability to see close up. Yet this is a controversial topic. Though various studies have found no clear benefit from eye exercises, many holistic practitioners and their patients say that vision can indeed be improved.

The challenge with aging eyes: Many people first become farsighted—meaning that nearby objects look blurry even though more distant objects are clear—starting in their 40s. This is due to *presbyopia*, a condition in which the aging lens of the eye becomes too stiff to focus clearly up close.

Detractors of eye exercise say that it won't restore lens elasticity. But supporters say that's not the point. Eye exercises can improve the strength, flexibility and adaptability of muscles that control eye movement and encourage a mental focus that helps the brain and eyes work better together. This can slow the progression of farsightedness and possibly improve vision.

So the answer to the question, "Can eye exercises help us say good riddance to reading glasses?" seems to be yes for some people—and it certainly can't hurt to try.

Four exercises can help improve close-up vision. While you do the exercises, remember to keep breathing and keep blinking. And smile! Smiling reduces tension, which helps your muscles work optimally and your brain focus on what's around you.

Try to do the exercises while not wearing any reading glasses—or if your close-up vision is not good enough for that, wear weaker reading glasses than you normally do. If you usually wear glasses or contacts for distance vision, it is OK to wear those while doing the exercises.

How long to practice: Do each exercise for three to four minutes, for a total practice time of about 15 minutes per session, at least three times weekly. If you get headaches while exercising your eyes, reduce the time spent on each exercise—and see your eye doctor if the problem persists.

•**Letter Reading**—for better scanning accuracy and conscious eye control when reading or using a computer.

Preparation: Type up a chart with four rows of random letters, just large enough that you can read them while holding the page at a typical reading distance (type size will vary depending on an individual's vision). Leave space between each row. In row one, type all capitals, one space in between each letter…row two, all lowercase, one space in between each letter…row three, all lowercase, no spaces…row four, wordlike groups of random letters arranged as if in a sentence.

Exercise: Hold the chart with both hands. Looking at row one, read each letter aloud left to right, then right to left. Then read every second letter…then every third letter. If your mind wanders, start over.

Over time: When you master row one, try the same techniques with row two…then row three… then row four. If you find that you have memorized parts of the chart, make a new one using different letters.

•**Near And Far**—for improved focus and focusing speed when switching your gaze from close objects to distant objects (such as when checking gauges on a car as you drive).

Preparation: Type a chart with six to eight rows of random capital letters, each letter about one-half inch tall (or as tall as necessary for you to read them from 10 feet away). Tack the chart to a wall and stand back 10 feet.

Exercise: Hold a pencil horizontally, with its embossed letters facing you, about six inches from your nose (or as close as possible without it looking blurry). Read any letter on the pencil, then read any letter on the chart. Keep doing this, switching back and forth as fast as you can without letting the letters blur.

Over time: Do this with one eye covered, then the other.

•**Pencil Pushups**—to promote eye teamwork. All you need is a pencil.

Exercise: Hold a pencil horizontally at eye level 12 inches from your face (or as far as necessary to see the pencil clearly). With both eyes, look at one particular letter on the pencil…keep looking while bringing the pencil closer to your face. If the letter blurs or doubles, it means that one eye is no longer accurately on target—so move the pencil back until the letter is clear once more…then try again to slowly bring the pencil closer while keeping the letter in focus.

•**The "Hot Dog"**—for improved flexibility of the muscles within the eye that allow the lens to change shape. No props are needed.

Exercise: With your hands at chest height about eight inches in front of you, point your index fingers and touch the tips together, so that your index fingers are horizontal. Gaze at any target in the distance and, without changing your focus, raise your fingers into your line of sight. Notice that a "mini hot dog" has appeared between the tips of your fingers. Still gazing at the distant object, pull your fingertips apart slightly—and observe that the hot dog is now floating in the air. Keep the hot dog there for two breaths…then look directly at your fingers for two breaths, noticing that the hot dog disappears. Look again at the distant object and find the hot dog once again. Continue switching your gaze back and forth every two breaths.

As your close-up vision improves, you may find that you need less-powerful reading glasses—or none at all—for your day-to-day activities.

Exercise Fights Glaucoma

Victoria Tseng, MD, PhD, ophthalmologist, UCLA Jules Stein Eye Institute, California.

The most physically active people (those who exercised moderately to vigorously 30 minutes a day, five days a week) were 73% less likely to develop glaucoma than the least physically active, according to a study that tracked 5,000 adults over several decades.

Theory: Exercise may change the blood flow to the optic nerve or affect intraocular pressure. More study is needed.

Aerobic Exercise Protects Eyes from Macular Degeneration and Other Retina Problems

Machelle T. Pardue, PhD, associate professor, and **Jeffrey H. Boatright, PhD,** professor, department of ophthalmology, Emory University School of Medicine, and the Atlanta VA Center for Visual and Neurocognitive Rehabilitation, both in Atlanta. Their study was published in *The Journal of Neuroscience.*

Even for people with healthy eyes, protecting eyesight should be a primary concern. That's because as we age, we are increasingly vulnerable to degenerative eye diseases such as *age-related macular degeneration* (AMD). These diseases can strike anyone…are very tough to treat…and can lead to severely impaired vision, or even blindness, sometimes with horrifying speed.

Good news: A recent study suggests a simple (and even enjoyable) way to help protect against AMD and other retinal problems. It's something that your eye doctor probably won't think to mention…but it might do your eyes a world of good by directly benefiting your retinas.

This new study used healthy mice. Some of the mice were given treadmills and trained to exercise for one hour, five days each week, at a moderate pace. For comparison's sake, other mice had identical living conditions—except that their treadmills did not move, so they were mostly inactive. After two weeks, the mice were intentionally exposed to a bright light for four hours. The light exposure was intended to damage the light-sensing photoreceptors of the retina in a way that's similar to the retinal neuron degeneration that occurs in humans who have AMD or a less common condition called *retinitis pigmentosa.*

Next, the mice were put back on the same exercise program (or lack thereof) for two more weeks. Halfway through and at the end of that time period, the researchers did some tests. *What they discovered…*

After being exposed to the damaging bright light, the mice that had exercised showed two times greater retinal function, based on measurements of electrical activity of the retina, compared with the inactive mice.

Examination of the retinas showed that, even though numerous photoreceptors had indeed been damaged by the bright light exposure, the mice that exercised had more than twice as many healthy photoreceptors as the inactive mice.

The fact that the test results remained consistent two weeks after the exposure to the damaging light suggests that exercise's beneficial effects have some power to persist…and may help slow the progression of vision-destroying degenerative retinal diseases.

EXERCISE'S EYE BENEFITS EXPLAINED

What could account for such dramatic vision benefits from exercise? Part of the answer may come from another portion of the experiment that involved measuring the levels of *brain-derived neurotrophic factor* (BDNF), a protein involved in nerve growth. In a different set of mice, some exercised for nine days and the others did not. Then researchers tested BDNF levels in the retinas, brains and blood of the mice—and found that, in all three areas, the active mice had significantly higher levels of BDNF than the inactive mice.

There's no known cure for AMD…and the treatments that can help slow its progress are anxiety-provoking and uncomfortable, involving injections of drugs directly into the eyes. Compared to that, aerobic exercise seems like a pleasurable walk in the park—quite literally!

Get motivated, get moving: This study makes a strong case that aerobic exercise directly benefits the retina and plays a significant role in protecting photoreceptors. Of course, an animal study can't prove that what's good for mouse eyes also is good for human eyes, particularly after just two weeks of regular aerobic exercise…but it certainly could be true. Besides, we do know beyond a shadow of a doubt that aerobic exercise is highly beneficial to people's bodies and brains. If you care about protecting your eyesight (and who doesn't?), let this study serve as yet one more excellent reason to add some aerobic exercise to your day-to-day routine (with your primary-care physician's OK)—whether or not your eye doctor thinks to recommend it.

PART III:

The Fit and Flexible Weight-Loss Guide

16

Better Ways to Weight Loss

8 Surprising Diet Mistakes That Exercisers Make

Nancy Clark, MS, RD, sports nutritionist with a private practice in the Boston area and author of the best-seller *Nancy Clark's Sports Nutrition Guidebook*. NancyClarkRD.com

If you're trying to lose weight or simply avoid creeping weight, you're likely adding exercise to your daily routine—good for you! Yet you notice a problem…the weight's not coming off the way you want it to or worse, it's sneaking upward. What's that about?

Here's one possibility: Research shows that many people overestimate the number of calories they burn through exercise and then eat back even more calories. But that's only one of the common mistakes at the intersection between exercise and eating that could explain why you're not reaching your weight goal, according to respected sports nutritionist Nancy Clark, MS, RD. *Here's the truth about exercise and calories—plus eight other mistakes that may be keeping your exercise from bringing the results you want…*

MISTAKE: **Overestimating the number of calories you burn through exercise and, as a result, eating more than you need.** Exercise has a ton of benefits ranging from boosting bone and brain

health to warding off diabetes and heart disease, but unless you're working out at a very high level for a very long time, you're not burning through a large number of calories. As an example, walking at a brisk 4 mph for 30 minutes burns about 200 calories (depending on your height and weight)—and that's the number of calories in just one ounce of some nuts—barely a handful.

Tip: Use a fitness chart or wearable fitness tracker to calculate what you're really burning off when you exercise, and factor that correctly into your diet strategy.

MISTAKE: **Counting on exercise alone for significant weight loss.** Using the same example as above, you can quickly calculate how many 30-minute walks it will take to burn off one pound, or 3,500 calories—yes, 17.5! For exercise to contribute significantly to weight loss, it needs to be coupled with cutting calories.

Tip: Although exercising more and eating less can combine to create the needed net calorie deficit, you really want to decouple the two things in your mind and put them into separate mental buckets. Exercising is vital for your health…and eating less is vital for losing weight.

MISTAKE: **Having a one-and-done approach to daily exercise.** If you work out for one 30-minute session per day and spend the rest of your waking hours at a desk or on the sofa, you aren't capitalizing on exercise as much as you should for weight loss and overall health.

Tip: Take a 24-hour view of activity and build on your formal workout. That could mean holding a walking meeting at the office instead of gathering around a conference table, adding an hour of gardening to your weekends, and jogging in place while you stream a TV show.

MISTAKE: **Working out too soon after a meal.** Exercise leaves many people hungry, and that can lead to eating more times during a day and taking in more calories than you had planned. Net result? You could end up with a weight gain, not a loss.

Tip: One way to account for post-exercise hunger is to make sure that your exercise session does not come soon after any meal—but rather, soon *before* a regular mealtime. That way you can satisfy your body's demand for fuel without adding extra calories (and in effect canceling out the calories you just burned). Just be sure to maintain—not add to—your food portion sizes.

MISTAKE: **Thinking you need to replace electrolytes with a sports drink.** Special "replacement" drinks are meant to boost fluid retention during heavy exercise, such as running a marathon. If you're exercising three hours or more in the heat, they may be helpful. Otherwise, they're not necessary. Electrolytes is essentially a technical term for salt. Chances are you're already getting plenty of that. (A slice of bread contains about as much salt as a 12-ounce sports drink.)

Tip: Water is all most people need to replace fluids after a typical workout, and it has no calories.

MISTAKE: **Eating the standard three meals a day.** Restricting yourself to breakfast, lunch and dinner is an old-fashioned way to fuel your body and can mean long stretches between meals. Instead, distribute your total daily calories somewhat evenly across four to six meals per day, depending on what works best for your schedule.

Example: Try a hearty breakfast at 7 am, lunch at 11 am, a "second lunch" (bigger and better than a snack) at 3 pm and a lighter dinner around 6 pm. You may find it helpful to work with a registered dietitian (RD) to design a food plan specifically for you, one that includes the most nutrient dense foods to keep you fueled and feeling full. The referral network at SCANdpg.org can help you find a sports nutrition expert near you.

MISTAKE: **Eating most of your protein at one meal.** The body makes fast work of this essential nutrient. Protein in your food is best used to build and repair muscle in the first four hours after you've eaten, so you should include a serving of protein at every meal. Protein is filling, so it will help you curb your appetite, too.

Tip: Plan on 15 grams (g) to 30 g protein per meal (with larger people needing more than smaller people) if you're eating four meals a day…or 10 g to 20 g per meal if you're eating six meals a day. Healthy choices include two or three eggs (6 g of protein per one large egg)…turkey or chicken (3 oz/24 g)…fish (3 oz/19 g)…and black beans (½ cup/7 g). Looking for more nonmeat protein choices? Enjoy a banana with peanut butter, a handful of (high-calorie but healthful) nuts, cottage cheese or Greek yogurt.

What don't you need? Protein shakes and bars, a source of unnecessary calories for the average person—even for people who exercise. What's more, packaged protein shakes are highly processed with added sugars, commonly contaminated with heavy metals such as lead and arsenic, and they're missing many of the nonprotein nutrients found in whole foods. If you enjoy smoothies, learn to make your own out of quality ingredients.

MISTAKE: **Eating a large meal close to bedtime.** Remember to think of food as fuel. You need more fuel during daytime hours when you are active and less when you are sleeping.

Tip: Front-load your day by having more of your calories at breakfast. Resist the urge to eat after dinner—move any calories you're in the habit of eating at night into the next day's breakfast.

Top Three Ways to Lose Weight

Anne McTiernan, MD, PhD, professor of epidemiology, Fred Hutchinson Cancer Research Center, and research professor in the departments of epidemiology and geriatrics, University of Washington, both in Seattle, Washington. Her study was published in *Journal of the Academy of Nutrition and Dietetics*.

L ots of people go on diets, but only a fraction of them are successful.

Why is it that some dieters meet their goals while others don't shed any pounds—or shed them and then gain them back almost immediately?

Researchers recently analyzed dieters over the course of one year—and then they looked at who lost the most weight and which strategies those people had in common.

It turned out that the people who whittled their waistlines most shared three particular tactics.

And they appear to be very simple!

DIETING DOS & DON'TS

The three tricks were…

1. Keep a food journal.

2. Don't skip meals.

3. Avoid eating out.

The study's senior author, Anne McTiernan, MD, PhD, professor of epidemiology at the Fred Hutchinson Cancer Research Center and a research professor at the University of Washington, reveals why these three methods worked best…

First, she explained how the diet in the study worked. Participants (who were all overweight) were instructed to eat between 1,200 and 2,000 calories a day. They were given a "food journal" in which they were told to record their daily eating habits, and they were also asked at the end of the study to fill out a 120-item questionnaire about how well they stuck to their diet. After analyzing the food journals, the questionnaires and how much weight each person lost, the researchers discovered the three shared strategies of the most successful dieters.

Let's learn more about each one…

A FOOD JOURNAL GIVES YOU AN EDGE

Dieters who used the food journals lost, on average, six pounds more than those who did not. Why does keeping a journal help? Dr. McTiernan said, "It's about accountability—knowing exactly how much you're eating." In other words, it's harder to fool yourself into thinking that you're making healthy choices when you have to write it all down.

To keep an effective food journal, record everything you eat and the calorie content of the foods. That includes side dishes, toppings and second helpings! It includes eating out, too. If you don't know the calorie content of a dish, look it up online. (Many restaurants post nutritional information on their websites or you can use CalorieKing.com). Whether you use a notebook or a smartphone app (such as Lose It! by FitNow), make sure that you record your food either during the meal or immediately after, so you don't forget. By looking at the journal at the end of the day, you'll know whether you're under or over your daily calorie limit. (Your daily calorie limit depends on your age, height, weight and gender and how much weight you want to lose—to get a ballpark idea, go to WebMD.com/diet/body-bmi-calculator, and for an exact amount, talk to your doctor.)

DON'T SKIP MEALS

It's tempting to skip a meal now and then, but ironically, the practice often leads to weight gain, not weight loss. The reason is that skipping a meal may make you so hungry that you'll overeat during your next meal. In the study, women who didn't skip meals lost, on average, about eight more pounds than women who did.

THE DANGERS OF DINING OUT

Nearly everyone eats out now and then, but the research showed that the less you do it, the easier it is to lose weight. For example, participants who ate out for lunch less often than once a week lost, on average, five more pounds than those who ate out for lunch at least once a week.

The figures show that it's much easier for dieters to go off track at a restaurant, where high-calorie dishes may be irresistible. It's also harder to know how those dishes are cooked, so unless the restaurant posts the calories on the menu or online, it's more difficult to know exactly how caloric the meal is. Plus, portions are usually much larger at a restaurant than what you'd serve yourself at home. So eat under your own roof—or eat food you've brought from home—except on special occasions!

To Lose Weight, Cut Carbs… Just Twice a Week

Louis Aronne, MD, professor of metabolic research, Weill Cornell Mediciine, director, Center for Weight Management and Metabolic Clinical Research at Weill Cornell Medicine and New York-Presbyterian, both in New York City.

There are many popular ways to lose weight. Lots of people try cutting calories across the board, but then they are hungry a lot of the time. Others dramatically cut carbs, which often helps with hunger, but that is hard to stick with if you love "carb-y" foods. Some people practice intermittent fasting, eating only 500 or 600 calories on certain days, but you might find that overly restrictive, too.

Fortunately, there is another, little-known approach that's just as effective as any of the above—and a whole lot easier for many people to stick with. Like intermittent fasting, it involves restrictive days, and like low-carb dieting, it involves drastically cutting carbohydrates.

But here's the big difference: All you do is go low-carb twice a week, without counting calories at all. The rest of the week you eat as much of a normal healthy diet as you want. It may work by "resetting" the brain so that you're not as hungry—not just on low-carb days but even when you go back to your "normal" way of eating the rest of the week.

Here's how to make it work for you.

THE TWO-DAY LOW-CARB DIET

At the Center for Weight Management and Metabolic Clinical Research at Weill Cornell Medicine, we became interested in this new approach when we reviewed a four-month British study of 115 overweight women. *The women were divided into three groups…*

- **Daily dieters cut their calories by 25% to an average of 1,500 a day on a balanced healthy Mediterranean-style diet.**
- **A second group did intermittent fasting on two consecutive days.** It was pretty intense—low-carb and no more than 600 calories a day…and then repeat the next day. The rest of the week, they ate as much as they wanted from a balanced diet.
- **The third group of women also went on an intermittent low-carb diet for two consecutive days, but they didn't have to restrict calories.** It was a big carb reduction—to just 40 grams, slightly less than the amount in one cup of rice. On those days, they were allowed unrestricted protein and healthy fats. The rest of the week they ate as they wanted from a balanced diet.

Results: The two-day-a-week low-carb dieters lost just as much weight as the intermittent fasters…and lost more weight than the everyday dieters. And besides losing more weight (11 versus eight pounds), the two-day-a-weekers also lost more body fat, becoming lighter and leaner.

What was even more intriguing was that just cutting carbs on those two days—and not counting overall calories—was as effective as intermittent fasting. In fact, neither group tended to overeat on days when they weren't, respectively, cutting carbs or fasting.

Could it really be that easy to lose weight—just cut carbs two days a week? Yes, it could—because carbs do some very particular things to the brain.

THE CARB-BRAIN-APPETITE CONNECTION

When you eat a lot of carbohydrates, especially simple starches and sugars, it can literally damage neurons in the hypothalamus, a part of the brain that helps regulate appetite. The nerve cells in the hypothalamus become surrounded by inflammatory cells, and then they don't function as well as they should.

Quality of fat matters, too. In animal studies, for example, high-saturated-fat diets—the kind of fats that are very prevalent in a typical Western diet—have also been shown to disrupt the appetite-signaling pathways. So the emphasis on healthy, mostly unsaturated fats in the diet may contribute to its effectiveness.

In effect, the brain becomes resistant to input from hormones, including leptin and ghrelin, which play key roles in regulating appetite. The hypothalamus mistakenly sends out signals to eat more. You feel hungrier, you eat more, and you create more damage—and so on.

The secret of the two-day-a-week carb-cutting diet is that the hunger-signaling pathway can be "reset" by giving the damaged neurons a break by cutting carbs, which also tends to cut calories, and by your eating healthy polyunsaturated and monounsaturated fats. When the oxidative load that's hitting those nerves decreases, the whole system can work much better.

That explains why people on this diet don't go crazy with overeating on their "off diet" days. Even after just one day of going very low carbohydrate, the signaling system between the appetite hormones and the hypothalamus works much more efficiently. That effect can last for a few days.

READY TO TRY THE INTERMITTENT LOW-CARB DIET?

In our clinical experience, we have found that there is no need to avoid carbohydrates two days in a row. We tell dieters that they are free to restrict their carbohydrates on any two days of the week.

For a lot of people, just eliminating bread, pasta and sweets (sugars are carbs) gets most of the job done. *But for a little more detail, here's a sample one-day low-carb menu…*

●**Breakfast.** Two or three eggs with spinach and mozzarella cheese, made with one teaspoon of oil.

●**Lunch.** A large vegetable salad with one-third of an avocado, five or more ounces of chicken or grilled shrimp or cheese, and one or two tablespoons of Italian dressing.

●**Snack.** Six to eight ounces of Greek yogurt (0% to 2% fat) with eight walnut halves.

●**Dinner.** Five or more ounces of grilled poultry, fish or red meat, roasted vegetables (such as cauliflower, Brussels sprouts or broccoli) with one or two tablespoons of olive oil, a tossed salad with one tablespoon of oil-and-vinegar and one cup of berries.

True, there's no linguine with clam sauce…no bread-and-jam. But it's only for two days a week—and on the other five days, you may find that you're not craving carbs as much as you do now. You're almost sure to lose weight.

How to Lose 12 Pounds… in Just 17 Days

Mike Moreno, MD, practices family medicine in San Diego, where he is on the board of the San Diego chapter of the American Academy of Family Physicians. Dr. Moreno is the author of *The 17-Day Diet.* DrMikeDiet.com

According to conventional wisdom, anyone who loses weight rapidly (more than a pound or two a week) will invariably regain the lost pounds because the diet will be too strict to maintain. But some researchers are now finding evidence that slow isn't necessarily better when it comes to weight loss.

New research: A 2010 study in the International *Journal of Behavioral Medicine* analyzed data from 262 middle-aged obese women.

Result: The fast weight losers dropped more pounds overall and maintained their weight loss longer than the gradual weight losers.

Good news: With rapid weight loss, most people can boost their metabolism, combat fat storage and help prevent obesity-related diseases, such as diabetes and certain types of cancer—all without feeling deprived of satisfying food.

Sound impossible? I've seen thousands of people lose weight by following what I call the *17 Day Diet.**

Why 17 days? This is roughly the amount of time it takes for your body's metabolism to adapt to a change in calories. By varying your diet at 17-day intervals, you "trick" your metabolism into functioning at its maximum efficiency to help you reach your target weight. *Four simple cycles to follow…*

*Be sure to check with your doctor before you start this or any other weight-loss program.

CYCLE 1: Cleanse Your System

For the first 17 days, the goal is to "cleanse" your system by eating lots of lean protein, such as poultry and fish. Lean protein requires more energy to digest than carbohydrates, so it burns additional calories and helps control your blood sugar. Because it's satisfying, protein also fights food cravings.

During this cycle, you're also allowed as many vegetables as you like. You will need to temporarily cut out all grains, potatoes, pasta and desserts. Doing this helps you avoid the dramatic fluctuations in blood sugar that fuel binge eating.

Note: Use olive oil for cooking during this cycle.

Fruit is allowed but only before 2 pm—when sugar (including natural sugar from fruit) is less likely to be stored as fat.

Good fruit choices: Apples, berries, oranges, pears, plums and red grapes. These fruits are relatively low in sugar and high in fiber, which slows digestion and helps you feel full. Avoid bananas and pineapple—both contain too much natural sugar.

During this 17-day cycle, people lose an average of 10 to 12 pounds (depending on their starting weights) while eating three to four meals daily plus snacks (for a total of 1,300 calories per day for men and women). Some of this weight loss will be due to water loss—but this is also beneficial because fluid retention can contribute to fatigue.

Sample day's meals: Breakfast—two scrambled egg whites…one-half grapefruit or other fresh fruit…one cup green tea. Lunch—fish, poultry or eggs…vegetables…one cup green tea. Dinner—fish or chicken…vegetables…one cup green tea. Snack—raw, cut-up veggies.

CYCLE 2: Reset Your Metabolism

During the second 17-day cycle, the goal is to reset the metabolism by alternating higher calorie intake (1,500 to 1,700) on even days with lower calorie intake (1,300) on odd days. Switching back and forth stimulates fat burning because it prevents your body from adapting to a certain level of daily calories.

Slow-digesting complex carbs, such as oatmeal, sweet potatoes and brown rice, are reintroduced during this cycle.

CYCLE 3: Good Eating Habits

By now, a little more than a month since you started, your body has undergone a significant metabolic shift that will allow you to reintroduce moderate portions—and no more than two to three servings per day before 2 pm—of carbohydrates such as whole-grain breads and pastas that may have made you feel sluggish or heavy before.

If you've reached your target weight, you may proceed to cycle 4, the maintenance cycle. If not, be sure to focus on portion control and continue to emphasize lean protein and nonstarchy vegetables, limiting carbohydrates after 2 pm until you reach cycle 4.

CYCLE 4: Weight Maintenance

During this cycle, which is followed indefinitely to maintain your weight loss, you are more strict with yourself throughout the workweek but relax your eating habits on the weekends. From 6 pm Friday to 6 pm Sunday, you can enjoy your favorite indulgences, such as pizza or hamburgers, as long as you maintain portion control and enjoy no more than three indulgences over a single weekend. This approach allows you to eat some favorite foods in moderation while also giving your metabolism the variety it needs to function efficiently.

Rule of thumb: Weigh yourself on weekends. If you gain five pounds or more over a week's time, return to any of the earlier cycles.

OTHER SECRETS TO WEIGHT LOSS

In addition to following the cycles described earlier…

•**Get more probiotics.** New research suggests that people who have an overabundance of "bad" bacteria in the intestinal tract are more susceptible to weight gain. But healthful bacteria, known as probiotics (found in such foods as certain yogurts, sauerkraut and miso soup), control the proliferation of bad bacteria and help fight infection—and ensure that your metabolism functions effectively.

My advice: Aim to consume two daily servings of foods containing probiotics.

Examples of one probiotic serving: Six ounces of fat-free plain yogurt or one-half cup of Breakstone LiveActive cottage cheese (which includes added probiotics).

Or: Take probiotic supplements, following label instructions.

•**Don't forget to exercise.** To avoid getting run down while you're scaling back on calories (especially the first few days of cycle 1), do only 15 to 20 minutes of walking a day.

Thereafter, aim for at least 30 minutes of aerobic exercise five days a week. Walking is a good choice, as is jogging, swimming, or using a stationary bicycle or an elliptical machine. For strength training, make the exercises as aerobic as possible using lighter weights and more repetitions.

Getting Off the Plateau

Mike Moreno, MD, a family physician based in San Diego and author of *The 17-Day Diet*. DrMikeDiet.com

If you've been dieting and hit a plateau in your weight loss, make a few changes in your exercise routine to "surprise" your body's metabolism. Also, stay hydrated—drink six to eight eight-ounce glasses of water a day, and limit alcohol and caffeine. Although fruit is a good source of vitamins, minerals and fiber, it can be high in sugar and other carbs. Limit fruit to two pieces each day. Check your portion sizes—no more than five ounces each of protein and whole grains a day for women ages 31 and older and six ounces each for men ages 31 and older. A serving is about the size of your palm.

Never eat carbs (including fruit) after 2 pm, since it is harder for your body to burn them off. For dinner, emphasize lean protein and vegetables.

And keep moving! You need at least 30 minutes of exercise every day, but the more you do, the more weight you will lose. Take the stairs, walk after lunch and dinner and/or try a new form of exercise, such as water aerobics or karate, to get other muscles moving.

For Lifelong Weight Control, Walking Beats the Gym

Study titled "Do All Activities "Weigh" Equally? How Different Physical Activities Differ as Predictors of Weight" by researchers at London School of Economics, School of Economics, University of Queensland, Australia and Indian Institute of Technology Kanpur, India, published in *Risk Analysis.*

When it comes to keeping your body weight in check, brisk walking almost every day is proving to be the best exercise.

In an analysis of a large British multiyear survey, men who engaged in brisk walking for 30 minutes or more a day about five days a week weighed about six pounds less—and women about 11 pounds less—than their sedentary counterparts.

By contrast, those who went to the gym or played sports just as frequently as the walkers didn't fare as well. Compared to the sedentary types, men weighed just 1.8 pounds less and women about six pounds less. Other activities done for the same time/frequency—heavy housework (moving furniture, walking with heavy shopping bags, scrubbing floors) or manual activities (digging, chopping wood, moving heavy loads)—were only weakly linked to a lower body weight.

It's just an association, not proof, but the research does suggest that the one exercise we can do almost anywhere, almost any time, for free, is a good lifelong defense against weight gain.

The Right Way to Walk for Weight Loss

Susan Besser, MD, board-certified family physician, Mercy Personal Physicians, Baltimore.

Walking to lose weight is so common that you'd think all you need to do is, well, walk to lose weight. Not true! Plenty of people walk and never see the results they expect. But we know the walking plan that will let you meet—and maintain—your weight goals…

How long to walk: The goal for losing weight is at least three hours of walking per week. Why? A review of 22 studies on walking for weight loss found that was the minimum number to decrease fat and lose, on average, 10 pounds over 12 to 16 weeks. While that's not even one pound lost per week, it's noticeable, and it was all due to the walking—in these studies, there were no changes to the participants' diets. If you walk and cut calories, you can lose weight faster. And if you walk more than three hours per week—ditto.

As you lose weight, your metabolism may slow, and you'll have to work harder to maintain the weight loss. In fact, try increasing your walking to five hours per week once you've reached your weight goal in order to keep the weight from coming back. You can break that up any way you like, such as five 60 minute-walks or even daily nuggets of 10-minutes six times a day.

How often to walk: If the only way you can fit in at least three hours a week is to walk, say, an hour and a half on Tuesdays and Thursdays, that's much better than nothing. But it's better by far to walk at least five days every week.

The reason: By walking regularly, you will more effectively raise your level of fitness.

And among the many benefits of being fit is this particular winner: A fit body tends to have more muscle, and muscle burns more calories than fat.

How fast to walk: Walk briskly—that means covering a mile in 15 minutes. Work up to that pace if you need to.

Here's an easy way to tell if you're going fast enough for your ability: You should be able to have a conversation while walking but not whistle or sing. And do the whistle test every two weeks or so. It will let you know if you're walking at a pace that's brisk enough to keep losing weight—speed up if whistling's a breeze.

To stay motivated, vary your walking route at least every two weeks. Challenge yourself periodically by walking additional hills or going a longer distance in the same amount of time.

Burn 100 Calories or More in 15 Minutes or Less

Lucas J. Carr, PhD, assistant professor in the department of kinesiology at the College of Health and Human Performance of East Carolina University in Greenville, North Carolina.

Didn't really need that extra handful of nuts or that scoop of frozen yogurt? Now how are you going to work off those surplus calories—and do it fast enough to fit into your super-busy schedules?

Lucas J. Carr, PhD, an assistant professor in the department of kinesiology at East Carolina University, describes ideas on how to burn off 100 calories or so in just 10 to 15 minutes…

● **Aerobic dancing of any type**—for instance, try belly dancing (take lessons so you'll be ready when you need it!).

● **Bicycling at a moderate intensity (12 mph).** You can hit the gym for some quick stationary cycling…or incorporate a real bike ride into your daily routine.

● **Calisthenics**—push-ups, pull-ups, jumping jacks—going full bore, like you used to in school. These can be done at home or even in the office.

● **Mowing the lawn** (with a push mower, not a ride-on) or raking leaves.

● **Playing basketball, tennis or even touch football** (no resting!).

● **Stair-climbing**—on a stair-step machine or a handy staircase at home or work.

● **Walking briskly at a continuous 4.5-mph pace**—do this first on a treadmill to see how fast this is.

● **Zumba, kickboxing or whatever other get-your-heart-racing moves you know and love from the gym.**

Simple Diet Strategies to Use with Your Workout

Leslie Bonci, MPH, RD, CSSD, LDN, owner of the Pittsburg-based nutrition consulting company Active Eating Advice by Leslie.

●**Have a small snack before exercising.** If you exercise on a completely empty stomach, your blood sugar will drop and you will feel hungrier afterward…and will be more likely to overeat.

●**Keep a food diary before eating, not after.** Writing down what you plan to eat encourages you to decide whether you are really making good food choices.

●**When you have a full meal, eat it soon after your workout.** People served 15 to 30 minutes after exercise tend to eat less than those who wait an hour or more for food.

●**Drink water regularly.** Water drinkers eat almost 200 fewer calories a day than people who drink only coffee, tea or soda.

The On-Again, Off-Again Diet That Works

Nuala Byrne, PhD, head of the University of Tasmania School of Health Sciences, researcher and coauthor of the study "Intermittent Energy Restriction Improves Weight Loss Efficiency in Obese Men: the MATADOR Study," published in *International Journal of Obesity.*

Do you feel that on-again, off-again dieting has become a way of life…with no pounds lost despite all your hard work? According to a new study, a purposeful twist on behavior that you likely see as dieting failure could be the key to weight loss—and weight loss that sticks!

The concept is surprising and surprisingly simple: Instead of trying to stay on a restrictive diet for a long stretch of time, follow a two-week on, two-week off plan. Called intermittent dieting, it involves alternating between distinct periods of weight loss and weight maintenance, each tied to a certain number of calories (yes, there's

a slight catch—more on that below), until you reach your goal.

The study: Forty-seven obese men, ages 25 to 54, participated in a study done at the University of Tasmania. The researchers separated them into two groups of similar weight loss needs. Half dieted for 16 weeks straight, reducing their normal calorie intake by one third during that time, and then they stopped dieting. The other half dieted during 16 weeks, reducing their normal calorie intake by the same amount (one third)—but it wasn't for 16 weeks straight. Instead, they dieted for two weeks, stopped dieting for two weeks, dieted again for two weeks, and kept repeating that pattern for a total of 30 weeks.

The results: After their 16 net weeks of dieting (spread out over 30 weeks), the intermittent dieters not only lost nearly 50% more weight than the continuous dieters did after their constant 16 weeks —they also lost more fat and were more successful at keeping weight off. The overall process was longer, but for the same 16 diet weeks both groups followed in total, the intermittent dieters saw better results. What's more, when researchers checked in with participants six months after dieting ended, the intermittent dieters had kept off more of the lost weight—almost 18 pounds more net loss, on average, from the start of the diet—than the continuous dieters. The researchers are currently testing the same intermittent dieting method on women, to see if it will work as well.

Now, before you stock up on ice cream and chocolate syrup for your next "two weeks off," know that the two-week diet breaks aren't meant to be a free-for-all—that's what causes true yo-yo dieting—but rather a careful maintenance period. During their off weeks, study participants divided maintenance calories according to typical dietary guidelines—25% to 30% of calories came from fat, 15% to 20% from protein, and 50% to 60% from carbohydrates…and just enough calories to maintain their weight—meaning that the number of calories eaten was the same as calories burned.

But even so, how could going off and on a diet lead to greater weight loss and fat loss than continuously dieting?

The body's metabolic processes and the human psyche both play a role. Even if you follow a conventional diet to the letter, the act of dieting alters a series of biological processes in your body, leading to slower weight loss over time and even potential weight gain. Simply put, your metabolism starts to work against you when you're on a diet. This is because calorie restriction causes what is referred to as the "famine reaction," a natural survival mechanism to slow weight loss when your food supply is reduced, left over from the hunter-gatherer days. Your metabolism overrides your own intentions, slowing down to conserve energy by burning fewer calories and storing food as fat because it thinks you're being starved by forces beyond your control.

The famine reaction can also result in an increased appetite—that explains why you might be disproportionately hungry when on a diet. But by taking a dieting hiatus every two weeks, you outsmart your body and prevent metabolism slowdown and everything that goes with it.

Another plus: Trying to stick to a strict diet—with no end in sight—is also mentally taxing. Taking a diet break every two weeks gives your mind a break from the stress of calorie restriction.

Here's how make a two-week-on, two-week-off diet work for you…

●**Do the math.** If you want to give this plan a go, your first step is to calculate how many calories your body needs to maintain your current weight, your daily "maintenance number"—and then reduce that number by one-third for the two-week periods you'll be dieting. Then, for each two-week break from dieting, increase your calories to your maintenance number minus 100 or so calories (to account for the weight loss of the previous two diet weeks). Keep repeating the cycle. The NIH provides a free body-weight planner that will help you figure out personalized calorie and exercise plans to reach your goal weight. Go to NIDDK.nih.gov/bwp.

● **Add exercise.** The study didn't measure physical activity, but dieters tend to do less physical movement across the day—such as walking and doing chores—than non-dieters. Being more active could enhance results.

●**Keep a food journal.** As with any diet, you might feel hungry and experience food cravings during each two weeks of calorie restriction. Logging these cravings can help you notice patterns, such as at what times of the day they normally occur, so that you can set aside some of your calories for then or even restructure your meals at these times when appropriate.

●**Up your protein.** Although more research is needed on this phenomenon, it's possible that increasing one's intake of protein above the USDA recommended daily allowance of roughly 48 grams for women and 68 grams for men during calorie-restriction weeks could help with weight loss. In general, high-protein foods take more work to digest and metabolize than carbohydrates, which means it takes more calories for your body to process them…providing more time before you're hungry again. Healthful protein sources include eggs, nuts, fish and lean meats.

Food-Free Stress Relief

Susan Albers, PsyD, psychologist, Cleveland Clinic, Wooster, Ohio. Dr. Albers specializes in eating issues, weight loss, body image concerns and mindfulness, and is the author of many books including *50 Ways to Soothe Yourself Without Food.* EatingMindfully.com.

Guess how much of the overeating people do is triggered by emotions—10%? 25%? Actually, it's about 75%, experts estimate. Considering how stressed out people today tend to feel, it's no wonder so many Americans are overweight!

Though macaroni and cheese, cake and ice cream, chips and other "comfort foods" may provide a temporary sense of relief from stress, in the long run, overindulging only makes you feel worse about yourself and your situation…and over time, the extra weight it brings can do serious damage to your health.

Fortunately, there are many enjoyable and effective ways to calm down that have nothing to do with eating. So whenever you feel tempted to eat, first ask yourself whether you are truly physically hungry. If the honest answer is no, try one of these tactics instead.

Do-anywhere techniques for when you're out and about…

●**Adopt a "blanket substitute."** You know Linus from the comic strip Peanuts? He uses his beloved blanket as a source of comfort whenever he feels overwhelmed or anxious. Of course, you're not going to drag a blankie around, but you can carry a small object—a smooth stone, a silk handkerchief—in your pocket or purse. When you feel the urge to eat emotionally, close your eyes for a moment and rub your fingers across the object, finding comfort in its familiar feel. This will help you not reach for food right away…and there's a good chance that the impulse to eat will pass.

●**Take a few cleansing breaths.** Inhale slowly and deeply through your nose…hold for a few seconds…then purse your lips and exhale through your mouth in short bursts as you imagine all your toxic thoughts or worries falling into a heap on the floor. This technique has been proven to calm the body and mind.

●**Go for a stroll.** This is not a power walk, and it isn't about burning calories or trying to outpace your cravings. Rather, it's a deliberate opportunity to notice and enjoy the scenery…the people…the sounds…the scents all around you. As you take time to fully experience the sensations evoked by your surroundings, thoughts of food will naturally be forgotten (provided you're not strolling past a row of restaurants, of course!). Though a 20-minute walk is ideal for curbing cravings, research indicates, even a quick five-minute stroll should help.

At-home tactics that can keep you from raiding the fridge…

●**Clean house.** It doesn't matter what you clean—the garage, the attic, your office, a closet (though the kitchen would not be your best bet)—because your actual goal is to scrub away stress. Try cleaning for 10 minutes, then see whether the urge to nosh has abated. If it hasn't, scrub for another three minutes.

Bonus: When you're done, your well-deserved sense of accomplishment will help keep comfort food cravings at bay.

●**Have a snooze.** Sleep-deprived people tend to eat more, probably in an attempt to increase energy levels. Ask yourself whether what your body really needs is a rejuvenating rest, and if the answer is yes, allow yourself a 30-minute nap. When you get up, chances are good that you'll no longer feel the immediate need to eat.

●**Take up a hobby that uses your hands.** Whittling, knitting, model building, painting and drawing are all good examples. Not only do they keep your hands busy so you can't reach for food, the hand movements themselves relieve tension…and your brain is pleasantly engaged, so you're not thinking about eating. Picking up your project-in-progress whenever the desire to comfort yourself with food arises will help you get through those moments of temptation…picking it up at other times will ease your stress level overall, reducing the likelihood of future food cravings.

●**Weed your garden.** Sure, digging in the dirt is good exercise…but more importantly, gardening helps to ease your mind, especially when you're stressed or angry. As you pull up each weed, imagine that you're pulling your negative or anxiety-provoking thoughts right out of your mind—and casting them away for good.

Your Lucky 13—The Best Secrets for Losing Weight Without Feeling Hungry!

Keith-Thomas Ayoob, EdD, RD, a nutritionist and associate clinical professor, Department of Pediatrics, at Albert Einstein College of Medicine, Bronx, New York. He is coauthor of *The Uncle Sam Diet: The 4-Week Eating Plan for a Thinner, Healthier America.*

When your stomach is sending out insistent, incessant "feed me!" messages, it's almost impossible to stick to a strict diet.

That's why the real key to weight-loss success is to shut down hunger and short-circuit food cravings—because then it is easier to cut down on calories. *Here are 13 simple strategies for slimming down without making yourself feel deprived*…

1. Have two servings of protein at breakfast. Proteins are natural appetite suppressants. This means that even if eating more protein ups your usual morning calorie count, you will feel fuller longer—so over the course of the day, you'll wind up eating less.

Breakfast combinations: An egg scrambled with an ounce of shredded cheese…or eight ounces of low-fat yogurt mixed with an ounce of slivered almonds. Do not just have coffee for breakfast—you'll feel ravenous later.

2. At lunch and dinner, consume items in order of least-to-most calories. Start the meal with your salad and vegetables…eat the grains next…and then work your way around the plate to the heavier foods, such as meat. By the time you get there, you're already starting to feel full—so it is easier to control your portions of those calorie-dense items.

Interactive tool: Gauge proper portion sizes based on your weight, height and exercise level at ChooseMyPlate.gov.

3. Don't think of snacking as cheating. Wisely chosen snacks keep hunger pangs at bay, so you won't overindulge later in the day. Have a midafternoon and an evening snack every day, combining two food groups.

Examples: Pair a vegetable with a whole grain (hummus or salsa with whole-wheat pita or crackers)…or pair fruit with dairy (pineapple with low-fat cottage cheese, a smoothie made with blueberries and low-fat yogurt). Prepare healthful snacks ahead of time so you'll reach for them—not candy or chips—when your stomach grumbles.

4. Choose foods that you can't eat quickly. Labor-intensive foods—pistachios in the shell, edamame in the pod, peel-and-eat shrimp—force you to savor each bite instead of shoveling everything down. This leisurely pace fools your brain into thinking that you're consuming much more than you actually are.

5. Drink water to squelch the munchies. People often mistake thirst for hunger—so downing eight ounces of water may quickly quell food cravings.

Also helpful: Make sure your diet includes high-water–content foods—cucumbers, lettuce, zucchini…oranges, peaches, strawberries, watermelon…low-fat broth and tomato-based soups.

6. Cut down on caffeine. Yes, caffeine gives a short-term energy buzz—but it also contributes to hunger.

Reason: Caffeine stimulates insulin secretion…which reduces blood sugar…which tells your brain that it's time to eat. Limit caffeinated coffee, tea and cola to two cups daily, consumed with meals, to see if this eases food cravings. Cut back further if you have insomnia.

7. Chew sugarless cinnamon gum. Of course, when there's gum in your mouth, you won't be tempted to put food in there, too—but there's more to this strategy. Chewing gum helps improve mental focus, so that you stay engaged in your activity and are less apt to hear the call of the refrigerator. Also, chewing gum helps relieve the stress that can lead to overeating. Why choose cinnamon? It retains its flavor longest.

8. Fill up on fiber. Soluble and insoluble fibers hold water and expand in your stomach, making you feel fuller longer.

Daily goals: Four cups of fruits and vegetables (assuming foods are small, such as berries, or chopped)…one-half cup of beans (which are highly nutritious yet underappreciated) or other legumes…and three servings of whole grains (brown rice, oatmeal, whole-wheat bread).

Party trick: Eat half an oat-bran muffin before you go out. Those 100 calories will save you hundreds more because you'll feel less enticed by the hors d'oeuvres.

9. Indulge in chocolate for dessert. One ounce of dark chocolate with 70% or more cocoa content has only about 150 calories. Savor it with a cup of decaf coffee or herbal tea—its big taste belies its relatively modest calorie count.

10. Fool the hunger hormone. Ghrelin, a hormone that stimulates hunger, drops about a half-hour after you eat—so nibble on a half-ounce of nutrient-rich nuts 30 minutes before dinner to make it easier to keep meal portions modest. If you're going out, carry nuts in your purse. (Recycle an Altoids mint tin—it's the perfect size for your portable nut stash.)

11. Shake your booty—or just take a brisk walk. Aerobic exercise lowers hunger-triggering ghrelin…increases levels of the appetite-suppressing hormone peptide YY…burns calories…and relieves stress.

Goal: At least 30 minutes of aerobic exercise (such as quick-paced walking) every day.

12. Retrain your palate. When you habitually consume lots of sugar, salt or fat, your taste buds become desensitized. Like addicts, they need a bigger and bigger "fix" to feel satisfied. But when you cut back on those three troublemakers, within a few weeks you regain the ability to detect and enjoy subtler flavors—and sugary, salty and fatty foods lose their appeal.

13. Move up your bedtime. People who sleep less than five hours a night have higher ghrelin levels—causing them to feel near-constant hunger. Sleeping for about eight hours per night helps normalize ghrelin levels. Also, fatigue increases stress and impairs judgment—so by getting more rest, you become better able to make sensible decisions about food.

Bonus: An early bedtime means that you won't be tempted to have a midnight snack, so you're likely to wake up weighing less—and feeling proud.

The Pleasurable Way to Lose Weight

Jena la Flamme, founder of Pleasurable Weight Loss and Madison Park Wellness in New York City, is a graduate of the Institute for the Psychology of Eating and the Institute for Integrative Nutrition. PleasurableWeightLoss.com

*F*ill in the blank: Successful dieting is about __ _____. Many of us would probably write willpower, discipline or saying no…but the best choice might be sensuality.

An appealing and effortless approach to weight control is possible, according to Jena la Flamme, founder of Pleasurable Weight Loss in New York City, who specializes in the psychology of eating. It's all about being attuned to your body's sensations and internal signals, she explained—because when that happens, you don't need to count calories or analyze what you eat in order to achieve and maintain a healthy weight.

Recent research supports the notion. For instance, a New Zealand study of 2,500 middle-aged women found that the more aware and responsive women were to their own bodies' signals of hunger and fullness, the lower their body mass index (BMI) was likely to be.

People think that pleasure is the problem when it comes to weight loss. They figure, "I'm having too much pleasure with food, therefore I'm gaining weight." But actually, it's the other way around, because your body is wired to need pleasure. So when you don't get enough pleasure—from the foods you choose and from things other than food—you're likely to overeat in compensation. That's when weight becomes a problem.

What this means: The more pleasure you can find in your food and in other areas of life, the easier it will be for your body to feel satisfied. You'll find that you take in fewer calories automatically, without needing to impose restrictions on yourself. Thus your pleasure increases even as your weight decreases.

When la Flamme discovered this for herself nine years ago, it was the end of her long-term battle with compulsive eating, excessive weight gain, constant fatigue, recurrent constipation and bloating. Since then, she has helped thousands of other women fill their lives with pleasure while dropping unwanted pounds.

Intrigued? Try these five easy steps…

1. Consider what you really want to eat. When you choose the food that will give you the most pleasure, you need less of it as a result. For example, a few spoonfuls of top-quality ice cream that is thoroughly enjoyed, without guilt, will be more satisfying and less fattening than a giant bowlful of fat-free, taste-free, fake "frozen dessert" eaten in a guilty rush. Treat yourself to the foods you truly enjoy and stay present to the pleasure each bite gives you. A week, a month or even a year later, you'll look back and remember how much you enjoyed them—and you'll have lost weight.

2. Before your first bite, take five slow, deep breaths to "charge" your metabolism. The idea is to consciously shift yourself into a more relaxed state. "Stress activates a response in the body whereby digestion is impaired, metabolism becomes sluggish and fat is stored rather than burned," la Flamme explained. You can counteract that by triggering the relaxation response. Think of your metabolism as a fire. Use your breath like a bellows, blowing air on your metabolism to stoke your digestive fire. This brightens your calorie-burning efficiency.

3. Actively engage all your senses in the experience of eating. This is the opposite of the mindless low-pleasure, high-volume eating that many people automatically slip into. Make a point of noticing the appealing appearance of your food…breathe in its unique aroma…revel in its texture on your lips and tongue…and ponder with appreciation the taste of each bite. When you're truly seeing, smelling, feeling and tasting your food, you activate the hormone *cholecystokinin*, which I call the "satisfaction molecule." It enhances your digestion and lets you know when you're full. Tuning into that feeling of fullness and satisfaction, you gain an intuitive sense of the portions that suit your needs. Soon you will find that you simply stop eating when you're no longer hungry, without ever feeling deprived. Weight loss will follow!

4. Destress with tea. If you do feel tempted to eat even when you know you're no longer hungry, stress is probably to blame. A nice soak in a hot tub is a good way to calm down, but of course you can't do that when you're out and about.

Convenient: Create a pleasure-filled ritual around a cup of regular or herbal tea. As you focus on the soothing warmth of the mug in your hands and the tea's complex fragrance and flavor, your cares and cravings will slip away.

5. Also seek out sensual rewards that don't revolve around eating. We are inherently sensual creatures, and if we don't make space for sensuality in other areas of our lives, then food fills the gap. So rather than relying on food as your sole sensory pleasure, find additional ways to satisfy your senses. Listen closely to a stirring piece of music…admire each detail of a beautifully decorated room…sniff appreciatively when you're near a fragrant bouquet of flowers…delight in the softness of the fabric caressing your skin. When you consciously take note of such things, food loses its power to control you and becomes just one more source of enjoyment amidst the myriad pleasures that surround you.

The 30-Second Food-Craving Cure

Study titled "Effects of simple distraction tasks on self-induced food cravings in men and women with grade 3 obesity" presented at the Obesity Week 2014 annual meeting of The Obesity Society.
Dawn Jackson Blatner, RDN, a registered dietitian nutritionist, certified specialist in sports dietetics and nutrition consultant for the Chicago Cubs, based in Chicago, and author of *The Flexitarian Diet.*

Got those late-afternoon munchies? Or late-night cravings? It can be tough to resist overeating between meals when mouthwatering images are so intense in your mind.

The quick and easy solution is at your fingertips…

What to do: Tap your head! With either index finger, tap your forehead for 30 seconds.

What it does: This simple motion will reduce the intensity of your food cravings. In a study of 55 obese people at Mount Sinai-St. Luke's Weight Loss Program in New York City, it was the most successful "distraction" tactic…better than tapping your toes, tapping your ear or staring at a blank wall (the control group). All worked, but forehead tapping was the most effective.

How it works: No one knows for sure. But it's possible that simply distracting yourself can be a brief time-out that lets your emotional urges calm down…plus, forehead tapping might stimulate an acupressure region that reduces stress hormone levels.

Easier Than a Diet…and Great for Your Health—Intermittent Fasting

Tina Marinaccio, RDN, integrative registered dietitian nutritionist and adjunct professor in clinical nutrition and food studies at Montclair State University in New Jersey. She leads the nutrition element of Dr. Dean Ornish's Program for Reversing Heart Disease. TinaMarinaccio.com

---

I am the first to admit that fasting sounds even worse than dieting. But some kinds of fasting can be easier than dieting—and have benefits that go well beyond weight loss. In fact, even people who are not overweight can get amazing benefits from fasting, including healthier hearts, stronger muscles and clearer thinking.

The technical term for what I'm talking about is "intermittent fasting," which means fasting for short periods—sometimes, just 12 hours—on a regular basis. Most intermittent-fast techniques are not daily, and many allow for some calories even on "fast" days. This is definitely not a hunger strike! Some researchers believe that these intermittent fasts are easier to maintain than daily "caloric restriction"—aka traditional dieting, which basically requires that you eat less than you want every single day forever. Intrigued? *Here's more on the benefits of intermittent fasting and how you could easily try it…*

WHY INTERMITTENT FASTING IS SO HEALTHY

Studies have shown that intermittent fasting can help people lose weight without losing muscle. Maintaining muscle is key to keeping weight off and healthy aging. People on intermittent fasts find it easier to control their appetite even on non-fasting days.

One reason: They are producing less insulin, a key "hunger hormone."

But there are many more benefits. These kinds of fasts have been shown to reduce blood pressure…

reduce blood glucose levels and improve insulin sensitivity…reduce levels of triglycerides (blood fats) and improve the cholesterol profile…reduce inflammation…enhance muscle endurance…and even improve learning and memory. In animal studies, intermittent fasting can reverse type 2 diabetes, slow the progression of cardiovascular disease and prolong life.

Why is this kind of fasting so good for the body? One hypothesis is that our gut biome—the mix of gastrointestinal bacteria that's key to health—needs a rest to function optimally. In addition, fasting has been shown to help the body get rid of damaged cells and regenerate healthy new ones. Humans likely evolved eating this way—food was scarce, and we couldn't spend every day eating and snacking every few hours like we can now. Periodic fasting respects—maybe even resets—our internal body clocks.

CHOOSING A WAY TO FAST

The best fast is the one that fits into your lifestyle. *Here are three options supported by scientific evidence…*

● **Time-restricted eating.** This is the easiest fast to pull off. Every day, you simply restrict eating to a specific stretch of the day. You'll get the most benefits by limiting yourself to eating during just an eight-hour stretch—say, 10 am to 6 pm. But time-restricted eating is something you can ease into—for example, by restricting your eating to 12 hours…and then gradually scaling back to eight hours. (See page 304, "The 8-Hour Diet," for more information.)

Eating at night, in particular, interferes with the body's natural day-night cycle, disrupting hormones in a way that favors weight gain. And there's psychology—choosing an endpoint to the day's eating helps eliminate nighttime eating.

Let's face it: No one is sitting in front of the TV at night eating carrot sticks. It's more likely to be ice cream or chips.

Tip: Get most of your calories early in the day, meaning you eat a big breakfast and a smaller lunch and dinner. It's fine to eat breakfast several hours after you wake up—that's healthy as long as it's not paired with late-night eating.

•**Periodic fasting.** On two consecutive days, you cut way back on calories—by 75%. The rest of the week, you eat in a normal fashion. The popular 5:2 Diet is an example of this approach.

•**Alternate-day fasting.** In this approach, you alternate days when you restrict calories—to perhaps 500 calories for the day—with days when you eat a normal, healthy diet. This way of fasting is one day on, one day off. It's effective, but some people find that they are too hungry on fasting days to sustain it.

Tip for periodic or alternate-day fasting: To meet your calorie goal and assure good nutrition on partial-fast days, make protein shakes with fruit and some form of healthy fat, such as ground flax or a no-sugar-added nut butter. A low-sugar plant-protein powder serves as the base. Two brands I like are Vega and Kashi GoLean (I'm fond of the Vanilla Vinyasa flavor).

Caution: Before you start any fast, discuss it with your health-care provider. That's especially important if you have a medical condition. For example, although fasting may help improve diabetes, people who take blood sugar–lowering agents need to be especially careful about low blood sugar. Plus, some medications need to be taken with food.

More tips for successful intermittent fasting…

•**See a registered dietitian (RD).** An RD can help you determine which of the eating patterns—if any—makes sense for you and help you put a plan into place. He/she can help you choose the most nutritious foods (especially important on days when you don't eat as much as you normally do)…and, if you need them, recommend nutritional supplements.

•**Be extra wary when you eat out on partial-fasting days.** Restaurants use more fat and sugar than you would at home, and portions are huge. It's easier to eat at home so that you know what you're taking in.

•**Consider professional metabolic testing.** How can you know what to eat to cut calories by, say, 75%? You start by calculating the calories you burn at rest—your resting metabolic rate, aka RMR—and then add everyday activities plus physical exercise. Online RMR calculators are notably inaccurate.

Better: An FDA-approved calorimeter, which measures your RMR when you breathe into it. These instruments are too expensive to make it worth buying one for home use, but many RDs have them in their offices.

•**"Cheat" with nonstarchy vegetables.** If you find yourself extra-hungry on a fasting day, don't suffer too much. The best way to "cheat" is with low-glycemic vegetables, many of which have lots of filling fiber and all of which have very little effect on blood sugar or insulin levels.

Examples: Salad greens, cruciferous vegetables (broccoli, cabbage, cauliflower, etc.), radishes, zucchini, summer squash, eggplant, tomatoes and mushrooms.

Bonus: These types of vegetables are especially good at feeding beneficial gut bacteria.

One caution, though: Don't pile on potatoes, winter squashes, corn, peas and the like—these are starchy vegetables that you shouldn't cheat with.

The 8-Hour Diet

Courtney M. Peterson, PhD, assistant professor, department of nutrition sciences at the University of Alabama at Birmingham.

Adena Zadourian, BS, clinical research coordinator in the department of medicine-cardiology at the University of California San Diego.

Could checking your watch instead of nutritional labels be the answer to losing weight, improving sleep, increasing energy and warding off chronic health conditions? That's been the promise of a diet strategy called time-restricted feeding or TRF, and now there's science behind it. It's a twist on fasting—you limit your eating to a set number of hours each day so that you are "fasting" during the other hours. And that period of fasting is longer than the amount of time most people tend to "fast" naturally each day—shortly before they go to bed and while they are sleeping.

This doesn't mean you will have carte blanche to binge during eating hours. What and how much you eat still matter, certainly for overall health reasons. TRF isn't meant to overcompensate for eating processed foods, for instance. Think of it as a beneficial addition to a healthy lifestyle or a simple, and quite clever, way to start a healthy lifestyle, says Adena Zadourian, clinical research coordinator at University of California San Diego, department of medicine-cardiology. In fact, even if all you do is change when you eat, you may still see benefits—that's because of your body's reaction to a longer time span without nutrients.

HOW TRF WORKS

Consuming food triggers the body's metabolism-digestion to start, Zadourian explains. When people are always eating, the body is constantly in digestion mode. But the digestive system was never meant to be "on" all the time. When you stop eating for a fairly long period each day—referred to as "intermittent fasting"—neuroendocrine hormones aren't signaled, so the metabolism-digestion mechanism isn't initiated. This gives the body a chance to rest from all the work it was previously doing to process food.

Practicing TRF is simple: Limit your eating to within a specific span of hours each day. Courtney M. Peterson, PhD, assistant professor in the department of nutrition sciences at University of Alabama at Birmingham, recommends "early TRF," or limiting eating to early in the day (with dinner by midafternoon) or to the middle of the day (with dinner by early evening). Such forms of TRF are based on the body's circadian system, the internal clock that influences everything from your sleep-wake cycle to eating habits to the release of hormones.

Work, play, family obligations—these can also influence when we eat or sleep, but they aren't always aligned with the body's natural timing for those activities, explains Zadourian, who is working on a three-year study of 150 firefighters to see whether TRF can improve their well-being. The theory is that intermittent fasting helps reset the body's clock to its natural rhythms.

There are many health benefits to the concept. Because your body is spending less time and energy digesting food, fasting gives the body more time to recycle damaged and worn-out tissues and to reduce a form of molecular damage called oxidative stress—in other words, time to rest, repair and rejuvenate, says Peterson. Her studies found that early TRF improves insulin sensitivity (the body's ability to process blood sugar), blood pressure, oxidative stress, hunger levels and fat-burning. Other research has found that it cuts diabetes risk (inflammation and oxidative stress directly increase blood sugar) and cardiovascular disease (caused by damaged blood vessels). Fasting also slows down the rate at which cells grow and divide, which reduces the risk for cancer. Studies done in the lab and with people have linked TRF with the prevention of digestive disorders, high cholesterol, liver disease and obesity.

And what about weight loss? In the first human study of early TRF, or eTRF, Peterson and her colleagues found that a daily 18-hour fast (yes, that means eating during a mere six hours a day, from 8 am to 2 pm) helped to keep appetite levels on an even keel throughout the day and to rev up fat-burning during the night. There were no hunger spikes that encourage unwanted eating and make it harder to stick to a weight loss diet. TRF also can boost metabolic flexibility, the body's ability to switch between burning fats and carbs, which is helpful for weight loss.

5 TIPS FOR TRYING TRF

Many people tend to eat at various times during a much larger chunk of the day—often about 12 to 14 hours, from breakfast at 7 am to an after-dinner snack at 9 pm. There's no doubt that cutting your daily chow time by a third or more can be a challenge. *These pointers from Peterson and Zadourian can help you stick with the plan…*

●**Start slowly.** Ease into a time-restricted diet to give your body time to adapt. Start by restricting eating to a 10-to-11-hour daily window. If you typically eat breakfast at 7 am, you'll have to shut off the kitchen lights by 5 pm or 6 pm. After two weeks, start shortening your eating period, scaling down to nine and then eight hours a day. (If you want to take the plunge and try a six-hour limit, you can, says Peterson, but she thinks that most of the benefits of TRF can be had with an eight-hour or nine-hour eating period.)

• **Find your own TRF "sweet spot."** There are variations on the TRF diet. For instance, during your daily fasting period, Peterson OKs consuming anything that has no calories—water, plain tea or coffee (but no cream, milk, sugar or honey…you get the idea) or sugarless gum. Zadourian, on the other hand, advises only water during the fasting times and suggests sipping hot water as a substitute for coffee or tea in the morning before you start eating.

Another difference concerns taking planned days off from the routine. Lab studies involving mice suggest that people will get nearly the same benefits in blood sugar control and cardiovascular health if they practice TRF only five days per week, says Peterson. This way, you can still enjoy going out to restaurants with others who aren't on TRF or entertaining in the evening at home. She generally advises that people experiment—after trying different eating periods for a while, pick the time frame that you can comfortably sustain for four to six days a week.

However, Zadourian suggests staying as consistent as possible with the eating time window and, rather than planning to take days off, thinking of off-days as things that happen on occasion (and are nothing to worry about).

• **Reframe your thinking.** If you want to stick with TRF, ban the idea of "falling off the wagon"—failing—from your mind. This is because it's bound to take trial and error to figure out how many hours you can go without eating each day without being unhappy.

• **Stock up on the right fuel.** Adapting to the no-eating period could make you physically uncomfortable beyond just hunger—for example, study participants have cited increased thirst and

headaches. Staying hydrated is key, so be sure to drink plenty of water, especially during your daily fasting period. What foods best work to prepare you for the daily fast? Scientists still are unsure, yet plenty of research shows that the super trio of healthful fats, fiber and protein can keep you fuller longer.

• **Track your experience.** Using a journal to log what and when you eat is a great way to measure your progress, reinforce good habits and stay motivated. Keep a written journal or consider participating in a study that gives you access to the free smartphone app MyCircadianClock developed by Satchin Panda Lab at the Salk Institute, MyCircadianClock.org. You'll be able to track your eating, sleeping, exercise and other activities and help scientists learn more about how circadian rhythms affect health.

The bottom line: While more research is needed, reducing your eating hours may help your waistline and your overall health.

Bonus: Fasting can remind us what it's actually like to feel satiated and to recognize real hunger cues as opposed to false ones—both crucial for a more mindful approach to eating.

Big Bellies Matter More Than Weight

Study titled "Normal-Weight Central Obesity: Implications for Total and Cardiovascular Mortality" by researchers at Mayo Clinic, Rochester, Minnesota, St. Anne's University Hospital Brno, Czech Republic and University of Ottawa Heart Institute, Ontario, published in *Annals of Internal Medicine.*

Mayo Clinic researchers examined data on about 15,000 adult men and women who were followed over 14 years. They had data not only on overweight/obesity as measured by the body mass index (BMI), but also waist-to-hip ratio, which measures how big your stomach is compared with your waist.

The healthiest combo, of course, was a normal weight and a flat stomach. But it's also possible for a normal weight man or woman to have a paunch—and some folks who are heavy carry their excess weight more on their backsides than on their bellies. *Here's where the results get interesting…*

•**Normal-weight men with big stomachs had twice the mortality risk of men who were overweight or obese but had flat stomachs.**

•**For women, those with normal weights but big stomachs were 40% more likely to die than overweight women with flat stomachs**—and 32% more likely to die than obese women with flat stomachs.

What's so bad about big bellies? A waist-to-hip ratio that's 0.85 or higher (for women) or 0.90 or higher (for men) is a sign of "central obesity"—the kind of fat that's inside the abdomen and other internal organs rather than just under the skin. This "visceral" fat accumulates around the pancreas, heart and other organs that aren't designed to store fat. That can lead to excess insulin, high blood sugar, high cholesterol and problems in the functioning of the heart. The result is an increased risk for heart disease, diabetes and other metabolic diseases.

Researchers have known about these increased risks of a big belly for a long time. But they thought it primarily a problem only if you were already overweight or obese. The new research suggests that a big belly is a serious problem whatever your weight.

To be sure, having a high waist-to-hip ratio is more likely if you are overweight or obese. Only 3% of women and 11% of men who were normal weight had central obesity, for example, compared to rates among the overweight of 12% (women) and 37% (men).

But it's clear that this is a risk factor that everyone who wants to live a long healthy life should pay attention to. Here's how to find out where you stand.

HOW TO MEASURE YOUR WAIST-TO-HIP RATIO

While medical facilities have sophisticated methods of measuring central obesity precisely, measuring your waist-to-hip ratio is proven to be accurate, and it's something you can do yourself…

•**First, find your true waist**—it's not necessarily where your belt falls. Locate your hip bone on one side, and then move upward until you can feel the bones of your bottom rib. Halfway between your hip and that first rib bone is your waist. For most people, it's where the belly button is.

•**Measure your waist with a tape measure.**

•**Measure your hip with a tape measure.**

•**Divide the waist measure by the hip measure.** For example, if your waist is 28 and your hip is 36, you'd divide 28/36 to get a ratio of 0.78.

Here's a shortcut: For most women, a waist of 35 inches or above, and for most men 40 inches and above, is a good quick indicator of central obesity, according to the American Heart Association.

If you do have a big belly, you know what to do—lose weight. The good news is that belly fat is the easiest to lose. It's the first to come off when you start to lose weight by changing your diet and exercise habits.

5 Ways to Get Rid of Stubborn Belly Fat

Timothy McCall, MD, a board-certified internist and medical editor of *Yoga Journal.* He is author of *Yoga as Medicine: The Yogic Prescription for Health and Healing,* in which he reports on the connection between stress and weight gain. His articles have appeared in *The New England Journal of Medicine* and *JAMA.* DrMcCall.com

Don't count on the latest diet to shrink an expanding waistline. Belly fat is stubborn. Unlike fat in the thighs, buttocks and hips, which visibly diminishes when you cut calories, belly fat tends to stick around. Even strenuous exercise might not make a dent.

The persistence of a belly bulge isn't merely cosmetic. Beneath the subcutaneous fat that you can pinch with your fingers, fat deep in the abdomen is metabolically different from "normal" fat. Known as visceral fat, it secretes inflammatory substances that increase the risk for heart attack, type 2 diabetes and some cancers. Even if you're not overweight, a larger-than-average waistline increases health risks.

Surprisingly, even thin people can have a high percentage of visceral fat. It might not be visible, but the risks are the same.

Weight-loss diets can certainly help you drop pounds—and some of that weight will come from the deep abdominal area. But unless you take a broader approach than the standard diet and exercise advice, it's very difficult to maintain visceral fat reductions over the long haul. *Here are better approaches to shrink your belly…*

●**Don't stress over losing weight.** Everyone knows about "stress eating." After a fight with your spouse or a hard day at work, food can be a welcome distraction. What people don't realize is that the struggle to lose weight may itself be highly stressful and that it can cause your belly fat to stick around.

How this happens: Cortisol, one of the main stress-related hormones, increases appetite and makes you less mindful of what you eat. It causes the body to store more fat, particularly visceral fat. People who worry a lot about their weight actually may find themselves eating more.

Take action to reduce stress by practicing yoga, meditation or tai chi for even just a few minutes a day. One study found that there was little or no obesity among more than 200 women over age 45 who had practiced yoga for many years. The key is regular practice—it's better to do 10 minutes of yoga a day than a 90-minute class once a week.

Also helpful: Belly breathing. Sit up straight in a chair or lie down on your back, close your eyes, and tune into your breathing. Breathe in and out through your nose slowly and deeply but without straining. You'll feel your belly gently moving out as you inhale and then in as you exhale.

This type of breathing is an effective form of stress control. Try it for one to five minutes once or twice a day…or anytime you're feeling stressed.

●**Cultivate mindfulness in your everyday life.** According to yoga and Ayurvedic medicine (a system of healing that originated in India), an overly busy mind can play as big a role in weight gain as diet or exercise. We all need to step back from the chaos of life and give our nervous system a chance to unwind. Take it one step at a time. Do less multitasking. Try to move a little more slowly and deliberately. Spend less time on the Internet and watching television—especially when you're eating. Although these activities may seem relaxing, they can stimulate the mind and the nervous system and lead to overeating.

Bonus: When you eat mindfully, you'll enjoy your food more and need less to feel satisfied.

●**Exercise, but don't go crazy.** Exercise, particularly aerobic exercise, can obviously be good for weight loss. But for many people, the intensity at which they exercise becomes yet another source of stress.

Example: One of my medical colleagues described a "Type A" patient who was an exercise fanatic. Despite her strenuous fitness program, she had a stubborn 10 pounds that she couldn't get rid of. He suggested that she might have more luck if she'd simply relax a bit. She ignored his advice—until she broke a leg and had to take a break. The 10 pounds melted away.

My advice: Get plenty of exercise, but enjoy it. Don't let it be stressful—make it a soothing part of your day. Go for a bike ride…swim in a lake…take a hike in nature. Exercise that is relaxing may burn just as many calories as a do-or-die gym workout but without the stress-related rise in cortisol.

Tip: If you've practiced belly breathing (see left), try to bring that kind of breath focus to your exercise. It's even possible to slowly train yourself to breathe through your nose while you exercise, potentially lowering cortisol levels and the rebound hunger that is so common after a workout.

●**Eat more fresh, unprocessed food.** What really matters for health and healthy weight is the quality of your food. Many diets that have been shown to be effective—such as the low-fat vegetarian Ornish program…the Mediterranean diet…and some high-protein plans—disagree with one another, but they all emphasize old-fashioned unprocessed food.

My advice: Worry less about micronutrients such as specific vitamins, minerals and types of fat or your protein/carbohydrate balance, and instead focus on eating more fresh vegetables, legumes, whole grains, fruit, nuts and seeds. If you eat animal foods, choose free-range and pasture-raised meat and dairy products, organic if possible.

●**Cut back on refined sugar.** If you follow the advice above and avoid processed foods, you'll naturally consume less sugar, refined grains (such as white bread) and other "simple" carbohydrates. This will help prevent insulin surges that can lead to more visceral fat.

As always, balance is important. I don't advise anyone to give up all sources of sugar or all carbohydrates. After all, a plum is loaded with the sugar fructose—and fruits are good for you! It's the added sugar in junk and fast food that's the problem. Just be aware that any processed food—including many snacks that are marketed as healthier alternatives—will make it harder to control your weight.

How a "Foodie" Lost 42 Pounds—No Dieting

Pam Anderson, a food writer, former executive editor of *Cook's Illustrated* magazine and a contributing chef at *Runner's World* magazine. She is the author of *The Perfect Recipe for Losing Weight & Eating Great.*

Pam Anderson, a food writer and cookbook author, faces challenges that would tax any dieter. She tests—and tastes—every recipe that she creates. She spends two or more days a week in a test kitchen, where she might sample three dozen versions of a chocolate cake or 16 versions of a pot roast recipe. That led her to her top weight of 192 pounds.

Over the years, she tried dozens of different diets, including Atkins and South Beach. She lost weight initially, but the pounds always came back.

●**Her "mirror moment."** Anderson took an exercise class that was held in a mirrored room. She didn't like the look of the overweight food writer looking back at her. At the same time, she experienced an intense longing for what she would like to become—thinner and healthier.

That morning in front of the mirror represented her first step in the healthier direction. It was another two years before she fully dedicated herself to healthier living. When she did, the results were striking. She lost 42 pounds in about eight months, without dieting, and has not gained it back.

The approach that worked for her…

●**Focus on your life, not your weight.** A few years after my "mirror moment," I saw an acupuncturist for shoulder pain. I left the sessions feeling centered and refreshed. That's when I realized that my weight was secondary. Changing my life was a necessary first step.

I started weekly therapy sessions with a psychologist, during which I came to understand that I have always shouldered too many responsibilities. As a working parent, I brought home a big chunk of the bacon, and I took on most of the household responsibilities. So in addition to my job, I shopped, cooked, oversaw the child care and housecleaning, took charge of the finances, planned vacations and organized the social calendar. It was too much. I unconsciously used food to "support" the many responsibilities that I carried.

Therapy didn't cause me to lose weight, but it did help me to understand that my life was out of balance. It helped me feel more in control and sure of myself, which allowed me to reduce the responsibilities that I had taken on.

●**Get physical.** I never exercised regularly until my husband and I took a trip to Italy several years ago. We walked miles every day. I was surprised to discover that daily exercise made me less hungry. At the same time, those daily walks burned a lot of calories. I wasn't trying to lose weight—I ate all the bread, pasta and desserts that I wanted—but by the time we returned, after two weeks, my clothes were looser.

After that, I kept up the habit of walking every day. I would walk briskly for a few miles in the morning and sometimes again in the afternoon. As

I got stronger, I alternated walking with bursts of running. I kept losing weight.

•Opt for casual calorie counting. Most diets incorporate nutritional rules. You're supposed to eat this many calories or limit yourself to these portion sizes. I don't bother with that. I've learned that food restriction only creates cravings and that strict portion control can leave you feeling hungry all the time.

I do have a sense of what I should and shouldn't eat and how much I should eat in a given day. I know from experience that I can maintain my current weight (about 150 pounds) on 2,000 to 2,500 calories a day. I'm in that range when I eat a big breakfast, a healthy salad for lunch and a light meal at supper, along with a few snacks. If I've been tasting a lot of new recipes, I cut back on calories somewhere else. I don't think about it very much. Calorie control becomes second nature once you know what "healthy" feels like. Now I'm rarely tempted to overindulge, because I feel so much better when I don't.

That's as specific as I get. I've developed a heightened awareness of what my body does and doesn't need at any given time. As long as I stay in this general calorie range—and burn roughly 450 calories a day with exercise—my weight naturally takes care of itself.

•Eat often. Most people get hungry every three to four hours. This is why doctors recommend "grazing," in which you eat five or six times a day. It's good for energy and healthy blood sugar levels, as well as appetite control.

I haven't given up my three main meals, but I supplement them with snacks whenever I'm feeling hungry. I make a ritual of afternoon tea, in which I'll have a cup of tea and something sweet, such as a small cookie. Then, before supper, I'll have an hors d'oeuvre—a deviled egg or a handful of nuts—along with a glass of wine.

•Look good, feel good. I got rid of the ugly sweatpants I used to exercise in. Now I have smart-looking spandex. After my workouts, I don't just shower—I fix my hair and put on makeup. The way we present ourselves indicates how we feel about ourselves. Looking good made me feel good—and the better I felt, the better I wanted to look.

I also go through my closet periodically and get rid of my "fat" clothes. I used to hang on to everything, probably because I knew in the back of my mind that my diets weren't going to stick. This new approach was different. I wasn't merely dieting, I was changing my life. I knew I wasn't going back.

•Personalize. One of the problems with weight-loss diets is that they force different people to follow exactly the same plan. But in fact, everyone has to figure out what works for him/her.

Example: I'm not about to give up my before-supper glass of wine, no matter how many calories it has.

I go to bed earlier than a lot of people, so I'm unlikely to snack after supper. But if you happen to be a night owl, you'll probably want to have a snack between supper and bedtime. Similarly, we all have our own favorites. I love pasta and couldn't stick with a diet that forced me to give it up. Maybe you crave a daily dessert or full-fat cream in your coffee. Don't give it up! Just make the necessary adjustments.

17

Power Food and Drink for Ideal Weight and Fitness

Foods That Rev Up Your Metabolism—Drop Those Extra Pounds for Good— and Get an Energy Boost to Boot!

Ridha Arem, MD, an endocrinologist, director of the Texas Thyroid Institute, an endocrinologist practice at Texas Medical center in Houston. He is a former chief of endocrinology and metabolism at Houston's Ben Taub General Hospital and is author of *The Thyroid Solution*. AremWellness.com

Forget about calories! Most people who are trying to lose weight worry too much about calories and not enough about the actual cause of those extra pounds.

The real culprit: Out-of-balance hormones.

Best approach for controlling weight: A diet that rebalances the body's hormones. Carefully chosen foods and food combinations rebalance levels and/or efficiency of metabolism-regulating hormones, such as ghrelin, leptin and thyroid hormone. You'll burn more calories, and your body will be less likely to store calories as fat. *Here's how…*

TWEAKING THE BEST DIETS

Hands down, the Mediterranean diet is one of the healthiest diets out there. With its emphasis on plant-based foods (such as vegetables, fruits, grains and nuts) and healthful fats (from fatty fish and olive oil), it is good for your heart and helps control blood sugar levels.

But for more efficient weight loss, you need to go a step further. That's where the Protein-Rich Oriental Diet, developed by Korean researchers, enters the picture. With its heavy focus on high-protein foods, this diet has been found to provide twice the weight loss offered by calorie restriction alone.

To achieve and maintain an optimal body weight: The diet I designed includes elements of both these diets—as well as some important additional tweaks such as timing your meals (see below) and consuming a mix of proteins in order to get the full complement of amino acids, which is essential for increasing metabolism and controlling hunger. On my diet, you will eat a combination of at least two proteins, good fats and vegetables at each meal. *For example…*

• **Fish, turkey and chicken contain all of the essential amino acids that are in red meat,** but with fewer calories and less saturated fat. They're particularly rich in arginine, an amino acid that increases the speed at which your body burns calories.

My advice: Aim for six to eight ounces of these foods as the primary protein for dinner. You also can include these foods at breakfast and lunch as one of your protein choices. (If you're not a fish lover, see below.)

●**Reduced-fat cottage cheese, ricotta, yogurt and goat cheese.** Certain forms of dairy are high in branched-chain amino acids, which suppress appetite and increase the ability of mitochondria (the energy-producing components of cells) to burn fat.

My advice: Each day, eat about a half-cup of low-fat or nonfat dairy as a protein.

●**High-protein beans, lentils and grains, such as black beans, kidney beans, quinoa and brown rice.** Eat one of these protein sources (three-fourths cup to one cup) at lunch—usually combined with a small serving of fish or lean meat. In addition to packing plenty of protein and fiber, these foods provide large amounts of amino acids that will help you get fitter and have more energy.

●**Egg whites contain all of the amino acids that you need for efficient weight loss,** and they are my favorite choice as a protein for breakfast. An egg-white omelet with onions, mushrooms and other vegetables can be prepared in just a few minutes.

LOW-GLYCEMIC CARBS

Carbohydrates that are digested quickly—mainly refined and processed foods such as juices, white rice and French fries—increase insulin and fat storage. Carbohydrates with a lower glycemic score are absorbed more slowly and don't cause unhealthy changes in insulin or fat storage.

Good choices: Whole oats, chickpeas and fruit (see below) at breakfast and lunch, and vegetables at each meal.

MORE FIBER

The fiber in such foods as beans and vegetables reduces appetite and slows digestion, important for preventing insulin "spikes." Research shows that people of normal weight tend to eat significantly more fiber than those who are overweight or obese.

For efficient weight loss: Get 35 g of fiber daily.

Fruit is also a good source of fiber. Just be sure that you choose fresh fruit that's low in natural sugar (fructose).

Good choices: Raspberries, strawberries, papayas, apples and cranberries. Avoid fruit at dinner to make it the lowest glycemic meal.

GREEN TEA

Green tea is high in epigallocatechin gallate (EGCG), a substance that can decrease the accumulation of body fat. It also increases insulin sensitivity and improves an obesity-related condition known as metabolic syndrome. Drink a few cups every day. Do not sweeten the tea with honey or other sweeteners—they are among the main causes of high insulin and weight gain.

FISH OIL SUPPLEMENTS

The omega-3 fatty acids in fish increase the rate at which calories are burned. However, even if you eat fish every day, it doesn't contain enough omega-3s for long-term weight control.

Solution: Take a daily supplement with 600 mg of EPA and 400 mg of DHA—the main types of omega-3s. Check first with your doctor if you take blood thinners or diabetes medication, since fish oil may interact with these drugs.

NOT JUST FOR WEIGHT LOSS

A hormone-balancing eating plan can rev up your metabolism even if you don't need to lose weight, giving you more energy and mental focus. If you aren't overweight and you follow this eating plan, you may lose a pound or two, but mostly you'll just feel better.

MORE FROM DR. AREM...

Timing Matters!

When you eat is almost as important as what you eat...

●**Plan on eating four or five daily meals—**breakfast between 6 am and 8 am...an optional (and light) late-morning snack...lunch between 11 am and 12:30 pm...a mid-afternoon snack...and supper between 5 pm and 7 pm.

• **Plan your meals so that you get more protein at supper.** It will stimulate the release of growth hormone, which burns fat while you sleep.

• **Avoid all food three hours before bedtime.** Eating late in the evening causes increases in blood sugar and insulin that can lead to weight gain—even if you consume a lower-calorie diet (1,200 to 1,500 calories a day).

Secret Weight-Loss Weapon

Cyril Kendall, PhD, nutrition researcher, University of Toronto, Canada.

What if there were a food that had an incredible power to help you lose weight or avoid gaining weight? You'd try it, right? Well, a new study shows exactly what that food is. It's beans and other legumes! To see what new benefits these nutrient-packed foods might have, researchers tracked adults who ate a daily serving (three-quarters cup) of beans, lentils, peas or chickpeas.

Result: They felt 31% fuller after meals than those who didn't eat legumes.

If you're trying to lose weight: Add legumes to your daily diet.

Seven Superfoods: Delicious Ways to Fight Disease

Mark A. Stengler, NMD, naturopathic doctor and founder of the Stengler Center for Integrative Medicine in Encinitas, California. He is author or coauthor of numerous books, including *The Natural Physician's Healing Therapies* and *Bottom Line's Prescription for Natural Cures.* MarkStengler.com

Nearly 2,500 years ago, Hippocrates, the father of modern medicine, said, "Let food be thy medicine and medicine be thy food." This is still true today—the right foods help you stay healthy and are powerful disease fighters. *Here are seven of the best…*

1. BEANS

Americans' consumption of beans has steadily increased over the past two decades, and that's good news because beans have tremendous healing power. Popular varieties include soybeans, garbanzo (chickpeas), pinto, kidney, lima, navy and black beans. Beans are a type of legume, a class of vegetable that also includes lentils and peas.

Beans are high in protein, low in fat and calories, and rich in complex carbohydrates, fiber, phytonutrients and several vitamins and minerals, including folic acid and other B vitamins, potassium, magnesium and iron.

In addition, beans are loaded with soluble fiber, the same type of gummy fiber found in the oat bran in oatmeal. This type of fiber helps bind and eliminate cholesterol and stabilize blood sugar levels.

A study conducted by the US Department of Agriculture found that beans—especially black, pinto and kidney beans—topped the list of vegetables that are rich in disease-fighting antioxidants.

Specifically, several studies have shown that regular consumption of beans significantly reduces the risk for cardiovascular disease. Recent studies now suggest that beans also have potent anticancer properties.

Recommended: Eat one-half cup of beans four times weekly. Beans make an excellent addition to salads, rice dishes and soups, and they can be pureed as a dip.

Helpful: Many people avoid beans because they experience gas after eating them. If this is a problem, take an enzyme product such as Beano, available at most grocery stores and drugstores. Follow directions on the label.

2. BROCCOLI

I am thankful that broccoli is such a popular food in my household—all three of my children like it. This king of the cruciferous family (other members include brussels sprouts, cabbage, kale, cauliflower and bok choy) is an excellent source of vitamin C, vitamin A, folic acid, calcium and fiber.

Broccoli fights cancer. It contains two classes of anticancer phytonutrients—isothiocyanates and glucosinolates.

Sulforaphane is an isothiocyanate that activates detoxifying enzymes in the body that prevent the formation of cancer-causing substances. Sulforaphane also has potent antioxidant properties.

Indole-3-carbinol (I3C) is a glucosinolate that has been shown to benefit women with early-stage cervical cancer and helps protect estrogen-sensitive cells, such as breast cells.

Broccoli also is rich in the carotenoid antioxidants lutein and zeaxanthin. Both are important in preventing ultraviolet damage to the eyes and can help prevent cataracts and age-related macular degeneration, the leading cause of blindness in people age 65 and older.

Recommended: Eat one-half cup of raw or lightly steamed broccoli daily (buying frozen broccoli is fine). Avoid boiling—it diminishes its nutritional value.

Broccoli sprouts, which are the newly sprouted seeds of broccoli, can be added to sandwiches or salads. They contain 30 to 50 times the concentration of protective phytonutrients that are found in mature broccoli plants. Broccoli sprouts are especially rich in sulforaphane. Because broccoli sprouts can be contaminated with bacteria, people with weak immune systems should check with their doctors before consuming them.

3. EGGS

The egg is an excellent source of protein, and it contains all the essential amino acids that your body cannot produce on its own. In addition, it is a rich source of vitamin K, cancer-fighting selenium, vitamin B-12 and choline, a nutrient required by cell membranes for healthy function. Some of these nutrients are found in the yolk, so egg whites alone are not as beneficial.

In the past, the egg got a bad reputation when it came to cholesterol and heart disease. However, multiple studies have now vindicated the egg.

A study in the *Journal of the American Medical Association*, conducted at Harvard School of Public Health, found no relationship between egg consumption and cardiovascular disease in a population of more than 117,000 nurses and health professionals who were followed for eight to 14 years. There was no difference in heart disease risk between those who ate less than one egg a week and those who ate one egg a day.

In fact, the protein in eggs appears to prevent blood clots. Eggs also contain the eye-protective nutrient lutein—and lutein from eggs is more easily absorbed than that from spinach (one of the richest sources) or from supplements.

In addition, in one Chinese study, women who ate at least six eggs a week lowered their risk of breast cancer by 44%, compared with no risk reduction in women who consumed two or fewer eggs a week.

Recommended: Eat one to six organic eggs weekly. Organic eggs don't contain hormone or antibiotic residues.

Caution: People with gallbladder disease should avoid eggs. Eggs may worsen symptoms, including pain and spasms, possibly due to the fat content.

4. BLUEBERRIES

One of nature's antiaging stars, blueberries contain a megasupply of powerful antioxidants known as anthocyanins, which help protect against cell damage. Anthocyanins have been shown to enhance the effects of vitamin C, improve capillaries so they're less likely to rupture and support the body's connective tissues. Anthocyanins give blueberries their blue-purple color. Blueberries also are a good source of vitamin C and vitamin E, manganese and fiber.

Blueberries contain the anthocyanin pterostilbene, a powerful antioxidant compound that is known to fight cancer. Animal studies have shown that pterostilbene also reduces cholesterol, improves memory and shortens recovery time from stroke. In addition, blueberries promote good eye health—they are particularly helpful in the prevention of macular degeneration.

Like cranberries, blueberries have been found to contain substances that prevent bacteria from adhering to the lining of the urinary tract, which may help guard against urinary tract infections.

Recommended: Eat one-half cup of blueberries five times weekly. Sprinkle blueberries, fresh or frozen, on cereal or add them to muffins and smoothies.

5. OATMEAL

Oatmeal, one of the most nutritious complex carbohydrates, contains several vital minerals, including manganese, selenium, magnesium, zinc and copper.

Oatmeal also provides protein and, as I mentioned earlier, is an excellent source of soluble fiber. Because this type of fiber stabilizes blood sugar, oatmeal is an excellent choice for people with diabetes.

The best-known benefits of this super food are its cholesterol-lowering properties. A type of soluble fiber known as beta-glucan (which also activates immune cells) and compounds called saponins bind dietary cholesterol and usher it out of the body unabsorbed.

A daily bowl of oatmeal can reduce total cholesterol by as much as 23%. It has also been shown to reduce the "bad" LDL cholesterol without changing levels of beneficial HDL cholesterol.

In addition, oats are a rich source of tocotrienols. These relatives of the vitamin E family guard against the oxidation of LDL cholesterol (thereby preventing LDL cholesterol from sticking to artery walls and causing plaque buildup) and reduce the production of cholesterol by the liver.

Recommended: Eat one cup of oatmeal three to four times weekly. When possible, choose the longer-cooking variety—instant oatmeal has a weaker cholesterol-lowering effect and often has salt and sugar added. Oatmeal is even healthier when sprinkled with a tablespoon of ground flaxseed and a teaspoon of cinnamon, both of which help lower cholesterol.

6. WALNUTS

Walnuts are the perfect snack. They are rich in omega-3 fatty acids, which reduce inflammation in the body. Walnuts also contain the minerals manganese and copper, both of which play key roles in the body's antioxidant network.

In addition, these tasty nuts contain gamma-tocopherol, a component of vitamin E that provides antioxidant protection, as well as the amino acid l-arginine, which improves circulation. Walnuts also contain the phytonutrient ellagic acid, which helps protect against cancer-causing free radical damage.

Walnuts also are a source of the sleep hormone melatonin. The amount is too small to promote sleep, but the melatonin in walnuts provides additional antioxidant activity.

Several studies have shown that the consumption of walnuts reduces the risk of coronary artery disease. One study found that a walnut-rich diet lowered levels of C-reactive protein, a marker of inflammation, which is strongly associated with atherosclerosis and heart disease. Walnuts not only increase levels of omega-3 fatty acids but also decrease the adhesion of cholesterol to the lining of the arteries.

A study conducted at the Lipid Clinic at the Endocrinology and Nutrition Service, Institut d'Investigacions Biomediques in Barcelona, Spain, showed that a walnut-rich diet reduced total cholesterol by 4.4% and LDL cholesterol by 6.4%.

Other studies have found that walnuts significantly increase the elasticity of the arteries, which is a marker for healthy blood vessels. The Food and Drug Administration allows walnuts to carry the health claim that "eating 1.5 ounces of walnuts per day as part of a diet low in saturated fat and cholesterol may reduce the risk for heart disease."

Recommended: Eat four to eight walnuts (approximately 1.5 ounces) daily in cereals, salads and yogurt—or eat them plain.

7. YOGURT

Yogurt is a fermented dairy product rich in "friendly" bacteria. These bacteria, such as *Lactobacillus acidophilus* and *Lactobacillus bulgaricus*, improve immune function. Yogurt also is a good source of calcium, phosphorus, vitamin B-2 (riboflavin), iodine, vitamin B-12, vitamin B-5 (pantothenic acid), zinc, potassium and protein. Several studies have shown that incorporating calcium-rich foods, such as low-fat yogurt and cheese, into a reduced-calorie diet is an effective weight-management technique.

Yogurt also suppresses the growth of Helicobacter pylori, the bacterium that causes most cases of stomach ulcer. Along with other dairy products, yogurt appears to protect against colon and rectal cancers—perhaps because of the calcium content. Studies also have found that yogurt reduces the compounds that contribute to bad breath, cavities and gum disease.

Recommended: Eat one-half to one cup of yogurt daily. Look for low-fat yogurts that list "live active cultures" or "living yogurt cultures" on the label.

Do not buy any yogurt that contains artificial color, flavoring or sweetener. Choose plain yogurt or flavored yogurt made by Horizon or other companies that don't use artificial ingredients. Opt for organic yogurt products to avoid hormone and antibiotic residues. Yogurt is delicious when used in place of milk in cereals or as part of a smoothie.

Caution: Avoid yogurt if you are allergic or sensitive to cow's milk—goat's milk yogurt is an option.

These 4 "Super Spices" Have Hidden Benefits

Joshua Levitt, ND, a naturopathic physician in private practice in Hamden, Connecticut. Dr. Levitt is a clinical preceptor for Yale School of Medicine and collaborates with the Integrative Medicine Center at Yale New Haven Hospital. He is author of *The Honey Phenomenon* and numerous other books and articles. WholeHealthCT.com

When it comes to "superfoods," fruits and veggies aren't the only heavy hitters. A handful of popular spices also have gained a rightful place on this list because of their own research-supported therapeutic effects.

Examples of the best known: Cinnamon for diabetes. Garlic for high cholesterol. Ginger for nausea. Cayenne for pain relief.

What you may not realize: Those same spices have even more benefits—little-known but powerful—that are also backed by scientific evidence. *How to use these spices for even greater preventive and curative effect…*

CINNAMON

A small daily dose of cinnamon has been proven in many studies to lower and help regulate blood sugar—crucial for those trying to prevent or manage type 2 diabetes.

Little-known benefit: Cinnamon also can lower high blood pressure.

Scientific evidence: In a recent study published in *Lipids in Health and Disease,* people who ingested 3 g (about two-thirds of a teaspoon) of cinnamon daily had a significant drop in blood pressure after four months—from averages of 136/88 to 122/80.

How to get more: Because cinnamon is so tasty, it's easy to include more in your diet. As a heavy cinnamon user, I buy organic Ceylon cinnamon (the highest quality) by the pound.

Note: Supermarket cinnamon is usually cassia (or Vietnamese), which contains a compound called coumarin that may damage the liver at high doses in susceptible individuals.

Cinnamon is great on roasted sweet potatoes and squash and adds delightful sweetness to pancakes and waffles. Plus, because it's such a powerful antioxidant, a sprinkle of cinnamon stops apple slices from turning brown—making the treat more delicious and more appetizing.

GARLIC

This potent spice—a rich source of many healing compounds—is proven to lower cholesterol, reducing your risk for heart disease.

Little-known benefit: Eating garlic regularly also may help reduce your risk for colorectal cancer.

Scientific evidence: When Italian researchers analyzed seven case-control studies on garlic consumption and colorectal cancer, they found that people who ate the most garlic reduced their risk for the disease by 37% compared with people who ate the least. These studies measured garlic intake in various ways, so there is no optimal intake. To be fair, there is also research showing no correlation between garlic and colorectal cancer risk, but even the potential benefit makes garlic a smart addition to one's diet.

How to get more: Lightly sautéed fresh cloves are likely the healthiest way to consume garlic, but you also can use garlic flakes or powder. I use garlic (usually combined with lemon) in nearly every cooking liquid, sauce and marinade that I make in my kitchen.

GINGER

Dozens of studies have proven ginger's usefulness in easing nausea and vomiting due to everything from chemotherapy to motion sickness to morning sickness.

Little-known benefit: Ginger also inhibits the COX-1 and COX-2 enzymes that play a role in the production of inflammation-causing compounds in the body. This means it works the same way as pain-relieving drugs such as ibuprofen (Motrin) and aspirin.

Scientific evidence: A study published in *Phytotherapy Research* found that ginger supplements are comparable to aspirin, ibuprofen, naproxen (Aleve) and other over-the-counter painkillers in easing muscle pain caused by exercise and other types of strenuous activity. Research also has shown that ginger is just as effective as the migraine drug sumatriptan (Imitrex).

How to get more: For a therapeutic, pain-relieving dose of ginger, take a 1,000-mg supplement, twice daily. For migraine, I recommend up to 1,000 mg at the onset of a migraine. If you want to use ginger to help prevent migraine, add fresh ginger to your daily diet or take a ginger supplement (250 mg to 500 mg daily).*

In the kitchen, add fresh ginger—finely diced or crushed—to sauces and marinades. Used three or more times a week, ginger in doses commonly consumed in the diet can have a mild pain-relieving and anti-inflammatory effect. Ginger is also great in smoothies.

CAYENNE

Cayenne is a powder made from dried, red chili peppers, and it's very hot when used to spice food. But the natural intensity of cayenne and its active ingredient capsaicin affect more than your taste buds.

*If you take blood thinners such as *warfarin* (Coumadin) or if you have gallstone disease, talk to your doctor before using ginger supplements.

It's the only natural compound that—when applied topically—can degrade substance P, a neurotransmitter that tells the brain to transmit pain signals. With less substance P, there's less pain—which is why capsaicin is a common ingredient in many creams, ointments and salves for pain problems such as arthritis, nerve pain, foot pain and back pain.

Little-known benefit: Cayenne can also help you lose weight. Capsaicin and other compounds in cayenne work because they have several effects that help you shed pounds—they suppress appetite…increase calorie-burning ("basal metabolic rate")…and burn up ("oxidize") body fat.

In a recent meta-analysis of nine studies on capsaicin and weight loss, published in *Critical Reviews in Food Science and Nutrition*, researchers concluded that the spice "could be a new therapeutic approach in obesity."

How to get more: For patients who want to lose weight, I usually recommend adding cayenne to the diet or using low-dose (2 mg) capsaicin supplements daily. (High-dose supplements can irritate the gastrointestinal tract.)

As a weight-loss aid, I recommend drinking one or more cups a day of warm water with a pinch of cayenne, juice from half a lemon, a teaspoon of honey and ground ginger (using a chunk of fresh ginger the size of half your thumb, from knuckle to tip). Cayenne is also excellent in marinades for fish and poultry and sprinkled on eggs. Plus, it adds a kick to salad dressings.

Grapefruit Does Aid Weight Loss

Ken Fujioka, MD, director, Center for Weight Management, Scripps Clinic Nutrition and Metabolic Research Center, San Diego, and leader of a study published in *Journal of Medicinal Food.*

Remember the grapefruit diet? There may be some validity to it.

Recent finding: Study participants lost an average of three-and-a-half pounds in 12 weeks by eating one-half a grapefruit with each meal, versus a group who followed the same diet but without the grapefruit.

Theory: Grapefruit lowers insulin levels, which helps prevent sugar from being stored as fat.

Caution: Grapefruit and grapefruit juice may interfere with some medications, such as statin drugs, so check with your doctor.

---

10 Hydrophilic Foods That Satisfy Hunger and Help You Lose Weight

Keren Gilbert, MS, RD, nutritionist and the founder and president of Decision Nutrition, a nutrition consulting firm in Great Neck, New York and Greenwich, Connecticut, and author of *The HD Diet: Achieve Lifelong Weight Loss with Chia Seeds and Nature's Water-Absorbent Foods.*

What if you could swallow a pill right before dining that would make your stomach swell like a balloon so you would feel artificially full? Well, such a pill is in the works, but there's a much better solution for you—hydrophilic foods. They attract and absorb water, which makes them swell in size—in a natural process—so you naturally feel satisfied and automatically consume fewer calories. Plus, unlike a weird new diet pill or other diet gimmicks, they are full of nutrients that your body needs. And besides helping you lose or maintain weight, hydrophilic foods—because they contain digestible soluble fiber—also help control blood sugar and cholesterol.

And it's all real food. What more could you want?

THE TOP 10 HYDROPHILIC FOODS

•**Chia seeds.** Chia seeds are the perfect example of a hydrophilic food. They start out as tiny, crunchy, nutty-tasting seeds (just a little bigger than poppy seeds), but each seed can absorb up to 12 times its weight in water, so they form a gel that's filling and extremely nutrient-rich—each seed is supercharged with omega-3s and packed with antioxidants, fiber, iron, magnesium, calcium

and potassium! So sprinkle a tablespoon into your smoothie for breakfast, add some to soups and porridges or even use them in place of breadcrumbs to bind meatballs. You can even make a simple and nutritious pudding by combining two tablespoons of chia seeds per cup of almond milk or other liquid, sweetening to taste and refrigerating overnight—no cooking needed.

•**Okra.** OK, okra might be a turnoff for some people because it gets sappy—or downright slimy—when cooked, but that texture speaks volumes about its soluble fiber, which, along with a host of vitamins and minerals, turns okra into a dietary powerhouse. Adding sliced okra to soups and stews, where the consistency doesn't stand out so much and, in fact, the okra acts as a natural thickener. Also consider cooking okra at high heat (in a wok, for example), or slicing it lengthwise and grilling it—both cooking styles will reduce the vegetable's slipperiness. To use it raw, slice and tossed into salads or dress with oil and vinegar all on its own. It's tasty, with a good crunch, and its slight sappiness enhances the texture of the dressing.

•**Oatmeal.** Oatmeal is a hydrophilic food you might already be filling up on since it's well-known for its cholesterol-controlling abilities. Just picture the way raw oats absorb water while they cook, and you'll understand why they make my top-10 list of hydrophilic foods. Don't like oatmeal? Maybe it's because the only kind you know is rolled oats—the kind that look flattened and may have even been partially cooked before you buy them. Rolled oats can cook up mushy and without much natural flavor. Try steel-cut oats. They cook up into a hearty, pleasantly toothsome and nutty-tasting dish.

•**Pears.** Pears are naturally full of *pectin*, a type of soluble fiber found in the walls of plant cells. If you've ever made jam, you've probably added pectin powder to thicken it. In addition to helping you feel full, pectin acts as a detoxifier, a gastrointestinal tract regulator and an immune system stimulant. Grab a pear for a juicy snack, or try these delicious ways to use them—add thin slices to sandwiches…toss into salads…or cut them in half, core them and either grill or roast them. To grill, simply place them, cut side down, on a lightly oiled stovetop grill until they are seared. To roast, place them, cut side down, in a baking pan, warm up a half cup of apple juice and a tablespoon or two of honey, pour the apple juice over the pears, and bake at 400°F for 30 minutes.

- **Barley.** Like oats, barley absorbs a substantial amount of water as it cooks—and like oats, it also expands further in your stomach, providing heart-healthy nutrition and natural fullness. Americans aren't very familiar with barley and don't use it very much in their kitchens—which is ironic since it was one of the original foods grown by the Pilgrims and may have been eaten at the first Thanksgiving. Beyond the standard beef-barley stew (which, by the way, can be a very healthful meal!), it's actually very easy to use and enjoy barley. Just follow cooking instructions on the package, and then use barley as the base in your favorite whole-grain salad recipe (instead of wheat berries, for example)...use it instead of small pastas in soups (it lends an earthier tone than pasta)...sauté it with some butter and sliced mushrooms, salt and pepper. You can even cook barley like risotto—barley's soluble fiber creates the right kind of creaminess for risotto-like dishes.

- **Brussels sprouts.** Serving for serving, Brussels sprouts are among the vegetables highest in soluble fiber. For a taste revelation, try tossing fresh Brussels sprouts with olive oil and salt, then roasting in the oven at 400°F for 30 to 40 minutes or until they are softened and caramelized...or shred them raw and use in slaw. You can also make an easy, delicious boiled Brussels sprouts dish. Cut the sprouts in half, then boil them with a variety of herbs such as garlic, basil, thyme, and rosemary in one part wine vinegar and one part water until they are tender. Drain, dress with balsamic vinegar and olive oil, salt, pepper and more herbs to taste. Let cool and serve at room temperature.

- **Kidney beans.** Like all beans, kidney beans soak up water as they cook and keep doing it after you eat them. I especially favor kidney beans because, their red color indicates a high level of disease-fighting antioxidants—the darker red, the better. Of course, they are a great addition to chilies, salads and soups such as minestrone. You might also like to partly mash a cup and a half of cooked kidney beans and mix them with olive oil, a dash of balsamic vinegar, salt, garlic and other spices to taste for a delicious bean spread served with crostini or Italian bread.

- **Chickpeas.** Also called garbanzo beans, these might be the single most easy and versatile food on this top-10 list. You know you can toss them onto any salad—but you don't even need the salad. You can simply open a can of chick peas, drain, add any salad dressing and start eating—and if you like this idea, don't miss trying them in Caesar dressing with Parmesan cheese sprinkled on top. If you have a little more time, purée chickpeas with garlic, cumin, tahini, olive oil and lemon juice for a healthy, homemade hummus. For a portable snack, toss chickpeas with a bit of olive oil and your favorite spice blend, then roast until irresistibly crunchy. Or make pasta e fagioli—the Italian version of "rice and beans"—by adding cooked chickpeas and small pasta to a saucy sauté of diced onions, carrots, celery or fennel, zucchini and stewed tomatoes and their juice.

- **Oranges.** That an orange easily fits in a purse or jacket pocket makes it one of my favorite snacks. Besides the famous vitamin C content, oranges are packed with soluble fiber. To get the most nutritional (and weight-loss) benefit, don't peel off all the pith—the white substance beneath the peel. It's got loads of pectin and almost as much vitamin C as the juicy fruit it covers.

- **Agar.** Unless you are really into baking or fancy cooking, agar (also called agar-agar) is the hydrophilic food you're least likely to have in your pantry, but you might want to consider stocking it. It's a gelling agent made from seaweed that has a whopping 80% soluble fiber with no fat and virtually no calories, carbs or sugar. If you want a homemade sweet, agar is the perfect ingredient for making custards, puddings and fruit gels. And it couldn't be easier to use—just substitute it for gelatin in recipes.

Bon appetit to your health and waistline!

Healthy Ways to Cook Potatoes, Pasta and Rice for Better Blood Sugar and Weight Control

Study of resistant starch content of potatoes by cooking method presented by researchers at the USDA Agricultural Research Service (ARS) Grand Forks Human Nutrition Research Center, North Dakota, and the University of Minnesota, Minneapolis and St. Paul, at the Federation of American Societies for Experimental Biology conference in Boston.

Study titled "Efficacy of increased resistant starch consumption in human type 2 diabetes" by researchers at University of Surrey, United Kingdom, published in *Endocrine Connections*.

Summary report of data on a study by researchers at the College of Chemical Sciences in Sri Lanka of how cooking methods affect resistant starch in rice, presented at the National Meeting and Exposition of the American Chemical Society in Denver.

To make potatoes and pasta healthier, cook in a way that increases the amount of "resistant starch," which raises blood sugar less than regular starch. *Here's how…*

Take a 100-gram serving of potatoes—about three-and-a-half ounces. Boil it, and you've got 2.6 grams of resistant starch…baked, 3.1 grams… chilled (either baked or boiled), 4.3 grams—good news for potato salad lovers. Chilled and then reheated potatoes do pretty well, too—3.5 grams. The same holds true for pasta—cooking and then cooling pasta increases the resistant starch modestly.

Does it make a difference? In a British study, people with diabetes who added 40 grams of resistant starch to their daily intake didn't improve their underlying diabetes but did have a reduced blood sugar spike after meals—a healthy thing. Whether there's any blood sugar benefit to taking in, say, an additional two or three grams of resistant starch in a meal, though, just isn't known.

So go ahead and enjoy your potatoes baked rather than boiled, and even better yet, cooled. But remember these foods already start with lots of easily digested, sugar-spiking starch, so cooking them in a way that boosts their resistant starch doesn't turn them into superfoods. A baked Russet Burbank potato has a "glycemic index" (GI), a measure of how quickly it raises blood sugar, of 111—more than white bread. So cook it right, but don't make it a daily staple—and add a healthful fat, such as olive oil, to further lower the GI.

Pasta, on the other hand, already has a lower GI than spuds, because the way it's made traps starch in a matrix that takes the body a longer time to break down into sugar. The GI range—30 to 60. So enjoy your pasta cooled in pasta salads…and if you like it hot, reduce its GI even more by cooking it al dente—slightly chewy rather than soft—and drizzling it with olive oil.

In the end, though, what matters more is how much you eat of these delicious but high-starch foods. Want to make a really healthy pasta salad? Start with whole grain pasta for extra nutrition, cook it al dente, and use just one cup of cooled pasta with three cups of chopped nonstarchy veggies with your favorite dressing. Now you're cooking.

NICE RICE

There is good science behind a rice-cooking technique that does cut calories—and makes rice less likely to spike your blood sugar levels.

Now that's healthy.

RICE RESEARCH

Researchers at the College of Chemical Sciences in Sri Lanka tested eight cooking variations on a variety of rice that's common in their country. One variation resulted in rice that had about 15% more resistant starch, a form of starch that our bodies can't digest, making it act more like fiber.

As a result, the rice cooked this way isn't likely to raise blood sugar as quickly as regular rice—a good thing, because rice, especially white rice, tends to send blood sugar up pretty quickly. Since resistant starch can't be digested, the new rice—at least the variety used in this study—also has about 10% to 15% fewer calories.

The 60% fewer calories claim? That came from the researchers speculating about what they might be able to achieve in future rice-cooking studies using other varieties of rice.

THE FORMULA

The successful technique is pretty simple: Add about one teaspoon of coconut oil to each half cup of dry rice, cook normally—and then refrigerate it for 12 hours.

The best part: You don't have to eat the rice cold. You can enjoy it reheated and get the same benefits.

The oil combines with the starch, and cooling the rice turns that starch into resistant starch. You could also use a different oil such as olive oil, although only coconut oil was used in this study. The cooling technique is well-known to food researchers—potatoes that are boiled then cooled tend to have more resistant starch, for example.

All in all, it's a pretty simple change that could have health benefits. Thinking of rice for tomorrow's dinner? You could cook up a batch tonight—and use it tomorrow. Any healthy recipe for leftover rice is a good place to start.

Five Rules for Healthful Snacking

Jamison Starbuck, ND, a naturopathic physician in family practice, Missoula, Montana, and writer and producer of "Dr. Starbuck's Health Tips for Kids," a weekly program on Montana Public Radio, MTPR.org. DrJamisonStarbuck. com

Do you like to eat a little something between meals? Here's a set of rules for healthful snacking—and a list of tasty, fun foods that make good snacks.

RULE 1: **Drink water first.** Often, we head for a snack when we're actually thirsty. Drink a 12-ounce glass of water and wait 10 minutes. If you are still hungry, select a healthful snack.

RULE 2: **Choose a snack food that still bears a resemblance to its original form.** Natural food—the most healthful food—comes from the earth or an animal. Lettuce grows in the dirt. Oranges and nuts hang from trees. Corn, wheat and oats grow in fields. The fillet or steak you're having for dinner was part of an animal before it landed on your table. When you apply this concept to snacks, it's fairly easy to make healthful choices. Cheetos, for example, are a long, long way from the corn from which they are made—many synthetic ingredients are added. An unsweetened rice cake, on the other hand, still looks quite a bit like rice.

RULE 3: **Avoid fat- and sugar-laden snacks.** If a sweetener or oil is the first or second ingredient on the label list, skip this snack.

RULE 4: **Keep portions small.** The more fat or sugar in the snack (cheese, nuts and dried fruit), the smaller the portion should be. Recommended snack size is one ounce of cheese…eight nuts…or two tablespoons of dried fruit. Watery, fiber-rich snacks, such as fresh fruit or vegetables, can be eaten in larger portions—½ cup to one cup is reasonable.

RULE 5: **Drink a cup of hot mint tea with your snack.** It aids your digestion, promoting absorption of nutrients, which improves the satisfaction you derive from the food. *My snack suggestions…*

Raw almonds, hazelnuts or pecans…whole fruit…celery sticks, carrots or a rice cake covered with a tablespoon of nut butter (almond, sesame, cashew) or hummus (mashed chickpeas flavored with lemon juice, garlic and oil)…whole-grain muffin (no bigger than a tennis ball) containing fruit, nuts and/or ground seeds and made with honey or cane sugar—not corn syrup…vegetable salads, such as cooked and chilled beets drizzled with olive oil and a sprinkle of goat cheese or coleslaw made with oil and vinegar rather than mayonnaise…air-popped popcorn—plain or seasoned with garlic or a pinch of sea salt…small baked potato, seasoned with herbs and a sprinkle of oil (put extra potatoes in the oven when you make dinner and refrigerate them for snacks that can be eaten later)…and rice—½ cup, with nuts and a dash of oil.

Experiment with different healthful and delicious oils—⅛ teaspoon of 100% virgin pistachio oil goes a long way to make a baked potato taste pretty special. Sesame, hazelnut and pumpkin seed oils are also tasty and add a special flavor to vegetable salads or whole-grain snacks.

The Real Secret to Lowering Your Blood Pressure

Janet Bond Brill, PhD, RDN, FAND, a registered dietitian/nutritionist and nationally recognized expert in nutrition and cardiovascular disease prevention. She is author of *Blood Pressure Down: The 10-Step Plan to Lower Your Blood Pressure in Four Weeks—Without Prescription Drugs.* DrJanet.com

Forget everything that you have read about the latest "superfood" for lowering blood pressure. While it's true that certain foods do provide this remarkable benefit, many people mistakenly assume that there must be one nutritional magic bullet that will do the job on its own.

Is it possible to control high blood pressure (hypertension) with diet alone? Yes, many people can—but only when they take advantage of the additive benefits from multiple strategically chosen foods.

Example: Suppose you eat a lot of bananas because you know that this food is high in blood pressure–lowering potassium. That's great, but you'll shave only a point or two off your blood pressure.

To really leverage your diet, you need to also regularly consume other foods that help control blood pressure. When combined, the nutrients in these foods work synergistically to give the greatest blood pressure–lowering effects. Then the benefits accrue quickly—for some people, a five-point drop may occur within a week.

Good news: By eating the right foods, losing weight if you're overweight and cutting sodium if you're salt sensitive (see next page), some people can achieve blood pressure drops that equal or exceed the effects of drug therapy—with none of the side effects. And if you must take medication, these foods may allow you to use a lower dose.*

Some of the best blood pressure–lowering foods are well-known—bananas, leafy green vegetables, etc. *Here are some lesser-known options to add to your hypertension-fighting diet…*

●**Beet juice/beet greens.** As a nutritionist, I usually advise clients to eat whole foods rather than

*Caution: If you take blood pressure–lowering medication, never change your dose or discontinue it without consulting your doctor.

drink juices because of the extra fiber. But beet juice is an exception. It's a concentrated source of nitrates, chemical compounds that quickly lower blood pressure.

When you drink beet juice or eat other high-nitrate foods (such as rhubarb, spinach, beet greens or chard), cells in the linings of blood vessels produce more nitric oxide, a molecule that dilates blood vessels and lowers blood pressure.

Scientific evidence: In a study that was published in *Hypertension* and looked at 64 adults with hypertension (ages 18 to 85), some of the patients drank a daily 8.4-ounce glass of beet juice, while others drank a juice with the active compounds removed (the placebo).

After one month, those given the real juice had average drops in systolic (top number) blood pressure of about eight points, while their diastolic pressure (bottom number) dropped five points. Blood pressure did not drop among those in the placebo group.

You can buy beet juice in health-food stores and juice shops. Or you can make your own by blending/processing cooked beets. To liven up the flavor, add a little lemon juice, ginger or a sweetener such as stevia.

Caution: If you have kidney disease, consult your nephrologist or a registered dietitian/nutritionist who specializes in kidney disease before regularly consuming beet juice—its high potassium level could worsen this condition.

●**Figs.** These delicious jewels are heart-healthy because they are super-high in potassium, with 232 mg in just two fresh figs. They also have a considerable amount of fiber and polyphenols, compounds that when consumed with additional blood pressure–lowering food can reduce systolic blood pressure by up to 12 points, in some cases.

Fresh figs are scrumptious, but dried figs are easier to find in grocery stores—and many people enjoy their intense sweetness.

What to try: Chop dried figs, and use them as a natural sweetener in oatmeal, pancakes, muffins or even soups.

●**Hibiscus tea.** If you enjoy chamomile and other herbal teas, you might like the delicate floral flavor of hibiscus tea, which is high in flavonoids, plant-based antioxidants with anti-inflammatory effects, and other heart-healthy compounds. One study, which compared hibiscus tea to *captopril* (Capoten), an ACE inhibitor blood pressure drug, found that the tea was just as effective as the medication.

•**Pistachios.** Even though most nuts are good sources of fiber, potassium and magnesium, pistachios are special because they are high in arginine, an amino acid that stimulates the production of nitric oxide (discussed earlier).

Important recent finding: A study at Pennsylvania State University found that people who ate 1.5 ounces of pistachios (about 70 nuts, unshelled) daily had drops in stress-related systolic blood pressure of nearly five points compared with those who ate nuts less than once a week.

Not fattening: Nuts are high in calories, but research has shown that people who eat them regularly actually tend to gain less weight than those who don't eat nuts—probably because the fiber and protein in nuts help dieters feel full longer. At roughly 260 calories per 1.5 ounces, you'll need to cut calories elsewhere to prevent weight gain but can likely do so easily because nuts give such a feeling of satiety.

•**Pomegranate juice.** Pomegranate juice contains many different flavonoids. The juice mimics the effects of ACE inhibitor drugs, such as *lisinopril* (Zestril, Prinivil, etc.), which dilate blood vessels and lower blood pressure.

A recent study found that people who drank a little less than two ounces of pomegranate juice daily for a year had average drops in systolic blood pressure of 12%.

The juice is tart, so some people buy sweetened versions.

My advice: Avoid the added sugar. Instead, add a little stevia or other natural sweetener. One pomegranate yields about half a cup of juice.

•**White beans.** Like many of the other foods described earlier, white beans are chock-full of potassium. One cup contains more than 1,000 mg of potassium. (A cup of black beans has about 800 mg.)

Potassium acts like a natural diuretic and removes sodium from the body. Many people are sensitive to sodium, which means that their blood pressure will rise if they consume too much (the standard recommendation is no more than 2,300 mg daily). Research has shown that one of the best ways to lower blood pressure is to increase your potassium–sodium ratio.

Purple Potatoes Lower Blood Pressure

Joe Vinson, PhD, professor of chemistry, The University of Scranton, Pennsylvania.

Recent study: 18 overweight people with high blood pressure ate about seven golf ball–sized purple potatoes twice daily for a month. The potatoes with skins were cooked in a microwave.

Result: The study participants' diastolic (bottom number) blood pressure readings dropped 4%, on average, and their systolic (top number) readings were 3.5% lower. None of the participants gained weight. Purple potatoes are available at specialty-food stores and some supermarkets.

Eat Nuts for Better Sex

Albert Salas-Huetos, PhD, postdoctoral researcher, University of Utah School of Medicine, Salt Lake City.

In a study of 83 men, eating just two ounces of an almond, walnut and hazelnut mixture (about 45 nuts) a day improved sexual desire and orgasm quality, even though they ate an otherwise unhealthy diet.

Theory: The nuts are rich in the amino acid *arginine*, a precursor of nitric oxide, which increases circulation by relaxing and widening blood vessels.

Important: There are about 320 calories in two ounces of nuts, so you may need to cut daily calories elsewhere.

More Coffee, Less Pain

Burel Goodin, PhD, associate professor of psychology, University of Alabama at Birmingham.

Caffeine is associated with lower pain sensitivity, according to a new study of 62 men and women who underwent heat and pressure tests after reporting their caffeine consumption from coffee, tea, soda and chocolate over seven days. Each extra 100 mg of caffeine consumed per day (about one cup of brewed coffee or two-and-a-half cups of tea) was linked to a reduction in pain severity that was deemed significant (the ability to withstand an additional 0.9°F increase in heat, a marker for pain tolerance).

Go Mediterranean for Healthy Eyes

Marc Grossman, OD, LAc, doctor of optometry and licensed acupuncturist in New Paltz and Somers, New York. He is coauthor of Natural Eye Care: Your Guide to Healthy Vision. A holistic eye doctor, his multidisciplinary approach uses nutrition, lifestyle changes and Traditional Chinese Medicine to tackle eye problems. NaturalEyeCare.com

The health-promoting effects of the Mediterranean diet—which emphasizes eating mostly vegetables, fruits, legumes, whole grains, nuts and seeds…and limiting animal products and sweets— are well-known. Yet few people realize that adhering to this eating plan also can greatly reduce their risk for age-related macular degeneration (AMD), the leading cause of irreversible vision loss and blindness after age 50. Most recently, a large-scale European study published in Ophthalmology investigated the connection between genes and lifestyle on the development of AMD and found that those who ate a primarily Mediterranean diet were 41% less likely to develop AMD than those who did not. Interestingly, it wasn't any of the specific components that lowered AMD risk. Rather, it was the overall pattern of consistently consuming a nutrient-rich diet that mattered.

The Incredible, Edible Egg Reduces Risk for Heart Disease and Stroke

No Longer a Forbidden Food

According to a recent study out of China that included more than 400,000 adults, individuals who ate at least one egg a day had an 18% lower risk of dying from cardiovascular disease than those who avoided eggs. Eggs balance good cholesterol with bad if not fried. Eggs also contain albumin, which is a healty protein that is easily absorbed.

Andrew Rubman, ND, founder and medical director of Southbury Clinic for Traditional Medicines in Southbury, Connecticut. He is author of Bottom Line's "Nature Doc's Patient Diary" blog. SouthburyClinic.com

Eggs Slash Stroke Risk

Eating up to one egg each day cut stroke risk by 12%—without increasing risk for heart disease—a study of more than 300,000 adults has found.

Theory: Eggs are rich in antioxidants (shown to reduce inflammation) and protein—both of which help lower blood pressure, an important risk factor for stroke.

Important: The new Dietary Guidelines for Americans eliminates restrictions on dietary cholesterol and notes that eggs are an inexpensive source of important nutrients.

Dominik D. Alexander, PhD, MSPH, principal epidemiologist, EpidStat Institute, Ann Arbor, Michigan.

Nutritionally Optimize Your Immune Function

Jacob Teitelbaum, MD, a Kona, Hawaii–based board-certified internist and nationally known expert in chronic fatigue syndrome, fibromyalgia, sleep and pain. He is author of numerous books, including *From Fatigued to Fantastic!.* Vitality101.com

The key nutrients for your immune system are zinc (15 mg a day), vitamin A (2,500 international units/IU a day), vitamin D (1,000 IU a day) and vitamin C (200 mg to 500 mg a day). But don't subscribe to a "more is better" approach. For example, doses of vitamin A over 8,000 IU a day can trigger birth defects.

Note: Use the retinol version of vitamin A (the type found in fish oil) for optimal results.

Two multivitamin supplements I like: ViraPro from Terry Naturally, and the Energy Revitalization System vitamin powder from Enzymatic Therapy—both offer optimal amounts of zinc, selenium and vitamins A, C, D and E.

Foods That Fight Specific Diseases

An overview of multiple research projects recently presented at a meeting of the American Society for Nutrition.

•**Eggs may help reduce risk factors associated with diabetes in overweight and obese people.**

•**Eating about 1.5 ounces of pecans daily cuts risk for both heart disease and diabetes in overweight adults age 45 and older.**

•**Yogurt protects against colorectal cancer.**

•**Vegetables and berries reduce risk for Parkinsonism** (a group of neurological movement-problem disorders similar to those seen with Parkinson's disease) and slow its progression.

•**Drinking three or more cups of coffee a day reduces the risk for liver disease.**

The Best Protein Powders

Tod Cooperman, MD, president, founder and editor in chief of ConsumerLab.com, a subscription-based website ($47.40 annually) that evaluates consumer products relating to health, wellness and nutrition. Consumer Lab.com recently completed an extensive product review of protein powders, shakes and drinks.

There was a time when bodybuilders and the elderly were just about the only people to use protein supplements. No more!

Now: There's an ever-increasing selection of protein powders available not just in health-food stores but also on the shelves of most US supermarkets and drugstores.

So which products contain the highest-quality ingredients at the best prices? For four top picks (see next page), we spoke with Tod Cooperman, MD, president and founder of ConsumerLab.com, which identifies the best health and nutritional products through independent testing.

WHY WE NEED PROTEIN

Our bodies need protein to build and maintain our muscles, bones and skin. Protein also helps keep our energy levels high and promotes weight loss in those who want to drop unwanted pounds.

Protein is especially important as we grow older. With each decade after age 30, we lose as much as 3% to 5% of our muscle mass, leading to weakness that also increases our risk for falls and broken bones. A recent report suggests that people with pronounced muscle loss, a condition known as sarcopenia, face more than twice the risk for a fall-related fracture.

Adults should get 0.36 g of protein per pound, according to the recommended dietary allowance. For example, someone weighing 150 pounds would need to get 54 g of protein daily. But research published in 2019 in *The Journal of Nutrition, Health & Aging* found that 30% of men and 45% of women ages 51 to 60 failed to meet this basic threshold… and 37% of men and 48% of women fell short during their next decade of life.

While foods (such as meat, seafood, dairy, legumes and nuts) should be our main sources of this vital nutrient, more and more people are turning to protein powders and drinks to help them get adequate levels in their diets. Such products are not only convenient, but also are free of the saturated fat and cholesterol that are often found in protein-rich foods.

Caveat: Protein—whether it's from food or a supplement—is not a miracle fix. Regular resistance exercise, such as lifting weights or using weight machines, is also necessary. As part of an overall fitness program, older adults should do strength training two to three times a week.

Strength-training regimens may include squats, wall push-ups and exercises, such as biceps curls, that use hand weights.

THE CHANGING FACE OF PROTEIN

The proteins found in powders and drinks are no longer your run-of-the-mill dairy-based products, derived from whey or casein. There's a recent push for more plant-based sources, including pea, hemp, rice, soy or other nondairy ingredients, which work well for people who are lactose intolerant.

Important: Because high protein intake can impair kidney function in people with kidney disease, they should talk to their doctors about how much and what types of protein they should consume. Some doctors advise increasing overall fluid intake when consuming a high-protein diet or protein supplements to help protect the kidneys, but this is probably not necessary if you have normal kidney function. Before adding a protein supplement to your diet, check with your doctor if you have any concerns.

ConsumerLab.com approves protein supplements based on their quality, value, taste and mixability. The products below also did not exceed contamination limits for lead, cadmium, arsenic or mercury. *Among the top low-sugar powders tested by ConsumerLab.com…*

MYPROTEIN IMPACT WHEY ISOLATE

• **Protein source: Whey.**

Price: 52 cents per 20 g of protein.

Why it's a top pick: Low in carbs and virtually fat-free, this whey isolate (it contains only 0.31 g of lactose per serving) has a slight powdered-milk taste and blends well into drinks. It provides 22 g of protein per serving and 12% of an adult's daily value for calcium. It's gluten-free.

NOW SPORTS PEA PROTEIN, NATURAL UNFLAVORED

• **Protein source: Pea.**

Price: 37 cents per 20 g of protein.

Why it's a top pick: Mixing easily and smoothly into liquids, this product enhances the taste of vegetable smoothies and provides 24 g of protein per serving. At 330 mg of sodium per serving, it's slightly higher in sodium than most protein powders but is gluten- and lactose-free.

NUTIVA ORGANIC HEMP PROTEIN

• **Protein source: Hemp.**

Price: $1.04 per 20 g of protein.

Why it's a top pick: With a bountiful 8 g of fiber per scoop—one of hemp's big benefits—this unsweetened supplement also has naturally high levels of potassium, iron, magnesium and zinc. Its complex but pleasant vegetable flavor is offset by a somewhat gritty texture that makes it less suitable for mixing with plain water but terrific in a smoothie. This powder provides 15 g of protein per serving. It has no measurable lactose but is not gluten-free.

GARDEN OF LIFE SPORT ORGANIC PLANT-BASED PROTEIN, VANILLA

• **Protein source: Mixed.**

Price: $1.35 per 20 g of protein.

Why it's a top pick: Primarily pea-based but also containing navy, lentil and garbanzo beans as well as cranberry protein, this powder mixes easily and evenly into water and other thin beverages. It provides 15 g of protein per serving and has a clean vegetable flavor with only a slight artificial-sugar sweetness despite its stevia content. This gluten-free powder has no measurable lactose.

Eat Nuts to Prevent Heart Disease

Frank Hu, MD, PhD, professor of nutrition and epidemiology, Harvard School of Public Health, Boston, and lead author of a 22-year study of 6,309 women.

Among women who have type-2 diabetes (which puts them at high risk for heart disease), those who ate five or more servings a week of nuts or peanut butter had a 44% lower risk for heart disease than those who rarely or never ate these foods, according to recent research.

Theory: Monounsaturated fat in nuts reduces cholesterol and inflammation.

Best: At least five times weekly, have one ounce of nuts or one tablespoon of peanut butter.

Better-for-Your-Body Beverages for When You Work Out

Laurie Steelsmith, ND, LAc, licensed naturopathic physician and acupuncturist in private practice in Honolulu. She writes Bottom Line's "Natural Healing Secrets for Women" blog and is coauthor of three books—*Natural Choices for Women's Health*; *Great Sex, Naturally* and *Growing Younger Every Day*. DrSteelsmith.com

---

Do you guzzle a sports drink after every workout? Depending on how you exercise, that drink may not be doing you much good… and depending on the beverage you choose, it could even contribute to health problems.

WHEN A SPORTS DRINK CAN HELP

Consider a sports drink when you are training hard or working out for more than an hour and sweating a lot—say, with a strenuous spinning session, marathon hike or Bikram "hot" yoga class. The reason is that electrolytes (minerals such as sodium, calcium, magnesium, potassium and bicarbonate) exit the body via sweat and a sports drink provides a convenient and concentrated source for replenishing electrolytes.

Why it matters: Electrolytes help maintain the body's fluid balance and prevent dehydration… carry electrical signals between cells… and help the muscles, heart and other organs work properly.

Before a big workout, drink plenty of water so cells are well hydrated. Then, when you are sweating heavily and need more than water to prevent dehydration, take frequent sips of a sports beverage during your workout to replace electrolytes as they are being lost, rather than waiting until you're done exercising.

When selecting a sports drink, be aware that commercial brands often contain high-fructose corn syrup (HFCS), which is just plain bad for you.

Better: Try naturally sweetened, HFCS-free sports drink brands, such as R.W. Knudsen's Recharge and Gatorade's G Natural line.

All-natural alternatives: Electrolytes also are found in fruits and vegetables—but of course it is less convenient to eat than to drink during a workout. And, fruit juice generally is not a great option during a workout because it naturally contains a lot of fructose, which can reduce the rate of water absorption into cells. Coconut water (the juice in young, green coconuts) or diluted vegetable juices, however, are good alternatives to sports beverages because they are naturally high in electrolytes and low in fructose.

WHEN TO SKIP THE SPORTS DRINK

If you are doing low- to moderate-intensity exercise for less than an hour and not sweating much, you are not losing many electrolytes. In that case, drinking plain water before and during your workout should keep you adequately hydrated.

How much water do you need? You may have heard that pale-colored urine generally is a sign of adequate hydration—but if you take a vitamin B complex supplement or a multi that contains B vitamins, your urine may be neon orange no matter how hydrated you are. In that case, a better rule of thumb is to divide your body weight (in pounds) by two… and drink that many ounces of water during the course of the day (so if you weigh 120 pounds, drink 60 ounces). Good hydration is important every day, of course, but particularly on days that you exercise.

AFTER YOUR WORKOUT

Whether you exercised moderately or intensely, afterward it is important to consume something with protein. This helps repair the micro-tears your muscles endured during your workout.

Surprising option: Low-fat chocolate milk. A recent study in the *Journal of Nutrition and Metabolism* found that adults who drank low-fat chocolate milk within an hour after working out had an improved VO2 max (a measure of how much oxygen you can use during intense exercise, which is a marker of athletic endurance), more muscle and less fat than their peers who consumed a beverage with no nutrients (such as water) or one with carbohydrates and some fat but no protein.

Some chocolate milk brands and chocolate syrups also contain HFCS—so if you opt for chocolate milk, choose one that is naturally sweetened. Or if you would rather avoid chocolate milk's sugar and fat, make a post-workout vegetable smoothie with added protein powder.

The Very Best Greens (Not Just Kale) for Your Health

Michael T. Murray, ND, a licensed naturopathic physician based in Paradise Valley, Arizona. Dr. Murray has published more than 30 books, including *Bottom Line's Encyclopedia of Healing Foods*, with coauthor Joseph Pizzorno, ND. DoctorMurray.com

Leafy greens are the superstars of the vegetable brigade. Kale, widely considered the reigning king, is unusually high in calcium, magnesium and vitamin K…and, like other greens, is loaded with disease-fighting phytochemicals, such as lutein and vitamin C.

But let's be honest—kale's somewhat bitter taste isn't for everyone…and even if you love this veggie, you're probably not going to eat it every day. What other disease-fighting greens do you need in your diet?

TARGETED NUTRITION

Basic nutrition is just one reason that experts advise Americans to eat at least five servings of greens and other vegetables daily. But if you're concerned about specific medical conditions, research has shown that some leafy greens are particularly effective. *For example…*

•**Arugula and cancer.** Arugula is a peppery green with a sharp taste that adds a distinctive zip to otherwise bland salads. The pungent flavor has earned it the nickname "salad rocket."

The zesty flavor of arugula is largely due to its high concentration of sulfur-containing compounds. We think of arugula as a salad green, but it's actually a crucifer—in the same plant family as superfoods such as broccoli, cabbage and kale. Like other crucifers, it contains a group of anticancer compounds known as glucosinolates, which have detoxifying effects.

How arugula helps: Compounds in arugula, including sulforaphane and indole-3-carbinol, increase the body's excretion of a form of estrogen that has been linked to breast cancer. A Chinese study found that women who regularly ate a daily serving of cruciferous vegetables were 50% less likely to develop breast cancer. Another study found that just one weekly serving was enough to reduce cancer risk (including oral, colorectal and kidney malignancies). Bonus: The sulforaphane in arugula has another benefit. It appea

Bonus: The sulforaphane in arugula has another benefit. It appears to help the body eliminate H. pylori, a bacterium that causes most peptic ulcers and greatly increases the risk for gastric cancer.

•**Spinach and macular degeneration.** As the US population ages, there's been a dramatic increase in age-related macular degeneration, a leading cause of blindness. Could a few weekly servings of spinach make a difference? There's good evidence that it might.

How spinach helps: Spinach is exceptionally high in lutein, a plant pigment that concentrates in the eyes and deflects damaging light from sunshine. Studies have found that people who consumed 6 mg of lutein daily—the amount in about one-half cup of cooked spinach—were 43% less likely to develop macular degeneration. Research published in *JAMA Ophthalmology* shows that people who consume generous amounts of lutein are also less likely to develop cataracts than those who eat less.

Important: Whether you prefer your spinach raw or cooked, be sure to have it with a little bit of oil or fat—a drizzle of olive oil is plenty—or a small amount of some other fat such as chopped nuts or avocado. Lutein is a fat-soluble nutrient, which means it is absorbed more efficiently when it's consumed with a little fat.

•**Parsley and UTIs.** Most people think of parsley as a colorful garnish—pretty to look at, but not much of a food. But around the world, parsley is found in tabbouleh, pesto (with or without basil) and other fragrant dishes…and it's a good green to eat if you get frequent urinary tract infections (UTIs).

About half of all women will eventually get a UTI…men get them, too, but less often. Patients with recurrent UTIs (defined as two separate infections within six months or three within one year) often depend on antibiotics—and resign themselves to the likely side effects of these drugs, such as diarrhea.

How parsley helps: It contains apigenin, a compound that acts as a diuretic and also has anti-inflammatory effects. According to a report in the journal Case Reports in Medicine, women who combined parsley with other herbal treatments (such as garlic) had an impressive decrease in urinary frequency and other symptoms—by 80%, in one case. Parsley's UTI-fighting effect is presumably because of apigenin's diuretic effect.

Another benefit: Reduced risk for cancer. Chlorophyll and other compounds in parsley have anticancer effects—including the ability to help inhibit the cancer-causing effects of fried foods.

Since parsley is so concentrated in nutrition and phytochemicals, just a few sprigs (or about one-quarter cup) consumed whenever possible provides exceptional health benefits. Chopped parsley can be added to salads, sauces, soups and grilled fish.

•**Kale and osteoporosis.** Kale's reputation as the king of veggies is based, in part, on its ability to promote bone health. People often think that milk is a great calcium source, but the absorption of calcium from kale and other leafy greens is actually higher—between 40% to 64%, compared with about 32% from milk.

And that's not all. In addition to being rich in calcium, kale also is an excellent source of vitamin K, a critical nutrient that helps anchor calcium into bone. One cup of raw kale supplies more than 600% of the recommended daily vitamin K intake. If you're concerned about bone health, you should definitely make an effort to eat more kale.

Another benefit: Improved heart health. Kale and other greens, as well as beets and celery, have been found to improve blood pressure and blood flow. While a high intake of fruit and vegetables is associated with healthy blood pressure and reduces risk for heart disease and stroke, kale and cruciferous vegetables are linked to even greater protection. A good goal: Three to four servings of kale and other greens a week.

Important caveat: In normal amounts, kale is among the healthiest foods you can eat. But some people go overboard. Too much kale, like other cruciferous vegetables, can cause flatulence (gas) for many people. Eating too much raw kale (for example, more than three servings a week) can also interfere with the production of thyroid hormone, leading to the formation of a goiter. And because kale is such a rich source of vitamin K, anyone taking *warfarin* (Coumadin), an important anticlotting drug that interacts with this vitamin, should consult a doctor before eating kale or any leafy greens.

Index